MOTOR DEVELOPMENT

Third Edition

Helen M. Eckert

University of California
Berkeley, California

Benchmark Press, Inc.
Indianapolis, Indiana

Copyright 1987, by Benchmark Press, Inc.

ALL RIGHTS RESERVED.

Library of Congress Cataloging in Publication Data:

ECKERT, HELEN, 1925–

MOTOR DEVELOPMENT
THIRD EDITION

Cover Design: Gary Schmitt

Copy Editor: Lynne Sullivan

Library of Congress Catalog Card number: 86–72313

ISBN: 0–936157–14–3

Printed in the United States of America
10 9 8 7 6 5 4 3 2

The Publisher and Author disclaim responsibility for any adverse effects or consequences from the misapplication or injudicious use of the information contained within this text.

Contents

Preface

Motor Development, third edition, incorporates research findings from many disciplines into a physical educator's view of motor development. It identifies developmental patterns of basic motor skills and structural components that influence the basic motor skills at all age levels.

The classic studies that identified the basic performance patterns have been retained and augmented by more recent research. Wherever possible, recent research which expands our knowledge of normative performance in the basic skills has been cited. However, it is not the purpose of this volume to provide the various scales for the assessing of normal development, as these are available from the originators. Rather, this volume is designed to illustrate normal developmental sequences and to highlight the many facets of structural and environmental components which may influence motor patterns and development.

This edition retains its view of the entire motor development process from conception through old age. It has been updated and expanded to integrate perceptual-motor development and physical performance. In addition, the discussion of structural and functional sensory development has been expanded. At the opposite end of the spectrum, separate chapters on adulthood and old age have been reorganized and considerably expanded to reflect increased research in these areas.

Physical educators, physical therapists, and others with a biological background may be especially interested in the growth processes and the interrelationship of structure to function. To psychologists, educators, and other students of behavior, the physical and motor development of the individual is an important aspect of human actions and interactions. Some suggestions have been made for activities to enhance motoric skill development.

Motor Development is designed to serve as a text for undergraduate students and as a source for more advanced students who may wish to pursue references in various areas. Many students have intentionally, or otherwise, served as judges for the selection of the content of this volume and indebtedness for their interest in human development is herewith acknowledged.

Helen M. Eckert

1

Heredity

All persons receive from their parents the greatest gift of all—that of life. Through the parents come also a multiplicity of hereditary factors which determine to a great extent physical appearance and maximum potential. Environment from the moment of conception modifies and interacts with **heredity*** to shape the individual and to control the extent to which the maximal potential will be realized. It is difficult, if not impossible, to assess the relative contributions of heredity and environment.

The great variability of physical appearances in the general population is obvious from a casual observation of persons encountered during a short walk down any busy street. Family resemblances are consistently present, however, and are a continuing source of interest. A boy may be the "image of his father," or perhaps he looks more like his mother or older brothers. If the offspring are identical twins, observers have the impression of seeing double. The duplication of what appears to be one individual has proven to be a fruitful model for research into the relative effects of heredity and environment. Such studies indicate that physical characteristics are determined to a great extent by heredity and are little affected by environment.

It is obvious that a child deprived of adequate food and shelter may be harmed physically. It is becoming increasingly evident that in our society no one can attain maximal potential in any respect if they do not grow up under favorable conditions. Children of parents of high intelligence tend to show higher intelligence than children of parents of low intelligence. At the same time, children of professional groups and those of higher **socioeconomic status** have the highest IQ's while children of unskilled laborers have the lowest. Relationships between the IQ's of the child and the socioeconomic status of the parents tend to increase with the age of the child. Maximal potential in intelligence is determined by heredity, but the extent to which it is achieved is limited by environment.

Human abilities and characteristics most affected by environment prove to be the ones in which increasing differences are observed as

---

* All boldfaced terms are defined in the glossary at the end of this text. Such boldfacing does not indicate emphasis by the author.

individuals grow older. Beliefs, values, and attitudes in which training and proximity are major factors have little or no hereditary basis. Temperamental characteristics in which glandular activity may be involved are somewhat dependent upon heredity. Scheinfeld (1939) indicates that intelligence, sensory discrimination, speed of reaction, and motor coordinations are among those facets of human behavior determined to a great extent by heredity. A study of monozygotic twins indicated that the percent distribution of slow twitch fibers in the vastus lateralis muscle was almost identical and only small intrapair differences were noted in measures of muscular power, running velocity, maximal heart rate, height, and weight. Maximal oxygen uptake was also more closely associated in monozygotic than dizygotic twins (Komi & Karlsson, 1979). The size of genetic effect for aerobic performance based on fat-free weight was estimated at 10 percent for maximal oxygen uptake and 60 percent for a 90-minute work output by Bouchard et al. (1986) using data from dizygotic and monozygotic twin brothers. Maximal heart rate was estimated at having approximately 50 percent heritability and the investigators concluded that a significant genetic effect was present in the population for endurance performance but a much lower heritability existed for maximal oxygen uptake. Winchester also points out that heredity determines the nature of many physiological reactions taking place in the body. Moreover, it plays an important role in determining aptitudes, susceptibility to disease, and even life span.

THEORIES OF HEREDITY

The inheritance of parental traits by offspring has fascinated the human race from earliest times, and there are many indications that attempts were made to influence heredity by selective breeding. The numerous strains of dogs extant today indicate the degree to which our ancestors were successful in breeding the types of animals best suited to their needs. Attention to the details of breeding in ancient times is indicated by a Babylonian stone tablet, evacuated in Chaldea and dated at approximately 4000 B.C., which shows the inheritance of head and mane characteristics in five generations of horses. **Flora** as well as **fauna** have been selectively bred to develop varieties more suitable to human needs. Archeologists have associated the improved yield of grains and maize with the rise of ancient civilizations. Early Chinese accounts indicate that superior varieties of rice were developed almost 6000 years ago, while ancient Egyptian paintings depict men cross-pollinating the date palm (Winchester, 1961).

Until relatively recently, human offspring were considered a mixture of the blood of their parents and hereditary traits were believed to be passed on in this blended blood from the parents. Hence the common referrals in literature to the blood of some renowned ancestor "flowing" in the veins of the hero or heroine. We still tend to use the term *blue blood* to refer to individuals who have a royal or noble ancestry although it is common knowledge that all blood is the same color and that blood is a product of each individual's body with not even a mother and her child having a single drop of blood in common.

Another inheritance theory that has been expressed in the past is the so-called jigsaw method of race inheritance whereby, for example, a child may be one-fourth Scotch, one-eighth Irish, one-eighth French, one-fourth Italian, plus others, and, of course, inherit frugality from his Scotch ancestors, emotionality from the French and Italian, and so forth. Scheinfeld (1939) gives a very succinct and realistic appraisal of the futility of assigning characteristics to races, and genetics, the modern study of heredity, makes it very clear that each offspring is an individual identity and not so many parts of this and that.

The applied science of heredity dealing with genetic aspects of reproduction in humans is called **eugenics** with emphasis placed upon **phenotypes.** The phenotype of an organism refers to its appearance, its physical and chemical properties, and/or its behavior. Because phenotypes are influenced by many **genes** and show continuous variation, the eugenicist must also be concerned with the contribution to population variance by genetic differences among individuals which is called **heritability.** Heritability is very different from Mendelian genetics, which are concerned with the passage of genes from parents to offspring and the transmission of genetic information from **DNA** to protein to phenotype. Since the task of isolating the **genotypic** differences between individuals within a population is immense but limited in its research potential due to moral reasons, factual confirmation of various eugenics theories is lacking (Woodward & Woodward, 1977).

MENDELIAN LAWS

A Moravian monk, Gregor Mendel, working with garden peas, discovered three relationships which have become the cornerstones of research in the field of genetics. The conclusions drawn by Mendel have since been referred to as the "Mendelian laws" of genetics and in modern terminology may be stated as follows:

1. Inherited characteristics are carried by genes that are passed along unchanged from one generation to another.
2. Genes are found in pairs in each individual. The two genes in a pair may be different in their effects and where this occurs, one

gene tends to dominate the other, in which case it is referred to as the **dominant** while the other is known as the **recessive.**

3. When reproductive cells are formed in any individual by the process of reduction division, the genes in each pair separate with only one of each pair going to each reproductive cell.

REPRODUCTIVE CELL DIVISION

A glance at the actual mechanism of **meiosis,** or reproductive cell division, indicates the complexities which stand in the way of any accurate predictions of the offspring of human parents. It has been clearly established that the normal human being has 46 **chromosomes** in the nucleus of the cell. The 46 chromosomes are made up of varying numbers of genes that are fixed in their effect and, in 44 of these chromosomes there are pairs, or **alleles**, of each of the genes that work together as single units in the effect that is produced, e.g., the action of paired dominant and recessive genes. In the female the remaining two chromosomes are also paired while in the male the Y chromosome is much shorter than the X chromosome so that a number of the X genes remain unpaired.

Normal body growth requires that cell division occur and also requires that the cells be duplicated in their entirety if the integrity of the structure is to be maintained. During the normal process of cell division, or **mitosis,** the number of chromosomes in the cell is the same before and after division. Reproduction, however, requires that the chromosomal number be reduced in half to allow for equal chromosomal contributions by each parent to the offspring.

Figure 1.1 illustrates, by the use of six chromosomes, how the **diploid number** of chromosomes (46) is reduced to the **haploid number** (23) with the maturation of the germ cells during the process of **oogenesis** (egg formation) and **spermatogenesis** (sperm formation). During the first step, or **prophase,** of meiosis there is a pairing of chromosomes with their **homologous** mates that is not present in the prophase of mitosis. By the time pairing is completed, the **chromonemata,** but not the **centromere,** of each chromosome has been duplicated to form two **chromatids** attached to the single centromere. It is at this time that the paired chromosomes may become entangled and a **crossing over** occur in the genes of the chromosomes.

The mechanism of crossing over in two paired chromosomes is illustrated in figure 1.2, where overlapping of one of the chromatids of each pair results in an interchange of the genes between the overlapped segments. Any amount of overlapping and interchange of the chromatids may occur so that in some instances both chromatids may be involved or both ends of the chromosome may be involved. In all cases, the reformed

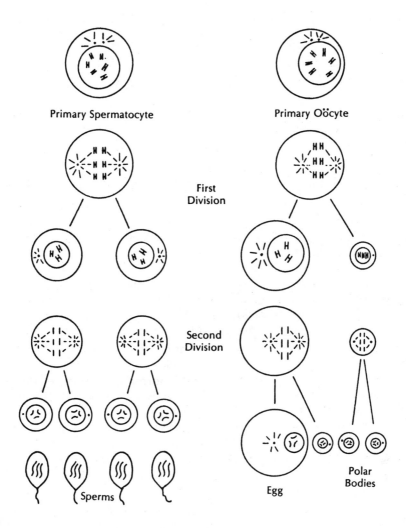

FIGURE 1.1. *Diagram of egg and sperm formation by meiosis.*

chromatids continue as a unit, comprised of the centromere with the remaining original genes and the crossed-over genes from the other chromosome, through the remaining phases of meiosis (Winchester, 1961).

Upon completion of the first division of meiosis, the diploid number of chromosomes has been reduced to the haploid number by one of each of the pairs of chromosomes being drawn apart to form a new cell. These new cells (secondary spermatocytes or oöcytes) contain 23 chromosomes with two chromatids but only one centromere (as in figure 1.2).

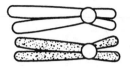 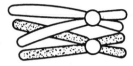 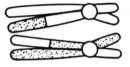

FIGURE 1.2. *Mechanism of crossing over. The chromonemata have been duplicated, but not the centromere.*

The second division in the process of meiosis is very similar to mitotic cell division with the centromeres also dividing into two parts and two new cells being formed with 23 chromosomes. In the case of spermatogenesis, four sperms are produced from one primary spermatocyte, two bearing the X chromosome and two the Y chromosome.

During oögenesis, the necessity of providing nourishment for the developing organism should the egg be fertilized results in the production of only one egg containing an X chromosome. The three polar bodies also produced are very small and soon degenerate so that they play no part in the process of reproduction (Winchester, 1961).

It should be pointed out that during the pairing up of the chromosomes in the prophase of meiosis such pairings are done in a haphazard manner with respect to the relative position of the pairs in relation to each other. That is, all the chromosomes inherited from the father do not line up on the right side while those from the mother do so on the left, or vice versa. Thus, the offspring may inherit a chromosome from the first pair from the mother, the next from the father, and so on, in any combination of dual arrangement of the 23 pairs. Moreover, it should be noted that the arrangement of the 23 pairs will probably be different in every germ cell during the course of its meiotic division. To this staggering number of possible combinations one must add the consideration that crossing over may have occurred in genes while each chromosome of a pair was composed of two chromatids, and, further, that this crossing over may occur in any amount in any of the paired chromosomes. Within each of the paired genes (alleles) of the 23 paired chromosomes there are, as will be seen later in the case of **brachyphalangy,** four possible combinations.

There are approximately 150,000 genes clustered in the 46 chromosomes within the nucleus of every human cell, and it has been estimated that the odds are about 1 in 200,000 trillion that the same parents will ever present the same packet of chromosomes to another child (Hicks, 1963). It is small wonder, then, that our prediction of the characteristics of human offspring is very unreliable, and we must content ourselves with the very general conclusion that heredity does tend to create likenesses in families.

GENETIC COMPOSITION

How, we may ask, do the genes regulate and order the growth and division of one single cell to eventually become the 26 trillion multi-differentiated, interrelated, and integrated cells that form the small human organism that we commonly call a baby? Biochemical analysis of the **chromatin** in the nucleus of the cells of higher organisms indicates that it is composed of DNA, chromosomal proteins, and a lesser amount of **RNA** (Stein et al., 1975). We know that all chromosomes are comprised of molecules of deoxyribonucleic acid (DNA) which are built up in an ordered linear sequence of nucleotides containing the same four bases in two linked pairs; namely, the base **adenine** paired with **thymine** and **guanine** paired with **cytosine.** This paired ordering of the base compounds of DNA is a mechanism which facilitates the accurate reproduction of the DNA chain within any one chromosome. The classic gene is a portion of the chromosomal DNA chain that has a specific function in the development process and/or maintenance of the cell with the number and arrangement of the paired nucleotides being specific to the function. Therefore, the substructure of DNA, with its paired nucleotides ordered in different combinations along different proportions of the chain within any one chromosome, has the capacity for the vast number of information requisites governing human reproduction, development, and maintenance.

The unique paired base structure of DNA allows for the exact duplication of the helix structure within any one chromosome in that each base will only combine with its respectively paired base during the process of **replication** (figure 1.3). Exact replication of DNA is vital during the second phase of meiosis, or reproductive cell division, and during mitosis, or cell division during normal growth. In addition, the DNA within the nucleus of a cell has the function of **transcribing** nucleotide sequences into complementary strands of ribonucleic acid (RNA) in which the base thymine acquires an additional oxygen to become **uracil.** It is believed that the chromosomal proteins, which are composed of **histones** and **nonhistones,** are prime determinants governing the replication and transcription processes of DNA. Stein et al. (1975) reports that histones are closely associated with DNA in the chromatin and that histone and DNA are synthesized simultaneously during replication. Nonhistones appear to be more closely related to the transcription process for it is hypothesized that they bind to a specific site on the histone-repressed DNA to cause **phosphorylation** of the histone-nonhistone complex and a displacement from that site on the DNA. The resultant area of DNA is thus freed of its inhibitory histone and can be transcribed into RNA.

Although the chromatin also contains RNA, the amount in the nucleus tends to remain small as the RNA produced during transcription

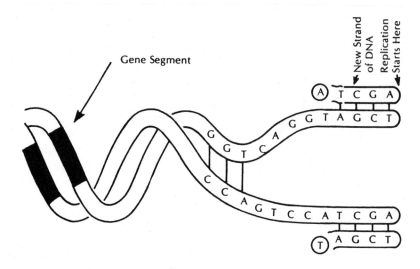

FIGURE 1.3. *Diagrammatic illustration of a gene segment on the helix structure of DNA and replication of DNA to form two identical helix strands.*

leaves the nucleus to interact with the 23 amino acids in the protein substrat of the **protoplasm** to produce the various types of proteins needed during the developmental and maintenance processes. It is the biological function of the **ribosome** to mediate the **translation** of the genetic code carried by the messenger RNA into the sequence of amino acids in a protein. The ribosome initiates the translation process by recognizing the starting point in a segment of messenger RNA and binding it to a molecule of transfer RNA bearing a single amino acid. Transfer RNA is comprised of three-unit code segments, and each molecule of transfer RNA has an affinity for a specific amino acid. The addition of amino acid bearing transfer RNA in single units appropriate to the coding sequence in the messenger RNA continues in the ribosome in an **elongation** process which terminates when the end of the genetic message is reached and the chain of amino acids folds spontaneously to form a protein. The protein synthesis within the ribosome is facilitated by a number of **catalytic proteins** (initiation, elongation, and termination factors) and by **guanosine triphosphate** which is a small molecule that releases the energy required for the process of translation (Engleman, 1976; Rich & Kim, 1978).

Although it is well established that chromosomal DNA contains the genetic coding for the reproduction, development, and maintenance of the individual, the foregoing processes indicate that there is a biochemical interdependence between DNA and other aspects of bodily functions. Sager (1965) has reported the existence of non-chromosomal genes carrying primary genetic information and cites work by David J. L. Luck and Edward Reich of the Rockefeller Institute which demonstrated the localization of extranuclear DNA in **mitochondria,** a feature common to all plant and animal cells. These findings indicate additional sources other than the chromosomes for transmitting the genetic information necessary for **morphogenic** development, which may play an important part in time differences and rate differences as well as in **organelle** differences in development. Considering the vast number of changes necessary in the developmental sequence whereby a single fertilized ovum eventually bcomes a fully matured human being, embryologists have questioned the possibility of such a vast storage of knowledge within the relatively small confines of 46 chromosomes. Moreover, different structural complexes appear at different times and with different rates of development; nor do they appear in full bloom but often require many adjustments before achieving their ultimate form.

Waddington (1962) points out that the **cytoplasm** of the **ovum** is not a homogeneous mass but contains many different types of protein which are in constant interaction as evidenced by the streaming of cytoplasmic material seen under a microscope. He contends that a certain amount of differentiation may occur in the ovum on the basis of the initial spatial distribution of these interactions with respect to the polarity of the cell. In the morphogenesis of masses containing large numbers of cells, Waddington (1962) indicates that the interactions of the chemicals of the cell membranes and the formation of attachment bodies, or **desmosomes,** may give rise to the mechanisms whereby the unification of the structure is achieved. Both of these types of interaction would require a feedback type of system rather than a one-way circuitry for effective operation. Similarly, if the gene-protein system incorporates some mechanism of feedback, an explanation is forthcoming for the ordered development of complex systems with different rates of development and in various time sequences. Waddington (1962) has postulated the existence of such a system which he has termed the *gene-action system* within which are incorporated short series of reactions leading from the gene to the first protein it determines and labeled *gene-protein systems.* Feedback from each gene-protein system, which in turn is in interaction with the cytoplasm, influences the gene-action system of which it is a part. Since the genes themselves are constantly interacting with one another, the feedback from the gene-protein system may result in intergenetic adjustments or serve as confirmation that "all is progressing as scheduled." Such an arrangement obviously incorporates a greater range of possibilities in the transmission of genetic information than a one-way copying system and also allows for minor deviations and variabilities from a set pattern for adjustment to external influences.

Glass (Shock, 1960) would seem to support the concept of genetic interaction, for he points to the abundant evidence from studies of suppressor genes indicating that the action of a particular gene may be turned on or off, without the gene itself being modified, by the action of a gene at another locus. He believes that this may be accomplished by controlling the flow of a limited amount of substrate through competing channels or by the provision of an alternate route, or bypass, for the formation of the chemical product of the particular gene-controlled reaction. Glass draws the conclusion that there is much evidence to support the theory that differentiation proceeds by controls over gene activity without altering the ultimate nature of the gene itself. With the development of chromosome banding and *in vitro* cell techniques, researchers have developed chromosome banding profiles and linkage groups for a wide range and number of genes. Homologous chromosome structures and gene arrangements have been identified in various species and have similar linkage groups in man (Evans, 1984). The linkage groups have been considered to be "master" genes which act like programming chips to control the genes that produce protein sequences. Thus, these master genes control such aspects of differentiation and integration as timing, position, and characteristics of the critical protein sequencings which are basic to development.

Studies on bacteria indicate that genes on chromosomes are in units known as operons which contain an **operator gene**. Operator genes stimulate adjacent **structural genes** to produce messenger RNA. At another location, a regulator gene produces a **repressor** molecule which inhibits the operator gene. In those situations where a noxious substance must be controlled or synthesized, the noxious substance becomes an effector and unites with the repressor molecule so that it no longer inhibits the operator. The operator gene then stimulates the necessary structural gene to produce the required messenger RNA. When the noxious substance has been used up, it no longer inhibits the repressor and the output of messenger RNA is stopped. This is called a positive feedback system (Winchester, 1979).

There are some chemical processes in the body that are regulated by a negative feedback system. One of these is the **thyroxine** level of the blood. In this instance the effector for the repressor molecule is thyroxine, but the thyroxine must reach a certain level before the repressor molecule inhibits the operator gene and the production of thyroxine is cut off. Both the positive and negative feedback systems are dependent upon the fact that **enzymes** break down within a short period of time. Although this means that a continuing supply of enzymes must be synthesized for the maintenance of bodily functions, it also prevents build-up of excess amounts of enzymes. It is the short duration of an enzyme that makes feedback control possible (Winchester, 1979).

DOMINANT AND RECESSIVE GENES

Despite the extreme complication of the genetic transmission process, we are, because of the dominant and recessive relationship between some pairs of genes, able to make reasonably accurate predictions of certain characteristics. In human beings, dominant and recessive genes control such physical features as eye shape and color, length of eye lashes, ear lobe attachment and size of ear, nose shape, hair texture and color, thickness of lip, and stature.

In some instances, the pairing of two recessive genes will produce a lethal combination resulting in death in early infancy. Such "killer" genes have been identified as producing glioma retina (eye tumor), amaurotic family idiocy, malignant freckles, and progressive spinal muscular atrophy in infants (Scheinfeld, 1939). Some dominant genes may be "intermediate lethals" in humans—they may pair with a recessive gene to produce nothing more than an abnormal effect, whereas the pairing of two such dominant genes will result in death. Such a gene exists for brachyphalangy, a condition in which the middle joint of the fingers is greatly shortened. A marriage between two individuals having this condition resulted in one of the four children, who was unable to survive, being born without any fingers or toes and with other skeletal defects. Of the surviving three children, one had normal fingers while the other two possessed short fingers. The exact 1:2:1 ratio was what could be expected if one considered the short fingers as being an intermediate expression of a dominant lethal gene (Winchester, 1979). A graphic illustration of this type of situation is presented in figure 1.4.

With brachyphalangy being produced by a dominant gene and the ratio of 2:1 tending to exist in surviving children of parents who both have brachyphalangy, one might well question why the abnormality is not more common. It is entirely possible that an individual with short fingers might have been so handicapped during the periods in our cultural

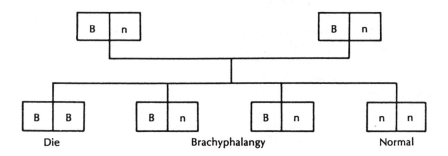

FIGURE 1.4 *Distribution of children from a marriage of two individuals with brachyphalangy.*

development when physical skill was a prerequisite to survival that few of them lived to reproduce. On the other hand, it is possible that brachyphalangy may be a relatively recent genetic mutation. In this case the possibility of marriage between two people having the condition is not very great and the ratio of brachyphalangy in the children of a marriage involving only one person with brachyphalangy would tend to be 2:2.

Genetic **anomalies** also occur when there are irregularities in meiotic cell division such as the lack of separation of the twenty-first chromosome pair during the reduction phase so that the offspring has three rather than a pair of the twenty-first chromosome. This condition results in Down's Syndrome and appears most frequently in births to women over 35 years of age. It is possible to determine prenatally the chromosomal array of the offspring by a process called **amniocentesis.** After the amniotic cavity has been formed during pregnancy, the fluid filling the cavity contains cells which have been shed by the developing organism. A sample of the cell-filled **amniotic fluid** is withdrawn by inserting a hollow needle through the abdomen of the mother. The cells are then cultured to encourage mitotic division so that the chromosomes can be microscopically analyzed. Most chromosomal aberrations can be detected by using amniocentesis and, in addition, more than 50 different metabolic disorders can be diagnosed by direct testing of the amniotic fluid withdrawn during the process. Genetic disorders involving the blood, such as sickle cell anemia, may be diagnosed from minute samples of fetal blood withdrawn from the fetal veins in the placenta by a procedure called **fetoscopy.** Such analysis enables the parents, in consultation with their doctor, to reach a decision as to whether pregnancy should be terminated or continued.

SEX-ASSOCIATED GENES

The foregoing discussion of dominant and recessive genes applies to all the paired genes in 44 of the 46 chromosomes in the human body. The remaining two chromosomes are the sex determinants of an individual and are called the X and Y chromosomes. The X chromosome has been found to be much longer than the Y chromosome, which means that a number of the genes in the X chromosome are unpaired in the male of the species (XY chromosome arrangement). Because the X chromosome in the male comes from the mother (XX), the son inherits all the effects of these unmatched genes regardless of whether they would be dominant or recessive in a pairing with the genes of another X chromosome.

Figure 1.5 illustrates the transmission of color blindness from mother to son while the daughters, although also having a color blind gene, do not have the symptoms. In this instance, the recessive gene on the X

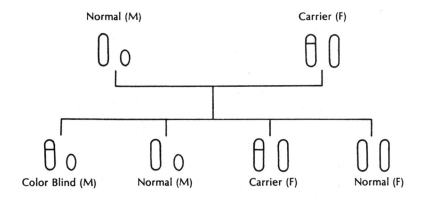

FIGURE 1.5. *Diagram of transmission of color blindness in humans.*

chromosome results in a color blind son and a carrier daughter with a recessive color blind gene. Only in the rare instance of a marriage between a color blind man and a woman with a recessive color gene, or even rarer, with a color blind woman, would there be color blind female children.

The same explanation applies to the other major X-linked abnormality, hemophelia. However, the nature of this genetic condition prevents it from being as common as color blindness. Only about one male in each ten thousand is afflicted with hemophelia, or the bleeder's disease. In females the disease is rare; the chance of a marriage between a man with hemophelia and a woman carrier is about one in 50 million. One half of the daughters of such a marriage could inherit the two recessive genes; this raises the odds to one in 100 million. However, when there is close inbreeding in families that carry the gene the chance of occurrence increases greatly for both sexes (Winchester, 1979).

Another type of sex-associated gene is the sex-limited gene which is normally expressed only in one sex but carried equally by both sexes. The sex-limited genes code the traits related to sex characteristics that include the primary sex traits directly related to reproduction and the secondary sex characteristics such as growth of hair on the face and differences in skeletal and muscular development. The expression of the sex-limited genes is affected by sex hormones, and abnormalities in sex hormone secretions may result in abnormalities in the expression of sex-limited traits (Winchester, 1979).

SEX RATIO AND MORTALITY

The imbalance of genes in the X and Y chromosomes seems to have effects beyond the determination of the sex of the individual with its numerous ramifications of biological sex development. The ratio of live births for males per 100 females range from 104.9 to 105.5 during the years 1940 to 1976 with the mean being 105.3. The excess of males over females at birth cannot be due to chance for our knowledge of meiosis indicates the production of an equal number of sperms with X and Y chromosomes by the male parent. One theory in explanation of this phenomenom concerns the difference in size of the sperms carrying the two types of chromosomes. The sperms carrying a Y are lighter in weight and smaller in size. It is believed this gives them a slight advantage in the race for the egg or, perhaps, in penetrating the cell wall of the egg. However, Winchester (1979) also reports that a number of investigations of the **karyotypes** of fetuses that were spontaneously aborted during very early pregnancy indicate a higher ratio of XX chromosomal array than of XY. This suggests the possibility that the sex ratio of conceptions may be approximately equal but that female losses are greater during the very early **embryonic period.**

After embryonic structural development of the sex organs, however, all data indicate that the male has a higher **mortality rate** than the female. Of the nearly 6000 spontaneously aborted embryos and fetuses in collection at the Carnegie Institute in Washington, the ratio of clearly recognizable males to females was 107.9 to 100 (Winchester, 1979). In addition, analysis of 2735 consecutive newborn autopsies by Naeye et al. (1971) indicated that the ratio of 128 males to 100 females differed significantly from that of 105:100 for all U.S. live births.

A survey of vital statistics data for fetal and early neonatal mortality in the U.S. from 1922 to 1936 and from 1950 to 1972 indicates that the sex ratio (male to female) of fetal deaths is highest from months three to five, lower from months six to eight, and increases at term with the sex ratio at conception being conservatively estimated to be 120 males to 100 females (McMillen, 1979).

In multiple births, the crowding and the reduced metabolic exchange per individual result in increased survival risks. Winchester (1979) makes note of the fact that the ratio of boys to girls in multiple births is lower than for single births and becomes increasingly lower with increases in the number of multiple births. In the United States, the ratio of twins is 103.5 boys to each 100 girls; for triplets, it is 98 boys to each 100 girls; while, for quadruplets, it drops to 70 boys for each 100 girls. Furthermore, it is pointed out that in regions where poor nutrition, insufficient medical care, and crowded conditions occur, there is a relatively lower birth ratio of males to females in comparison to areas having a high standard of living.

Although the sex ratio favors the males at birth, the higher mortality rate for males results in the sexes being nearly equal in number at 20 years of age. The higher mortality rate is particularly marked for infants under one year of age where the rate per 1000 was 17.6 for males and 14.2 for females in 1976. The improvements in medical and postnatal care that have occurred since 1940 have reduced the greater sex differential and the previously higher infant mortality rates of 61.9 for males and 47.7 for females (U.S. Bureau of the Census, 1978). However, the mortality rates remain higher for males at all age levels and later in life women outnumber men. By the age of 50, women outnumber men by about 100 to 85 and at 85 years of age are approximately twice as numerous as men (Winchester, 1979). Landreth (1958) cites the fact that, along with a higher mortality rate at all age levels, males are more likely to have congenital deformities.

GENETIC ALTERATIONS

Until recently, the appearance of **mutations,** which involve chemical changes in genetic structure that are capable of being transmitted to future generations of offspring through the germ cells, was the only known method of genetic alteration. Although we are not aware of all the factors which may cause mutations, we do know that mutations are more likely to occur in the germ cells of older fathers and that high levels of radiation will contribute to the increased appearance of mutations in both sexes. The latter knowledge has been of utmost importance in world affairs since the development of the atomic bomb. At a 1978 international meeting of geneticists, it was estimated that the percentage of children born with **congenital** defects had doubled within the previous 25 years. The proportion of children born with congenital defects was estimated at over 6 percent (*This World,* 1978b).

A mutation which received a great deal of political prominence in the early part of the century was the appearance of hemophelia in the offspring of Queen Victoria. Because of the custom of intermarriages among royal families and the practice of assigning prime inheritance to the male offspring, the sudden appearance of this mutation had serious repercussions in the royal families of Germany, Russia, and Spain. Edward, Queen Victoria's father, was 52 years old at the time of Victoria's birth and it is conjectured that his chromosome was the site of the mutation (McKusick, 1965).

Although its biochemical mechanism of operation has not been understood until relatively recently, the importance of heredity has long been appreciated by man with research efforts focused not only on the identification of genetic structure but on the modification of that structure with the aim of eradication of genetic anomalies. The development of the electron microscope, laser, and atomic reactors and accelerators has opened the immense field of biophysics to the geneticist and medical researcher. Such efforts have resulted in research on recombinant DNA where pieces of genes from widely dissimilar species of living organisms are combined to create new hybrid genes that may potentially synthesize disease specific antibodies, hormones such as insulin, or enzymes to correct genetic defects. Some genes with simple genetic coding have been synthesized and a few nonhistone proteins, which regulate the expression of specific genes, have been identified in nonhuman chromatin.

The control as well as moral problems associated with genetic engineering place constraints upon the applications of this type of research. It would seem that genetic counseling imposes fewer constraints on the aim of eradication of genetic anomalies. However, the success of such counseling depends upon the identification and cataloging of genetic information. Chemical and laser technology have made the task of sorting and cloning genetic material a faster and easier process so that approximately 17 "libraries" of human genetic material have been created. These libraries contain the genetic coding and locations for about 5000 of the approximately 50,000 active genes in the human body. Included are the genes believed to be responsible for such inherited ailments as Down's Syndrome and Huntington's chorea. The genetic aspects of cystic fibrosis and Alzheimer's disease are also being investigated. These libraries of genetic information are constantly expanding their compiled knowledge of both harmless normal variations in human chromosomes as well as harmful anomalies and the potential exists that, in the future, chromosomal analysis may be as common as blood tests for individuals who are planning to be married.

SUMMARY

1. The genetic blueprint for living matter is contained in the compound deoxyribonucleic acid (DNA) and in humans the DNA is contained within the 46 chromosomes in the nucleus.

2. The 46 chromosomes are organized into 23 pairs, each of which have similar DNA composition and function with the exception of the 23rd pair (X and Y chromosomes) which are the sex determining chromosomes.

3. In the reproductive cells (sperm and egg), the number of chromosomes is reduced to 23 (haploid number) and, with the fusion of the sperm and egg during conception, the number again becomes the normal 46 (diploid number).

4. Each chromosome contains segments of DNA which act as a unit called a gene. In association with its paired gene, each gene may have a dominant or recessive characteristic which determines how this gene will influence the development of the individual after conception.

5. During the developmental process, some genes (master genes) have the function of controlling the differentiation and timing processes that change the single celled organism into a multicelled structure. Other genes produce the proteins from which the body cells are constructed.

6. Increasing knowledge of genetic structure (DNA arrangement) is constantly increasing information about normal and abnormal gene structure.

7. In general, genetic material (which is transmitted to the offspring by the mother and father) determines the physical structures and most cellular functioning of the offspring. The degree to which the child attains the optimal development of these inherited characteristics is determined by the environment in which the child develops.

2

Prenatal Maternal Influences

With the maturation of the reproductive germ cells into the egg and sperms, as the case may be, the hereditary contribution of the parents to the potential offspring is completed. If no union is effected between the egg and a sperm, the egg disintegrates. However, fertilization of the egg by the penetration of its wall by a sperm marks the conception of a new offspring and from this moment the environment in which the individual grows and develops influences the extent of attainment of the hereditary contributions.

PRENATAL DEVELOPMENTAL PERIODS

When, in the course of its progress down the fallopian tube from the ovary to the uterus, the egg is fertilized, the haploid number of chromosomes in the **gametes** (sperm and egg) combine to form a cell with 46 chromosomes. This initiates the **germinal period** and triggers off the processes that result in the development of a human individual. The wall of the **zygote** (fertilized ovum) becomes impermeable to additional sperms and mitotic cell division begins. During the three or four days it takes the fertilized egg to travel down the fallopian tube to the uterus, mitotic cell division has transformed the single cell into a solid, spherical cluster of cells called a **morula.** Test-tube babies, where conception takes place by exposing a mature egg to sperm and then providing laboratory conditions suitable to the division of the embryonic cells, are injected into the mother's uterus in a simulation of the timing of natural progress down the fallopian tubes (*This World,* 1978a). In the uterus, where the developing organism floats about for a few days, it continues cell division and its structure changes to that of a hollow sphere with a tiny protuberance, called the **inner cell mass,** at one spot along its inner wall so that it is now called a **blastocyst.**

The outer cell layer of the blastocyst is called the **trophoblast** and this develops small burr-like tendrils on the outside which are utilized in the process of burrowing into the prepared wall of the uterus. Implantation usually occurs from seven to 10 days after fertilization with the blastocyst positioned so that the side with the inner cell mass lies in contact with the uterine lining. Some of the cells of the trophoblast begin to differentiate to form villi which work their way into the uterine wall to become closely associated with the maternal blood vessels in the uterus and thus form the placenta during later pregnancy (figure 2.1). It is believed that a hormone produced by the fetal part of the placenta plays a part in **damping** the **thymus-lymphatic system** of the mother so that the embryo, which is a foreign body, is not rejected by the mother (Tanner & Taylor, 1965). Additional trophoblastic cells differentiate to form the protective layers of the chorion and amnion, the allantois, and the umbilical cord that houses the blood vessels carrying nutrients from the placenta to the developing organism and waste products back to the placenta.

As the amniotic membrane enlarges it becomes filled with amniotic fluid which has a definite chemical make-up and specific gravity of 1006-

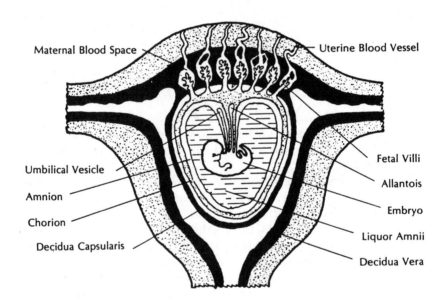

FIGURE 2.1. *Diagram representing the relationship between the uterus, the membranes, and the embryo during pregnancy. (From L. Carmichael, The onset and early development of behavior. In L. Carmichael (Ed.), Manual of child psychology (2d ed.). New York: John Wiley & Sons, Inc., 1954. By permission of the publisher.)*

1081 (Feldman, 1920). The amniotic fluid provides a cushioning effect for the developing embryo and, because of the consistency of its chemical composition, lends itself to analysis for purposes of identifying prenatal anomalies. The two-week period from conception until the formation of the blastocyst and connections have been completed with the wall of the uterus is known as the **germinal period.**

The inner cell mass is the segment of the blastocyst that develops into a recognizable human being during the next six weeks known as the period of the embryo. The **primitive streak,** a group of **ectodermal** cells which emerge at one end of the embryonic disc at about the twelfth day after conception, appears to be the organizer for embryonic develop-ment. **Mesodermal** cells develop from the primitive streak and form the **notochord** and **somites.** The notochord organizes the rest of the embryo so that the adjacent upper ectodermal cells multiply to produce a thick-ened strip which becomes the neural groove, then neural tube, and ulti-mately the spinal cord and brain. In addition, the notochord causes the mesodermal cells on each side to be arranged in paired blocks (somites) which eventually develop into the vertebrae and muscles of the back (Tanner & Taylor, 1965). (The differentiation and integration of the sensory-motor system is examined in greater depth in another section.)

The layer of cells of the inner cell mass which faces the cavity of the trophoblastic sac is called the **endoderm** and it combines with the other types of cells, primarily mesodermal, to form the organs of the body. For example, the digestive system begins as a tube of mesodermal cells lined with cells from the endoderm. In general, the ectoderm of the embry-onic disc continues its development to differentiate into the epidermis of the skin, nails, hair, **cutaneous** glands, oral glands, enamel of teeth, lens of eye, and the entire nervous system including the sense organs. The **mesoderm** eventually forms the dermis, or inner layer of the skin, con-nective tissue, all types of muscles, blood and the circulatory system, the skeletal structure, kidneys and excretory organs, and the lymphatic sys-tem. The endoderm differentiates to produce the lining of the digestive tract and associated glands, the respiratory system, the liver, and various glands of internal secretion.

The six week span of the embryonic period is remarkable for the rapid and marked changes that take place as, from a pin-head size cluster of relatively undifferentiated cells, there develops a miniature individual approximately 1½ to 2 inches in length complete with all essential inter-nal and external features, some not yet functional, encased in a protec-tive world of its own making. During the third week after conception, small blood vessels begin to form within the placental villi which are pro-liferating rapidly. By the fourth week, the heart tubes have fused and the U-shaped heart begins to beat in its position outside the main body cav-ity, but the primitive nervous system with the two-lobed brain must be

greatly refined before it becomes functional. The embryo's blood is produced by the yolk sac at this time for the internal mechanisms for blood
manufacture are not yet available and will not be functional until the
sixth week when the liver takes over blood manufacture after which the
process is eventually assumed by the bone marrow.

The fourth week also marks the appearance of limb buds but neither
limbs nor digits achieve form until 8 weeks of age. The internal organs
also begin developing at this time so that by the beginning of the eighth
week the stomach secretes gastric juices even though it contains no food.
By the eighth week, the major musculature has been formed and the
elastic cartilage of the skeleton is beginning to be replaced by bone
tissue. The head is recognizably human with eyes, ears, nose, and mouth
all present. In short, the embryonic period marks the period of greatest
structural differentiation and integration for the developing organism
and culminates with appearance of all essential structures.

The development of the placenta and umbilical cord early in the
embryonic period makes maternal nutrients available to the organism. A
discussion of nutrition later in this chapter will emphasize the importance of adequate maternal nutritional intake during this crucial period
of structural differentiation and integration. It is important to note that
there is no direct connection between the fetal and maternal blood vessels and that food and oxygen for the embryo and waste products from
the embryo must be filtered through a living membrane. There are also
no neural connections between the mother and the fetus, which rules
out the possibility, as is sometimes believed, that the nervous condition
of the mother will directly affect the child.

The period of the fetus (**fetal period**), which extends from the end of
the second month until birth, is one where development consists mainly
of changes in relative or actual size and of refinement of existing structures rather than the appearance of new parts. The rapid physical growth
that occurs during the fetal period is marked by differential growth rates
in body parts. During the early part of this period there is rapid increase in
body length, but as the growth rate in this dimension begins to decline, a
rapid increase in limb length occurs. A sevenfold increase in trunk length
and an eightfold increase in limb length alter the body proportions. The
head, which was 1/3 of the body length at the end of the embryonic
period, becomes less than 1/4 and the trunk less than 1/2 the total length,
while the limbs are a little more than 1/4 of the body length at the time of
birth.

Although not marked by the appearance of new parts, the fetal period is characterized by the completion of integration and the stabilization
of function of essential life structures and by the first appearance of
sensory-motor behavior. The functional development of the individual is
examined in greater detail in another section. So rapid is this functional

development that, by the end of the seventh lunar month, the fetus has reached the state of development that would make survival possible should birth occur at this time. This is referred to as the age of **viability.** However, the body is not completely formed until the end of the next month and chances of survival increase as the age of the fetus approaches that of the normal full term. The last two months of pregnancy contribute to maturation of lung tissue, increased functional levels of the reflexive system, increased muscular and fat deposition, and the acquisition of immunities from the maternal system.

TERM OF PREGNANCY

Although the normal term of pregnancy is usually placed at 280 days, Needham (1931) has summarized the estimates of a number of investigators and found them to vary from 270 to 284 days. Another survey (Landreth, 1958) indicates that two-thirds of all pregnancies terminate within two weeks, plus or minus, of 279 days. Although the opinion has been expressed that it may be possible to successfully rear premature infants who have passed less than 180 days in the mother's body, the average lower limit below which viability cannot be maintained is usually taken to be 180 days (Hess, 1922).

The weight of the infant is also important in premature viability and survival is doubtful if the child is under three pounds at birth. However, the establishment of special neonatal care centers is increasing the viability percentages for premature small-for-age infants such as Tammy who weighed one pound and eleven ounces at birth (*University Bulletin,* 1972a). The smallest known surviving infant is Marion Chapman who weighed 10 ounces and was 12½ inches long when born on June 5, 1938 in Northwest England. She was born unattended and subsequently fed hourly through a fountain pen filler by Dr. D. A. Shearer. By her first birthday she had attained a weight of 13 pounds 14 ounces, and weighed 106 pounds on her twenty-first birthday (McWhirter, 1978). In the United States, the smallest known infant, Jacqueline Benson, weighed 12 ounces when born in Illinois in 1936, spent 4½ months in an incubator, and grew to normal womanhood. Tanner and Taylor (1965) speculate that Jacqueline's birth probably occurred during the sixth month of pregnancy when the respiratory and reflex systems had developed sufficiently to sustain life in the cloistered environment of an incubator.

Premature infants with insufficiently developed lungs are subject to a severe respiratory condition called **hyaline membrane disease** (HMD). Mature lungs have a substance called **surfactant** which forms a film on the surface of the lungs and helps the lungs retain some residual air to prevent collapse during exhalation. Prior to birth, the level of surfactant in the fetal lung can be determined by testing a sample of the amniotic fluid of the expectant mother. In instances where the test shows that respiratory problems are imminent, lifesaving treatment can be made available and initiated immediately after birth. One of the techniques is Continuous Positive Airway Pressure, which involves placing a tube in the baby's trachea and forcing a steady stream of air into the lungs. Usually between the third and fifth day after birth the cell lining of the lungs begins to produce the vital surfactant and the pressure is reduced as the lungs improve. The use of this technique has sharply decreased the incidence of side effects, such as mental retardation, blindness, and cerebral palsy occurring in the survivors of HMD, in addition to substantially increasing the survival rate (*University Bulletin,* 1972b).

At the postmaturity end of the scale, Ballantyne and Browne (1922) indicate that 334 days may be the longest legally considered period for the fetus to have remained inside the mother's body and still be delivered alive. Our knowledge of labor-inducing hormones has increased considerably since publication of Ballantyne and Browne's survey of the problems of fetal postmaturity so that it has become common medical practice to utilize such hormones to assist in the inducement of labor for women whose pregnancy is exceeding that of the normative term of pregnancy.

MULTIPLE BIRTHS

Sometimes, rather than the usual single egg, two eggs may be present in the fallopian tubes and each of these may be fertilized by a different sperm. In this case, the development of both fertilized ova would proceed as if only one ovum were present except for the restrictions that the uterine cavity would have to be shared by the developing individuals as would the nourishment available from the mother. The space limitations would impose restrictions upon the size and activity of the two developing fetuses while the food and oxygen limitations would also affect size and activity. Twins produced from the fertilization of separate ova by separate sperms are called nonidentical, or fraternal twins, and have no greater genetic similarity to each other than to their other brothers and sisters. Furthermore, they may be of either sex. They tend, however, to show greater similarity in acquired characteristics than do ordinary siblings because of the greater similarity in their experiences as they grow up together.

It is also possible that, instead of dividing and maintaining a cohesion between the two new cells during the first mitotic division, a fertilized ovum may divide so that no cohesion exists between the two new cells.

These new cells in turn continue to divide and develop independently into two separate individuals who have a common genetic background. Winchester (1961) cites a simple but dramatic experiment to illustrate this process. If a fertilized salamander egg is pinched in two along the line of demarcation between the cells after the first mitotic division, the two separated cells will continue to divide and differentiate until eventually each develops into a complete salamander. Human twins formed by this cleavage process are identical with respect to their genetic inheritance and are consequently always of the same sex. They also have identical hair-whorl patterns; the same color and pattern in the iris of the eyes; the same hair texture; and similarly shaped ears, lips, and eyebrows. Physiologically, they have the same blood type, subtype, and **Rh factor**, and it has been found that skin grafts and kidney transplantations may be successfully made from one identical twin to another.

Approximately once in every four identical twin births, a phenomenon called mirror-imaging occurs. In this instance, the physical characteristics of one side of one twin's body are reflected in the opposite side of the other twin so that if one twin's hair spirals clockwise, the other's hair does so in a counterclockwise direction; one twin's heart and appendix are on the left side, the other twin's are on the right; dental irregularities appear on opposite sides while opposing eyes are dominant. Since one's impression of one's personal appearance is gained from observation of one's image in a mirror, it is easy to believe stories of mirror-image twins talking to their reflection in an unexpected mirror in the belief that it is their mirror-image twin (Hicks, 1963).

Multiple human births may also occur in threes, fours, fives, and even sixes. The likelihood of occurrence of twin births is once in approximately 85 births; triplets, once in 7225 births, quadruplets, once in every 614,125 births; and quintuplets, once in every 52,200,625 births (Hurlock, 1953).

There have been fewer than 50 recorded cases of the birth of quintuplets with the Dionne quintuplets, who are identical, being the first set to survive to adulthood. The Diligenti quintuplets of Argentina were the second group to survive; they are a fraternal set composed of two boys and three girls (Hicks, 1963). Of the less than 10 authenticated cases of the birth of sextuplets, the Rosenkowitz sextuplets, who were delivered by **Caesarean**, are the first set to survive. The South African sextuplets are comprised of three boys and three girls whose weight at birth ranged from 2 pounds, 12 ounces to 4 pounds, 8 ounces for a total weight of all infants of 26 pounds, 1 ounce (*National Enquirer*, 1974). A second set of sextuplets also delivered by Caesarean and weighing from 2.2 pounds to 2.75 pounds were reported as being in very good condition in Leyden, Netherlands (*This World*, 1977). In this instance, as in the case of septuplets who did not survive (*Oakland Tribune,* 1966), the mothers had been treated with fertility hormones. Early detection of multiple births by such recent technological advances as ultrasound (or **sonography**) and increasing medical knowledge of hormonal interactions during pregnancy are tending to enhance the survival potential of multiple birth children.

From the preceding discussion, it is obvious that both fraternal and identical twins may be found in all categories of multiple births. With triplets, there can be three different combinations. (1) A single egg fertilized by a single sperm divides and one of the resulting two eggs divides again. This results in identical triplets. (2) Two separate sperms fertilize two separate eggs of which one divides to form twins. This results in two identical twins and one fraternal twin. (3) Three separate eggs are fertilized by three separate sperms resulting in fraternal triplets. Similarly, there can be five different combinations with quadruplets and seven with quintuplets.

The age of the mother seems to have some influence on the likelihood of the occurrence of multiple births. Older women are more likely to have twins than are younger women. A woman of 40 is three or four times as likely to have twins as a woman 20 years old. The maximal twin frequency occurs when the mother is in her 37th year. The age of the father has no effect on the twin rate. Furthermore, the tendency towards identical multiple births may be inherited from either parent, whereas the tendency towards fraternal twins is carried principally by the female. There are some remarkable family histories such as those of a Sicilian woman who produced 11 sets of fraternal twins in as many years and an Australian woman who is reported to have borne 69 children including four sets of quadruplets, seven sets of triplets, and 16 sets of twins (Hicks, 1963).

PRENATAL MATERNAL INFLUENCES

Even within the mother's body, survival is beset with numerous problems. During the period of the ovum, the yolk must have enough nourishment to enable the zygote to complete its journey down the fallopian tubes to the uterus or it will die. If the uterus has not been properly prepared to receive the ovum, implantation cannot occur and the fertilized egg disintegrates from lack of nourishment (Hurlock, 1953). Although the living membrane in the placenta acts as a filter through which food and oxygen pass to reach the developing individual, it is also permeable to alcohol, nicotine, drugs, and some viruses and bacteria. If the mother's diet is insufficient to meet the demands of the developing fetus, the latter exerts a parasitic effect in various ways, for example, the robbing of the mother's teeth of calcium. Certain glandular conditions of the mother may indirectly affect the fetus as hormonal secretions filter through the placenta. Thus violent emotional states of the mother may be reflected in unusual activity of the fetus. The embryo seems to be particularly susceptible to maternal conditions. The first six weeks after implantation is the period of rapid differentiation of the various organs of the body and as such is the most crucial and vulnerable period in an organ's development.

NUTRITION

The nutritional adequacy of the expectant mother's diet seems to have a very definite effect upon the condition of the newborn infant, its size, and the length of its term. A study made by Burke et al. (1943) reports that where the mother's diet was excellent, 95 percent of the children were born in excellent condition whereas in instances where the mother's diet was poor, only 8 percent of the infants were in excellent condition. Furthermore, a positive correlation of .80 was found between the length of the infant and the protein intake of the mother.

Since proteins are necessary for human growth and are obtainable in quantity and quality only in the more expensive foods such as meats and fishes, it may be assumed that they would tend to be in inadequate supply among low income groups and, as such, affect the condition of the infants in these groups. This surmise tends to be confirmed by the results of a study by Baird (1945) of the relationship between prematurity and the income of the family, with observations indicating that the percentage of prematurity was twice as high in the lower income groups of Scotland than it was among those groups of higher status, both economic and social.

Since the developing fetus is dependent entirely upon maternal nutrition supplied through the placenta, the condition of the placenta is of crucial importance to the development of the organism. Winick (1967, 1970), noting that placentas from infants with "intrauterine growth failure" showed fewer cells in comparison with controls, found that 50 percent of the placentas from an indigent population in Chile had a decreased number of cells and placentas from a malnourished population in Guatemala had fewer cells than the norm. The effects of poverty on the weight of organs and body measurements of stillborn infants or infants who had died within 48 hours after birth was examined by Naeye et al. (1969). The families of 49 of the autopsied infants were classified as poor, whereas 203 were in the nonpoor classification. The poverty infants had decreased total birth weights and decreased size and weights of organs such as brain, internal organs, and skeletal bones. There was a significant difference between the 2.0 millimeter mean thickness of the abdominal **subcutaneous** fat of the poor infants and of the 4.5 millimeter mean thickness of the nonpoor.

The noted decrease in skeletal bone size for autopsied poor children supports the findings of Scott and Usher (1964) who X-rayed the knees of 30 markedly malnourished infants and 18 **controls** (normally nourished infants) within the first six days after birth. The mean diameter of the distal femor at its largest point was 3.8 millimeters in the malnourished whereas it was 5.9 in the controls. Similarly, the average diameter of the proximal tibia was 1.6 millimeters in the malnourished and 4.8 millimeters in the controls. Scott and Usher also examined the development of, or absence of, the **epiphysis**. In interpreting this data it should be kept in mind that the developing bone begins its growth in the center of the bone and growth of new bone tissue progresses to the extremities of the bone until the epiphyseal layer, which is the last segment where bone growth may occur, is reached. It was noted that the distal femoral epiphysis was absent in 37 percent of the malnourished infants but was present in all the controls, whereas the proximal tibial epiphysis was absent in 84 percent of the malnourished infants and in only 17 percent of the controls. In addition to indicating that bone development is affected by nutritional status, these results also illustrate the **proximal-distal** direction of skeletal development. As the correlation between epiphyseal size and birth weight was .835 and with body length was .651 but only .137 with gestation age, it may be concluded that epiphyseal development is much more dependent on birth weight and length than on gestational age and that fetal malnourishment produces a striking delay in skeletal maturation.

The birth weight of infants also appears to have some relationship to behavior. Drillien (1972) assessed behavioral neurological signs on the basis of abnormalities of movement and posture, of reflexes, and of retardation in development, especially postural. Of the 35 infants with a birth weight of 1250 grams or less, 52 percent exhibited moderate or severe abnormal neurological signs during the first year of life. There was a gradual decrease in the incidence of abnormality with increasing birth weight so that only 18 percent of the 102 children weighing 1751-2000 grams at birth had moderate to severe neurological signs. Drillien also examined the neurological status of the children at 2 and 3 years of age on the basis of presence or absence of moderate or severe **dystonia** during the first year of life. He concluded that children who exhibited moderate or severe transient dystonia in the first year of life may have more difficulties in both mental and motor performance at school age than children who did not exhibit such symptoms. It is also possible that some low birth weight infants may be more prone to becoming "clumsy children." An incidence of 3.5 percent has been reported among 165 very low birth weight children born during 1961-70 (Davies & Tizard, 1975) and clumsiness has been observed in experimental adult animals following undernutrition during their prenatal period of rapid growth of the **cerebellum** (Dobbing & Smart, 1974).

In a summary of the characteristics of the population associated with low birth weight infants, Davies and Stewart (1975) indicate that low socio-economic status is a prime factor with the poor childhood status of the mother correlating most closely with low birth weight. Mothers of low birth weight infants tend to be above average age or very young, to smoke, to be single, and to eschew antenatal care. In addition, they often have a history of reproductive failure, involving infertility, recurrent abortion, stillbirths, or previous low birth weight infants. Davies and Stewart point out that the chance of survival of low birth weight infants has increased during the past 10 years owing to a better understanding of their illnesses and to technological advances in perinatal care with the improvements in survival rates being greatest in centers specializing in such care. However, the most desirable approach to the problems of prematurity and low birth weight is prevention, and this is markedly enhanced by maintenance of a nutritionally adequate diet for the expectant and nursing mother.

MATERNAL INFECTIONS

It has been found that when rubella, or German measles, is contracted in the first month of pregnancy, the expectant mother has a 50-50 chance of delivering a defective child. Even in the second or third month contraction of the disease presents an 8 percent chance of delivery of a deformed child, with the defects including congenital deafness, cataracts, abnormal heart formation, and mental retardation (Cooper, 1966). Since the early differentiation of the organs most affected by the disease takes place during this time, it would appear that these organs tend to pass through a critical period in development in which they are most susceptible to certain environmental influences. The possibility for malformation of the child is very great for the expectant mother who contacts rubella especially during the early weeks after conception before the woman even realizes that she is pregnant. Therefore, all females should be vaccinated for rubella prior to childbearing age or else the woman should avoid all contacts with the disease in situations where there is even the slightest possibility of pregnancy.

As well as causing deformities during early pregnancy, some maternal infections may be transmitted to the unborn child and result in its birth with the infectious condition or its death. Some of the infections that may result in the death of the infant are influenza, smallpox, typhoid fever, chicken pox, measles, and syphilis, with the latter disease also presenting the alternatives of blindness or other abnormalities, as well as prematurity and stillbirth. Other maternal infections which, through the condition of the mother, will usually result in the death of the unborn child are cholera, erysipelas, and malaria.

DRUGS

As with infections, some drugs cause fetal malformations when the drug is ingested or injected, in even small amounts, during the early formative period of pregnancy. Laboratory testing of drugs may not reveal their potential effects on fetal development since laboratory animals do not respond in exactly the same way as humans; moreover, there is also considerable variability of response among humans.

The problems associated with drug use and potential effects on fetal development are illustrated by the highly publicized accounts of the use of the tranquilizing drug, **thalidomide.** It was found that a high incidence of malformed births occurred when the drug was taken by an expectant mother in the early stages of her pregnancy, with the most obvious defects being congenital deformities such as paddle appendages or lack of limb development as well as heart and other internal organ deformities. In West Germany, where the drug was easily available from 1957 to 1962, an estimated 5000 malformed births were attributed to the drug with about 2000 of these babies dying as a result of their deformities. In the United States, however, later release and more stringent controls of the drug resulted in only 14 cases of gross deformities of newborn babies directly traceable to thalidomide. The publicity surrounding the discovery of the deforming effects of thalidomide resulted in its withdrawal from the market and pointed up the dangers associated with the administration of drugs to pregnant women.

In a survey of adverse drug reactions to the fetus, Shirkey (1972) states that any drug administered in proper dosage and at the appropriate stage of development may cause embryonic disturbances. This investigator points out that there are many sources of potential danger such as prescribed drugs, drugs obtained from other sources, food additives, and environmental hazards. Although the tranquilizer drugs are under high suspicion for causing malformations and injurious effects, the common drugs with a long history of use are not absolved. The standard treatment for malaria, quinine, may result in deafness in the newborn child. Even such a common medication as aspirin may depress the formation of fibrinogen (an agent in the clotting of blood) so that its use during the last three months of pregnancy may result in an increase in the length of labor and an increase in clotting time.

Alcohol, consumed in excessive amounts by the mother during early pregnancy, may result in death or malformation. Children of alcoholic mothers are sometimes born with a pattern of birth defects that is called *fetal alcohol syndrome*. The most prominent aspect of this syndrome is growth retardation and early death (The National Foundation/March of Dimes, 1977). Some of these infants may also suffer from withdrawal as do the infants of mothers engaged in narcotic drug consumption, such as heroin, cocaine, or morphine. Here, drug consumption by the mother may result in the child entering the world as a drug addict and subjected to withdrawal symptoms in addition to the adjustments of the change from uterine to postnatal environmental conditions.

The nicotine from smoking has been found to have the same stimulating and depressant effects on the child as it does on the mother but to a larger magnitude since the same amount of nicotine is available to the much smaller body area of the fetus. The National Foundation/March of Dimes (1977) indicates that women who smoke heavily (a pack a day or more) tend to have low-birth weight babies of 5½ pounds or less. A study by Sexton and Hebel (1984) reports pregnant smokers who received smoking intervention had, for single, live births, children whose birth weight was 92 grams heavier and were 0.6 centimeters greater in length than infants born to the control smoking mothers. Thus, some fetal growth retardation can be overcome by providing antismoking assistance to pregnant women. Stillbirths and early infant mortality also occur more frequenty among babies of women who smoke during pregnancy. The degree of the effect of these factors seems to depend upon how much the mother smokes and it is not known if it is the nicotine that is responsible for the growth changes or whether it is the smoking-related constriction of the placental blood vessels which deprives the fetus of adequate nutrients. Smoking is expecially harmful during the second half of pregnancy when the central nervous system is developing rapidly and the fetus gains markedly in weight.

Exposure, over varying periods of time, to some types of agricultural pesticides or to industrial processes and/or wastes may cause prenatal complication because substances such as lead, mercury, or arsenic will filter through the placenta to the fetus. One of the most widely known incidents of industrial pollution is that of the poisoning of the offshore waters of Minamata, Japan, with mercuric waste products. In this instance, consumption of great amounts of fish and shellfish caught in Minamata Bay resulted in central nervous system damage to individuals at all age levels including fetal. Neural damage was centered in the **cere-**

bral cortex and cerebellum resulting in varying degrees of mental retardation and motor impairment (Murakami, 1972).

Rh INCOMPATIBILITY

An intrauterine problem that may cause complications during pregnancy is the incompatibility of Rh blood types between the mother and her developing child. Although, as previously mentioned, there is no direct exchange of blood between the mother and her child, there may, toward the end of the pregnancy when the weight and the movements of the fetus cause some capillary breakage in the placenta, be some seepage of blood from the fetus to the mother. In instances where an Rh negative mother is carrying her first Rh positive child, this seepage results in the prodution of antibodies in the mother's blood. Because it has no **Rh factor,** her body therefore treats the Rh factor in the blood that has entered her system from the child as a noxious substance. Since this seepage usually occurs towards the end of pregnancy and it takes some time for the mother to develop antibodies to the Rh factor, this process usually has no effect upon the first Rh positive child born to the Rh negative mother. However, the sensitization that has been produced in the mother may have been great enough to develop a **titre** of antibodies that may be sufficiently high to affect the blood cells of the embryos of any future Rh positive pregnancies. In this instance, the second, or any subsequent, Rh positive child will be born with **erythroblastosis fetalis,** a condition which is characterized by immature, nucleated red blood cells that are inefficient carriers of oxygen, and with anemia and jaundice (Winchester, 1961).

Since 85 percent of the population has Rh positive blood and the foregoing situation only occurs in instances when marriage involves an Rh positive man and an Rh negative woman—the gene for the Rh factor is dominant—some indication is given as to the likelihood of Rh incompatibility resulting from a marriage. Surveys indicate that approximately 12 percent of marriages involve Rh positive males and Rh negative females. Of the total number of children of these marriages, a study in England found that one child in every 23 had erythroblastosis. However, this total included first born positive children as well as all Rh negative children so that, while the overall chance appears low, it masks the truth with respect to subsequent Rh positive children born to Rh negative mothers. Here the danger is very great and a physician can be readily alerted to possible incompatability, if the mother has been found to be Rh negative, by testing blood samples from the father and all previous children or by the previous births of children with erythroblastosis. In the event of the live birth of a child with erythroblastosis, the child may be saved by draining off some of the damaged blood and replacing it with transfusions of compatible Rh positive blood immediately after birth and during the first few subsequent days (Wincheser, 1979).

For an Rh negative woman bearing her first Rh positive child, an injection of **rhogam** immediately after the birth of the child will prevent the formation of antibodies from any possible Rh positive blood seepage into the maternal blood stream. Rhogam is the **gamma globulin** fraction of the blood from an Rh negative person who has previously been sensitized to the Rh factor. As the injected rhogam neutralizes the Rh factor from the fetal blood, the Rh negative mother never builds up a titre of antibodies. This process must be repeated for each Rh positive pregnancy and is not applicable once the Rh negative mother has built up antibodies to the Rh factor (Winchester, 1979).

POSITION OF FETUS

Another factor in the intrauterine environment of the fetus that affects its development is its position in the uterus. It has been found that pressure on the tips of the bones stimulates ossification of the bone. However, the fetus must relax in order to accommodate to its cramped quarters in the uterus so that, in instances of excessive relaxation of the hip ligaments, it is possible that the lack of pressure will result in the birth of a child with a congenital cartilaginous dislocated hip. Such a defect may be remedied by medical treatment after birth (Landreth, 1958).

Although maldevelopment of the limb bud may also be the cause, it is possible that clubfoot may be due to the position of the child in the uterus. Since correction involves the stretching of muscles and ligaments and the realignment of bones, treatment must begin early and is usually prolonged to prevent recurrence. In instances of multiple births, the cramped quarters and the more limited food supply available to each developing child tend to restrict motility and size of the infants and are more likely to produce deformities of the cartilaginous tissue.

Experiments with animals tend to indicate that cleft lip and palate may also be partially attributable to the position of the embryo or the blood supply in the uterus as well as having genetic components. Although a cleft palate will also occur in 70 percent of the one in approximately every 1000 white births with a cleft lip, the two conditions are not genetically related; cleft palate appears less frequently. Investigations of the relationship of these conditions with regard to paternal age indicates that the risk of producing a child with cleft lip and cleft palate is increased in older parents (Woolf, 1963). Today many operative techniques are available for repairing these defects. Cleft lip, or more commonly, harelip, is repairable during the first few weeks after birth, and cleft palate is repairable before the child is 14 months old in the majority of cases.

AGE OF PARENTS

Parental age would seem to have a very decided effect in instances where chromosomal changes or errors are responsible for mutations, as previously mentioned with regard to hemophelia in Queen Victoria's offspring and for abnormalities such as Down 's Syndrome where all individuals have chromosomal error; namely, 47 chromosomes or the equivalent instead of the normal complement of 46 chromosomes. In all instances of chromosomal error, the cause can, of course, be either hereditary or environmental, or both. However, the high incidence of Down's Syndrome, an average expectation of about one child in every 50 births for women 45 years and over, in contrast with the expectancy of about one child in 2000 births for women of 25 years of age, certainly indicates that the environmental factor—in this case, age—plays a very important role. Since Down's Syndrome has an occurrence of one in 600 for all ages it would seem the incidence may also be higher at the younger age limits. Certainly, statistics for all birth defects show that mothers under 18 years and over 35 years of age have a higher proportion of children with birth defects than those between the ages of 18 and 35 years (The National Foundation/March of Dimes, 1977).

HORMONE DEFICIENCIES

Prior to 18 years of age, women are probably still undergoing physiological adjustments associated with increased **estrogen** production, whereas women over 40 years tend to have a decreased estrogen production. Therefore, it seems highly likely that hormonal imbalance is an adjunct of the age relationship to birth defects. Mothers of Down's Syndrome children tend to have a history of threatened abortions, impaired hormone regulation, menstrual irregularities, ovarian abnormalities, menopausal symptoms, or difficulties in becoming pregnant. It is also believed that a deficiency of maternal thyroxine during the early development of the embryo or of iodine in the later stages of pregnancy may be the cause of **cretinism**, which occurs in approximately two children in 10,000 births. No cure is known for cretinism or Down's Syndrome (Landreth, 1958).

SUMMARY AND DISCUSSION

With the exception of the last two items in table 2.1, the selected birth defects are ordered in terms of the highest to lowest annual incidence at birth. Muscular dystrophy and diabetes occur in childhood or later but are reported as having a prevalence of 200,000 and 90,000 re-

TABLE 2.1. Selected birth defects, U.S.A.*

Birth Defects	Type	Cause	Treatment
Prematurity/markedly low birthweight (4 lbs. 6 oz. or less)	Structural/functional: organs often immature	Hereditary and/or environmental	Intensive care of newborn, high nutrient diet
Congenital heart malformations	Structural	Hereditary and/or environmental	Corrective surgery, medication
Clubfoot	Structural: misshapen foot	Hereditary and/or environmental	Corrective surgery, corrective supports, physical exercises
Polydactyly	Structural: multiple fingers or toes	Hereditary: dominant inheritance	Corrective surgery, physical exercise
Erythroblastosis (Rh disease)	Blood disease: destruction of red blood cells	Hereditary and environmental	Transfusion: intrauterine or postnatal
Spina bifida and/or hydrocephalus	Structural/functional: incompletely formed spinal cord; water on the brain	Hereditary and environmental	Corrective surgery, prostheses, physical exercises, special schooling for any mental impairment
Down's syndrome	Functional/structural: retardation often associated with physical defects	Chromosomal abnormality	Corrective surgery, special physical training and schooling
Cleft lip and cleft palate	Structural	Hereditary and/or environmental	Corrective surgery
Cystic fibrosis	Functional: respiratory and digestive malfunctions	Hereditary: recessive inheritance	Treat respiratory and digestive complications
Sickle cell anemia	Blood disease: malformed red blood cells	Hereditary: incomplete recessive	Transfusions
Hemophilia	Blood disease: poor clotting	Hereditary: X-linked recessive inheritance	Clotting factor
Muscular dystrophy	Functional: impaired voluntary muscular functioning	Hereditary: often recessive inheritance	Physical therapy
Diabetes mellitus	Metabolic: inability to metabolize carbohydrates	Hereditary and/or environmental	Oral medication, diet, insulin injections

* Adapted mainly from Birth Defects, Tragedy and Hope. The National Foundation/March of Dimes, 1977.

spectively for individuals less than 20 years of age. For Americans of all ages, 4 million are estimated to be afflicted with diabetes (The National Foundation/March of Dimes, 1977).

The annual incidence of prematurity and/or markedly low birth weight is, at 50,000, twice as high as that of the next most frequently occurring birth defect, namely, congenital heart malformation. In the 9000 to 6000 annual incidence range are clubfoot, polydactyly, erythroblastosis, and spina bifida and/or hydrocephalus. The remainder of the birth defects listed in table 2.1 range in annual incidence from less than 6000 to more than 1000 (The National Foundation/March of Dimes, 1977).

An examination of causes of the most frequently occurring birth defects indicates that both hereditary and environmental influences are contributing factors. Genetic services are available to provide analyses of karyotypes and genetic counseling for the prevention of most genetic anomalies. However, the environmental factors are not marked with such definite indicators as may be gathered from the previous discussion. The most obvious environmental factors are the noxious substances that filter through the placenta and the lack of a sufficient supply of the proper nutrients in the maternal diet to nourish the developing organism. This means that the expectant mother must be exceptionally careful to maintain a well-balanced nutritious diet, refrain from smoking or alcohol consumption, and only take medication prescribed by a doctor. An average weight gain of 24 pounds, a gain of about one pound per week during the second half of pregnancy, is considered to be reasonable and commensurate with the most favorable outcome of pregnancy (Working Group, 1970).

The ramifications of low birth weight appear to go beyond the structural features of smaller size for all organs and higher incidence of lesser maturity. Dobbing (1971) makes the statement that there is no longer any doubt that growth restriction resulting from malnutrition at certain ages is associated in many children with irreversible deficit in higher mental function. His investigations lead him to conclude that there is a need to maintain a good growth rate at least until the 18th month of postnatal life. Neuronal cell division to adult numbers is complete in the brain during the first half of pregnancy but the main growth spurt does not begin until the second half of pregnancy and continues in intensity until 18 months after birth. There is a marked increase in the weight of the brain which is probably growth in cell size and includes the all-important special growth of neuronal processes and their interconnections. This period also includes marked myelination of neurons.

Rydzynski (1971) in support of Dobbing's findings, notes behavioral disturbances in Jewish and Polish children born and reared in marked deprivation conditions during World War II. The psychological and psychiatric state of the children was similar with all showing great disturbances of both recent and reproductive memory. In addition, they had great difficulty in concentration and an apathetic and anxious mood with a tendency to irritability, explosiveness, and fear reactions. The intelligence of these children was frequently normal or a little below the standard.

In a survey of literature pertaining to malnutrition and intellectual development, von Muralt (1975) states that malnutrition not only delays the maturation of the brain and distorts the biochemical pattern, but it has lasting and irremediable effects even if the nutrition is normalized in later life. A follow-up study that was conducted by Monckeberg (1975) on 14 children who had suffered severe marasmic malnutrition during infancy indicated that the average Binet intelligence quotient for the children was 62 and in no case above 76. On the Gesell test, which included motor, adaptive, language, and personal-social areas, only one child was able to reach normal limits in all four areas. The 14 children in this study consisted of five males and nine females ranging from 3 to 11 months upon admission to the metabolic ward and were between 4 and 7 years of age when the follow-up tests were made.

On the other hand, Read (1975) makes a distinction between severe and moderate (or chronic) malnutrition effects. He concludes that severe malnutrition during prenatal life and/or infancy has been shown to decrease the number of brain cells significantly and to alter brain structure. These changes are associated with mental retardation and behavioral change, which also appear to be permanent and nonreversible. The effects of moderate malnutrition are not so clearly established with reports suggesting that the adverse effects of chronic undernutrition are more in the areas of attentiveness, activity, curiosity, and social responsiveness rather than in the cognitive domain. In addition, there are indications that the malnourished individual may be particularly susceptible to social stresses and deprivations.

In summary, Read (1975) comments that the effects of malnutrition constitute a continuum from permanent neurological defects to consequences arising from personal interactions between the child and his environment and are dependent upon the timing and the severity of malnutrition. It would appear that medical programs initiated after the occurrence of severe malnutrition cannot overcome the resultant deficits in development. Therefore, programs of prevention involving both education and dietary intervention would seem to be vital to reducing birth defects due to malnutrition.

3

Differentiation and Integration of the Sensory-Motor System

With the fusion of the ovum and sperm, the destiny of the new individual becomes a product of the genetic information stored in the fertilized egg and the environment in which it develops. Cell division begins to take place immediately and involves not only multiplication of existing cells to enlarge the organism but also differentiation to alter the form and function of cells to create new structures. During embryonic development in particular, it is vital that these processes balance each other in order to supply both the diverse types of cells required for the efficient functioning of a multicelled organism and maintenance of the inherited integrity of the fertilized ovum for future transmission to offspring. There must be an orderly cell division, differentiation, unification, and integration to the end that the structuring and functioning of the organism can be classified **phylogenetically** as human.

It is well established that genes located in chromosomal DNA have the role of planners and supervisors of the replication, multiplication, and differentiation processes (Tanner & Taylor, 1965). It is possible that the non-chromosomal DNA found in mitochondria (Sager, 1965) may also influence these processes through enhancement, control, or feedback mechanisms. So complex is the process of organized differentiation that DNA, despite its remarkable properties, cannot be the sole determinant. Researchers have observed that the tying off of various amounts of cellular material during cell division will have different effects on the resultant cells (Tanner & Taylor, 1965), so that the spatial cytoplasmic distribution with respect to the polarity of the cell would appear to be a factor in some types of cell differentiation (Waddington, 1962).

During the early embryonic period, the developing organism receives its nourishment **osmotically** so that the metabolic status of the cell may be a factor in the differentiation process (Landreth, 1958). Similarly, variability of pressure, depending upon structural location with respect to surrounding structures, may be instrumental in causing differentiation of structures (Landreth, 1958). Experiments with embryonic chicken skin cells which show that these cells will not differentiate into feather cells in the absence of nerve cells indicate that the process of induction is vital to embryonic differentiation (Tanner & Taylor, 1965). The interactions of chemicals in the cell membranes and cell junctions may be a factor in both cell differentiation and in the unification of similar ends in multi-celled structures (Staehelin & Hull, 1978). This was indicated by Moscona's experiment in which the nearly mature kidney tissue of a chick embryo, when broken up into a disorganized group of cells, soon regrouped to form a new tissue remarkably like the original (Tanner & Taylor, 1965).

The position of a differentiating structure in relationship to other parts of the organism would seem to be a prime factor in structural and functional alteration of cells. The role of the notochord as an organizer and differentiator of the surrounding tissues during early embryonic development was mentioned previously. Position undoubtedly also plays a role in the differentiation of the limb buds into either arm or leg depending upon location. Similarly, the movement of cells is vital to the formation of a differentiating structure such as the central nervous system, the development of which is discussed later. The movement of cells which sculptures the various forms during the formative period is probably the result of differential growth rates. This timing aspect of the growth process is crucial to the development of the individual during the entire life span.

In addition to the crucial timing of the appearance of new structures during the embryonic period, the differential growth rates of various body parts during the adolescent growth spurt sculpture the conformations of the body into the adult physique and gerontological theorists hypothesize that the rate and number of cell replications may be a determinant of the aging process. Although the **anabolic** processes predominate during the periods of incremental cell production, there is some **catabolic** activity even during the embryonic period. During this period, the death of cells is a part of the sculpturing process of such structural developments as the fingers where some of the epidermal tissue between the developing digits dies to allow for a separation rather than a webbing which might otherwise remain between the fingers (Tanner & Taylor, 1965). The period of adulthood is usually considered to be a balanced period with respect to metabolic activity whereas the catabolic processes tend to predominate during the later years.

NEURAL DEVELOPMENT

The uneven growth rate of the neural plate, which forms from ectodermal cells along the mid-dorsal line of the embryo, causes the developing neural tissue to fold into a groove at the time somites are also appearing. The groove continues to deepen and thicken until the folds meet and fuse **dorsally** to form the neural tube which develops into the brain in the head region and the spinal cord in the trunk. Prior to the closure of the groove, the neural crest begins to form within the **concavity** of the neural folds and develops into the **primordial ganglion.** With the formation of the tube, the neural structures become detached from the ectoderm which subsequently continues its differentiation into epidermal tissue (figure 3.1).

The primordial ganglion develops into the spinal ganglion which contains sensory **neuroblasts** (embryonic sensory cells) that grow processes which terminate in the dorsal part of the neural tube and also peripheral processes which leave the ganglion at the dorsal root. At the same time that the sensory neuroblasts are developing processes, the motor neuroblasts, located in the ventral section of the neural tube, send out ventral root fibers that will become the **axons** of mature motor

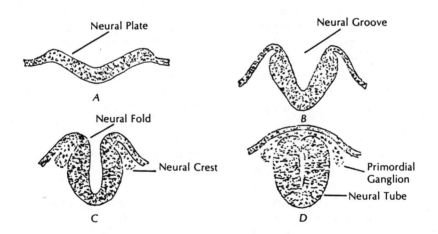

FIGURE 3.1. *Origin of the neural tube and neural crest, illustrated by transverse sections from early human embryos. (From L. B. Arey,* Developmental anatomy. A textbook and laboratory manual of embryology. *Philadelphia: W. B. Saunders, 1946. By permission of the publisher.)*

nerves. **Commissural neurons** that will subsequently make connections within any one level or up and down the spinal cord also develop at this time.

The nervous system is the mechanism by which the organism is made aware of its external and internal environment and whereby it transmits its reactions to such stimuli. Because of its complexity and the primacy of its role in the viability of the individual, the functional integration of the nervous system has been subjected to considerable investigation. Growing neuroblasts must frequently traverse long distances to reach their peripheral connections, such as from the **lumbo-sacral** plexus to the foot, and researchers have been intrigued by the fact that each fiber follows a specific path. It has been found that growth takes place only when the nerve fiber is in contact with a supporting surface and never just in a homogeneous media (Harrison, 1914). Various structures, even those as small as delicate interfacial films or even ultramicroscopic particles of **interstitial fluid** will deflect or channel the fine filamentous pseudopodia of the advancing nerve fiber tips (Weiss, 1941a). This indicates the importance of mechanical factors in the guidance of growing nerves toward their destination.

A considerable body of evidence has been accumulated to suggest that chemical forces are even more important in impelling a nerve in a specific direction. Nerve generation studies, especially on amphibians, have supplied the major portion of our knowledge in this area. Piatt (1942), for example, observed that retarded invasion of nerves into a previously innervated area proceeded in a normal fashion. He grafted limbs, which had grown on **parabiotic** salamander twins to an advanced stage of development in the complete absence of innervation, in place of the corresponding limbs on the otherwise normal twin counterpart. The resultant nerve pattern formed by the invasion of the host nerves into the developed limbs that had not previously been innervated was found to be remarkably normal. Many features of the process, such as the entrances of the nerves into their muscles at their customary points, the penetration of the cartilage masses by the nerves, and the tunnelling of the **ulnar** nerve through the belly of the **ulno-carpal** muscle instead of coursing around it, indicate the vitality of the process and suggest that the different nerve fibers are prone to grow preferentially along pathways with specific chemical properties.

In some instances nerves seem to be able to induce the appropriate end organs to develop at their terminal points. The theory has been advanced that this is brought about by a high degree of **biochemical specificity** (Speidel, 1946; Olmsted, 1931; Bailey, 1937). A somewhat lesser degree of biochemical specificity is exhibited by the nerve fibers of the general cutaneous system, as these terminate freely without inducing any specialized endings (Speidel, 1948). Occasionally nerve fibers can be forced to form **atypical** terminations but at no time do **adrenergic** fibers form functional connections with **cholinergic** endings or vice versa. Sensory nerve fibers are also unable to form transmissive junctions with motor nerve fibers (Langley & Anderson, 1904; Weiss & Edds, 1945).

Further support to theories of neuronal biochemical specificity is lent by studies in which atypical connections have been induced by surgery. Following surgical rotation of the eye of the frog combined with severence of the spinal cord, Sperry (1942, 1943, 1944) made a histological examination of the optic axons at the point of regeneration. He found that, although the axons became thoroughly disarranged during the course of regeneration, the reassociation of the various fibers during regeneration was not achieved in a random manner, since there was a persistent systematic reversal of the visuomotor reactions directly correlated with the rotated position of the retina after recovery.

Further studies by Sperry and colleagues show clearly that this specificity is present in the very early stages of the development of the organism and cannot be changed by surgical rearrangement. Transplantation of skin flaps with their original innervation intact across the midline of the metamorphosing tadpole before it has had any experience with localizing responses results, in the adult frog upon stimulation of the displaced flaps, in wiping reactions to the original site of the skin flaps (Sperry, 1951). For example, when the belly skin which had been displaced to the back of the frog was stimulated by a drop of mild acid, the frog performed the wiping actions with its leg at the site where the skin would normally be located on the belly of the frog.

In another study, the dorsal roots of the hind limb nerves of a frog were cross-connected with those of the opposite side of the cord (figure 3.2). After regeneration of the nerves, the **proprioceptive** reflex actions were restored in a selective manner. Sperry found that the reaction of the **contralateral** limb, to which sensory input was diverted, was conditioned by the position of the stimulated limb. For example, if the stimulated right limb is extended, a stimulus applied to this foot will result in flexion of the left leg, whereas if the stimulated right limb is in a position of flexion, the stimulus will result in extension of the left leg. The position of the left limb had no effect on the nature of the response as proprioceptive sensory input from this limb had been severed (Sperry, 1959).

These studies suggest that, where functional specificity is required, in such senory systems as the visual, vestibular, cutaneous, and proprioceptive, the end organ tissue undergoes primary differentiation and then induces local specificity into whatever sensory fibers come in contact with them. Therefore, it appears that the sensory neuroblasts, upon achieving connections with peripheral sensory end organs, undergo a differentiation (or biochemical specificity) that parallels in miniature that of the body surface. Subsequent selective chemical affinities within the

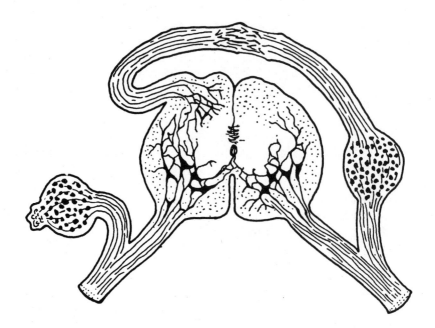

FIGURE 3.2. *Contralateral cross union of dorsal roots. When the dorsal roots of the hind-limb nerves are crossed in the manner indicated, the regenerating sensory root fibers establish functional relations with the spinal centers of the contralateral limb similar to those that they establish with the* **ipsilateral** *limb centers. This selective formation of the central reflex connections cannot be attributed either to mechanical guidance or to functional adjustment. (From R. W. Sperry, Mechanisms of neural maturation. In S. S. Stevens (Ed.),* Handbook of experimental psychology. *New York: John Wiley & Sons, Inc., 1951.)*

central nervous system are adjusted accordingly so that the sensory cortex of the brain forms a map-like projection of the body surface (Sperry, 1959). In other sensory systems, specificity is neurally induced. In both instances, patterns formed at the neural centers remain fixed despite any subsequent forced atypical connections.

Although the chemoaffinity theory of neural organization proposed by Sperry has been widely accepted to explain most aspects of neural connectivity, Easter et al. (1985) have proposed that the specific connections in vertebrates also involves competition between axon terminals, trophic feedback between pre- and post-synaptic cells, and modification of connections by functional activity. In support of their hypothesis, they cite the fact that, during initial outgrowth, more axons project to the target structure than are present in the adult and many of these supernumerary axons are eliminated during the phase of segregation. Also experiments performed in the developing and adult central nervous systems in mammals show that connections can be substantially changed when one input to a given target is deleted or when the target is surgically altered. On the basis of these observations, the investigators suggest that the development of neuronal connections in the central nervous system of vertebrates is a dynamic process of rearrangement of connections rather than simply a wiring of rigidly identified elements.

There is a great deal of variation in the rate of development of the cortical regions of the human brain. Most of the general cytoarchitecture of the brain, including the six cortical layers, is recognizable by the seventh month of fetal life. From this time on the definition of the various structures of brain becomes clear in all areas. However, the development of the cerebellum is unique and much delayed relative to the rest of the brain. This structure, which is closely associated with the coordination of movement, undergoes most of its development in the first postnatal year of the infant (Parmelee & Sigman, 1983).

MOTOR NEURON DEVELOPMENT

Although it is possible that a similar mechanism of selective axon outgrowth to their proper **peripheral** connections may operate with regard to motor neurons, studies seem to indicate that, in amphibians, the outgrowth and termination of spinal motor neurons is entirely nonselective in both development and regeneration (Weiss 1937a, b, and c; Piatt, 1940). Saunders (1947) has expressed the opinion that some selectivity of motor axon termination is assured, under normal conditions, by the chronological order in which the neurons differentiate and send forth their axons and by the proximo-distal order in which the limb segments develop. Weiss (1936, 1941b) on the other hand, maintains that a considerable amount of freedom remains to the motor neurons invading any limb segment since the proper muscular coordination is achieved even with highly random outgrowth and termination in the periphery.

Weiss (1941b) also noted that the adaptation of the timing of the central motor discharge was not achieved by a learning process for, even when the limbs of amphibians are transplanted to the contralateral side and reversed in such a way that the resultant movement of the limbs tends to push the animal backward when it attempts to go forward and vice versa, the individual movement patterning of the limbs persists despite its obvious malfunctioning. When similar limb transplants are made in prefunctional stages of the amphibian's development, similar effects are obtained indicating that these relations are patterned initially through developmental forces and not through any kind of functional adjustment. Additional studies showed that these motor patterns developed in the same systematic way in the absence of sensory innervation and, furthermore, they persisted in the animal after decerebration and cord transection down to the levels of the cord just rostral to the limb segments (Weiss, 1937c). These results ruled out the possibility that learning or any type of functional adaptation may have produced specificity in the patterning of the peripheral neuromuscular relations.

There must be some sort of central discrimination of motor neurons according to the muscles they innervate because the timing of the central discharges is always adjusted on this basis. Since Weiss only disturbed the end-organ, or peripheral, connections in his experiments, he concluded that the motor neurons possess some constitutional, presumably biochemical, specificity induced in them by their muscles. It follows, then, that each muscle must have biochemical properties of its own. This explanation would also serve to account for the differentiation of the limb musculature during its morphogenetic development. If one accepts the hypothesis that biochemical muscular specificity induces biochemical specificity in motor neurons, then it becomes possible to explain the relationship between peripheral motor connections and the sensory and central nervous systems in terms of the general **chemoaffinity** theory of **synaptic** patterings (Sperry, 1959).

Under the connectionist theory, synaptic connections in the central nervous system are made on the basis of selective chemical affinities. When the growing fibrils of the motor neuroblasts hve reached their terminal muscles, the neuron becomes a mature motor nerve by becoming biochemically specific to that particular terminal muscle. Connections in the spinal cord and higher levels of the central nervous system are made accordingly. Similarly, when the growing processes of the sensory neuroblasts reach the peripheral sensory end organs, the sensory nerve becomes biochemical specific to locale of the sensory end organ, and central nervous system connections are made accordingly.

When forming synaptic connections, the afferent sensory fibers from each muscle exhibit a special affinity for those motor neurons biochemically specified by the same muscle. They also show some degree of affinity for the motor neurons of the most closely related muscles. Such simplicity of interneuronal connections as the two-neuron arc are rare, however, and it is highly probable that the same proprioceptive root fibers may form connections on a different basis on other levels of the cord (Shepard, 1978). So complex is the problem of sensory-motor innervation and so painstaking the research in the area that, although the concept of reciprocal innervation was advanced by Sherrington in 1906 to account for the action of the agonists and antagonists in muscular action, we are still not sure of the neural basis of reciprocal innervation (Eccles, 1965; Wilson, 1966).

A neural network, such as reciprocal innervation, involves synaptic stimulus transmission using chemical substances called **neurotransmit-**

ters. Approximately 30 neurotransmitters have been identified; the location of the synapse and the biochemical composition of the neurotransmitter determines whether the stimulus transmitted is excitatory or inhibitory. The duration of the action is dependent upon the presence of enzymes and other agents (deactivators) that terminate the activity of the neurotransmitters to permit multiple stimuli to be transmitted per second. The types of neurotransmitters present and the strength of their deactivators change with maturation and normal behavioral development appears to be dependent upon the progressive maturation of the biochemistry of synaptic transmission (Parmelee & Sigman, 1983).

MUSCLE STRUCTURE AND INNERVATION

The relationship between the developing somite, spinal cord, and sensory ganglion is illustrated in figure 3.3. The close proximity of these developing structures and the timing of the structural differentiation of organs, such as limb buds, would seem to be major factors in the integration of function of the bones and muscles and of innervation of these structures (Waddington, 1962).

As indicated previously, somites differentiate from embryonic mesodermal cells on both sides of the developing spinal cord. Continued differentiation of the somites results in the formation of **myoblasts** which will form muscle cells (composed of actin and myosin); of **fibroblasts** which will form connective tissue; and of precartilage cells which will form cartilage and **osteoblasts** with the latter having the function of

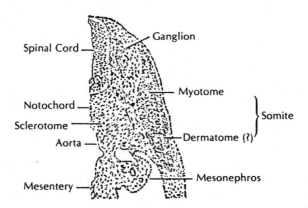

FIGURE 3.3. *Human spinal cord, sensory ganglion, and somite (myotome and dermatome), shown in transverse section at 7 mm. (From L. B. Arey, Developmental anatomy. A textbook and laboratory manual of embryology. Philadelphia: W. B. Saunders Company, 1946. By permission of the publisher.)*

depositing bone matrix. In its more mature form, bone consists of an outer covering called the periosteum; the bone matrix containing Haversian systems; a central cavity of bone marrow; a layer of cells towards each extremity of the bone called the **epiphysis** where longitudinal growth continues until adulthood; and a covering of cartilage over the articular ends of the bone. It serves as the anchor point of the tendons of the muscles and provides the rigid levers necessary for bodily movement.

A gross muscle is made up of numerous muscle fibers separated from each other and into various sized bundles by connective tissues. The smallest unit, the muscle fiber, varies greatly in length and diameter among muscles but is relatively consistent within each gross muscle. In the adult human being, **striated** muscle fibers vary from 1 millimeter in the **stapedius** muscle to 34 centimeters in the **sartorious** muscle; the smaller fibers are generally associated with finer movements. Diameter sizes, ranging from 10 to 150 microns, also show this type of distinctive association with movement, for the greater diameters are found in the larger muscles such as the gluteus maximus (Harrison, 1962).

The connective tissue surrounding each muscle fiber is called the **endomysium,** and the connective tissue surrounding the small bundles or fasciculi, in which the muscle fibers are arranged parallel to each other is called the **perimysium.** The **fasciculi,** also called bundles of the first order, or primary bundles, contain from 10 to 300 muscle fibers depending upon the type of muscle. These primary bundles are, in turn, arranged in parallel with several other primary bundles to form bundles of the second order. This structural arrangement is followed until the final bundle consists of the entire gross muscle itself which is covered with connective tissue called the **epimysium.** This abundance of connective tissue is important in the structure of the muscle and it serves as the harness against which the force of contraction of the muscle is directed. Various arrangements of the connective tissue, therefore, will result in diversification of movement.

Changes in the structural development of the muscle fibers and connective tissue continue until well after birth. The thickness of the muscle fiber increases unevenly in the postnatal period with a considerable increase from 1 to 7 years which results in an approximate doubling of fiber thickness. At about 14 years a more pronounced increment occurs in thickness of the muscle fiber which persists up to 25 years of age. In the adult body, fiber thickness is influenced by the body loading (i.e., exercise component). The elastic fibers in the connective tissue also increase gradually in density, thickness, and length during the entire age range to 25 years. At first the elastic structures are found only in the perimysium externum, then gradually penetrate the internal perimysium and the endomysium. Networks composed of elastic fibers were not observed before 4 years of age (Baum, 1967).

Diversification in the contractive force of the gross muscle is mediated through the *motor unit*—the term given to the functional unit of muscular contraction comprised of the motor neuron and the muscle fibers activated by that neuron (Liddell and Sherrington, 1925). For the eye muscles, it has been found that approximately five to eight muscle fibers are innervated by one motor nerve fiber. Similarly, approximately 25 muscle fibers have been found to be innervated by one motor nerve fiber for the **platysma** muscle; approximately 95 muscle fibers to one motor nerve fiber for the first **lumbrical** muscle; approximately 609 muscle fibers to one motor nerve fiber for the **tibialis anterior** muscle; and approximately 1775 muscle fibers to one motor nerve fiber for the medial head of the **gastrocnemius** muscle. Innervation of the muscles indicates fewer muscle fibers per motor nerve fiber in the motor units mediating finer movements than in the motor units mediating gross movements. The muscle fibers of a motor unit are confined to an oval or circular area which is only a small fraction of the total cross section of the muscle and the territory encompassed by the motor unit does not seem to vary with the degree of development of the muscle. Furthermore, the territories encompassed by separate motor units overlap one another. Of a maximum of six units that have been found to overlap, two or three of the motor units have been found to overlap each other entirely so that their muscle fibers are assembled within the same region of the cross section of the gross muscle (Harrison, 1962).

After observing the reactions of the **vastocrureus** muscle in the decerebrate cat, Liddell and Sherrington (1925) concluded that the motor unit acted in an all-or-none fashion when its motor nerve was stimulated. The motor units, however, have gradient thresholds so that some motor nerves require minimal stimulation to trigger off the firing that causes muscular contraction whereas others do not fire until stronger stimulation triggers off the motor unit when stronger contractions are required. The strength of muscular contraction, then, is determined by the frequency and the number of motor units firing—a greater number of units are involved in a stronger contraction. However, the synchronous use of all the motor units in a gross muscle occurs very rarely, if at all. It appears that an exceptionally strong emotional stimulus would be necessary to trigger off the synchronous firing of all motor units. That such instances do occur is illustrated by stories of feats of exceptional strength under unusually strong emotional stimuli.

MYELINATION

The sheathing of the nerves with myelin is the final stage in their morphological development. The general correlation that has been found between the order in which nerves become functional and the order of the appearance of stainable myelin tends to suggest that there may be a relationship which is, however, not simple and tends to be of a reciprocal nature. Central nervous tracts become myelinated in a definite sequence that shows a considerable constancy in all the mammals and which tends to roughly follow the order in which tracts are developed phylogenetically. In the human fetus, the neural fibers involved in the earliest reflexes are not myelinated until some time after they begin functioning (Timiras et al., 1968).

While the absence of function does not prevent the laying down of or decrease the ultimate degree of myelin (Romanes, 1947), it has been found that the laying down of myelin is stimulated and accelerated by function (Langworthy, 1933). Although Langworthy has shown that fairly complex activity can be carried out prior to myelination, functions, in general, have been found to show a considerable improvement in speed, precision, steadiness, and strength coincident with the laying down of myelin. Timiras et al. (1968) report that there is increased conduction velocity, lower threshold, shorter latency, and a higher amplitude coincident with the time appearance and the degree of myelination. It would appear, then, that myelination and the order of its appearance is an inherently determined process capable of proceeding in the absence of function in the usual sense but is also a process that is stimulated and accelerated by the presence of function.

This reciprocal mechanism which results in an acceleration in the laying down of myelin with increased function and in improved function as a result of increased myelination is only effective within the limits of myelination set down within the genetic inheritance of the individual. During the period of development of myelination, the interrelationship of the myelination-function process makes it difficult to assess the extent to which improved motor development is due to this process or to other maturational processes that may be going on simultaneously. In addition, the establishment of such relationships is complicated by the fact that composition of myelin changes in terms of basic proteins and proteolipid proteins during human development (Norton, 1971). However, the degree to which myelination has been completed offers an excellent method of assessing the degree of maturation of the nervous system and, as such, is an indicator of the order and the degree to which various parts of the system become functional.

The functioning of the neural tissue, especially the brain, can be assessed by EEG activity which shows variations in evoked potentials for various areas of the brain with maturational changes. In addition, positron emission tomography (PET) has marked potential for providing information about brain metabolism under varying conditions of stimulation (Parmelee & Sigman, 1983). Although anatomical studies of structure and structural maturation in association with observed functioning have been the basis for most of our understanding of neural functioning in the past, the use of non-invasive techniques should greatly enhance our understanding of neural functioning in the future.

SUMMARY

1. Neural tissue develops from ectodermal cells along the mid-dorsal line of the embryo to form first the neural plate and then, successively, the neural groove and neural tube. The neural crest also develops to subsequently form the primordial ganglion.

2. Motor neuroblasts grow out from the ventral section of the neural tube to make connections with muscles and sensory neuroblasts grow out from the primordial ganglion to make connections with sensory endings.

3. Sperry has proposed the chemoaffinity (biochemical specificity) theory to explain the integration of connections between the developing sensory neurons and end organs and between the motor neurons and muscles. The theory proposes that the biochemical specificity of the end connections adjusts the chemoaffinity of the more central connections so that the connections in the motor and sensory areas of the cortex of the brain reflect a topographical map of the body structure.

4. The somites which form along the side of the neural groove during the embryonic period develop from mesodermal tissue and further differentiate into myoblasts which will form muscle; fibroblasts which will form connective tissue; and pre-cartilage cells which will develop into cartilage and osteoblasts for bone formation.

5. Whole muscles are composed of muscle fibers covered with en-doysium and arranged in bundles, or fasciculi, which are enclosed by perimysium, whereas the covering for groups of muscle bundles is called epimysium and is connected with the tendon attached to the bone.

6. The motor unit is comprised of various numbers of muscle fibers innervated by a single motor nerve. For areas where fine muscle movements are required each motor nerve controls fewer muscle fibers (i.e., more control per fiber) than where less precise movement is required.

7. Although neural connections are completed well before birth, myelination continues at varying rates in various parts of the nervous system well after birth. The degree of myelination is associated with the amount of function (i.e., the amout of use) but the maximal amount of myelin is determined by heredity.

8. Increased myelination is associated with increased conduction

velocity, lower threshold, shorter latency, and higher amplitude of neural response.

9. The degree of myelination provides a means for assessing the level of structural maturation of the nervous system, whereas EEG and PET provide evidence of changes in the functioning of the brain.

4

Prenatal
Development

Moral considerations and principles prevent us from conducting experimental studies in human embryology. Our limited knowledge of human prenatal development comes from premature fetuses that have not survived or those which have been surgically removed from the mother for medical reasons and have had no chance of survival. In these instances, it is obvious that behavior, if it can be elicited, will occur under a failing oxygen and food supply as well as under environmental conditions differing from the constant temperature, composition, and comparatively stimulus-free environment within the uterus. However, it has been found that there are stages in the morphological development of fish, amphibians, reptiles, birds, and infrahuman mammals which are similar to those in man so that it is possible to draw some inferences from studies of these creatures to augment and provide clues to the development of human behavior.

PRENATAL DEVELOPMENT IN INFRAHUMANS

As early as 1885, Preyer studied the development of trout (Coghill & Legner, 1937). A few days after fertilization of the egg he liberated the tiny fish from their coverings and continued at successive periods to do so with others of the organisms. He noted that movements became more and more regular and specific and increased in strength with age. After disappearance of the yolk sac, definite changes in behavior were observed.

Exhaustive work has been done by Coghill (1929) in tracing the motor development of the salamander amblystoma. This investigator was the first to chart the relationship between detailed growth of the nervous system and the consequent alterations which occurred in behavior. A study of the neural structures in association with stages of development of the "S," or swimming reaction, in the salamander, for example, showed that certain structures of the nervous system made possible specific types of behavior. The "S" reaction is clearly seen in the swimming of the lower vertebrates but is obscure in the locomotion of four-legged mammals and even more so in the biped locomotion of human beings. However, Coghill believes this fundamental pattern may be a significant stage in the behavioral development of all higher organisms. He cites as evidence supporting his theory that when both sets of limbs first appear in the metamorphosing amphibian they move only with the trunk in swimming. Gradually the front legs achieve independence of action from the larger trunk movements and this is followed in turn by independence of limb action of the hind legs. The cephalocaudal progression of development of independent limb action repeats the cephalocaudal progression of trunk movements seen in the "S" reaction. Eventually the alternate positioning of the limbs in walking synchronizes with a reduced "S" reaction of the trunk during locomotion. Thus the "S" reaction is seen as a phylogenetic feature in the development of all vertebrates.

Some supporting evidence for the primacy of the "S" reaction may be found in the marsupials who give birth to their young in a condition equivalent to that of a very immature fetus in comparison with mammals. The fetal kangaroo and opossum travel directly from the vulva to the maternal pouch without any aid from the mother. Only the arms which are strongly developed are used to propel the body with the lower trunk merely trailing during the journey. This type of overhand swimming motion is reminiscent of the "S" reaction of the larval salamander.

This "S" type of reaction is not evident in the fetuses of four-legged mammals such as the guinea pig which have their limbs fully formed before the occurrence of the first behavioral responses or reflexes. A very definite progression of stages in development can be traced, however. Bridgman and Carmichael (1935) found that myogenic responses could be elicited in the fetal guinea pig from certain muscles prior to the onset of behavior. "True" behavior, defined by these investigators as the responses resulting from stimulation, was next in order of appearance. These true behavior responses were sufficiently different in character from the earlier myogenic contractions to indicate that stimulation had induced a neural discharge to trigger off the muscular contraction. The first active responses of the fetal guinea pig were found to involve movements of the head caused by contraction of the neck muscles and movements of the four legs. They concluded that these earliest responses might advantageously be described as reflexes because of their simple and specific nature. They did not identify a gradual progressive individuation of specific responses out of a total pattern but rather identified the specific responses as primary.

Coronios (1933) made extensive studies on the fetal development of the cat. He formulated seven generalizations which typify the course of fetal development in infrahuman organisms.

1. Before birth, there is a rapid, progressive, and continuous development in the behavior of the fetus of the cat.
2. The development of behavior progresses from a diffuse, massive, variable, relatively unorganized state to a condition where many of the reactions are more regular in their appearance, less variable, better organized, and relatively individualized.
3. In the early stages of prenatal development the behavior appears to be progressing along a cephalocaudal course.
4. The development of the sensitivity of the reflexogenous zones passes through a continuous and transitional development from a time when a rather vigorous stimulation of any "spot" of the body within a large area serves to elicit variable, diffuse, uncoordinated patterns of behavior to a later time when a weak stimulus becomes adequate, within a much more circumscribed area for precise, well-coordinated, uniform, and less variable patterns of behavior. The direction of such development is cephalocaudal.
5. The "primitive" reactions of breathing, righting, locomotion, and feeding are the products of a long and continuously progressive course of prenatal development.
6. Behavior development appears first in the gross musculature, and later in the fine musculature.
7. Behavior develops in each of the limbs from a proximal to a distal point, that is, the entire limb is first involved in the response and then gradually the more distal joints become, as it were, independent of the total movement.*

PRENATAL HUMAN DEVELOPMENT

Investigations into the field of prenatal human behavior are beset with numerous problems which were controlled or partially overcome in reported studies of infrahuman mammalian fetuses. Even when human fetuses become available for observation, it is difficult to assess the age of the fetus and this is very important both for comparative purposes and for formulating longitudinal concepts.

The starting point for the development of the new individual is taken to be the moment of fusion of the nuclei of the sperm and the ovum. However, this moment generally cannot be accurately determined so

---

* From J. D. Coronios, Development of behavior in the fetal cat. *Genet. Psychol. Monog.*, 1933, 14, 283-386. By permission of the publisher, The Journal Press.

that the numerous methods have been used to calculate fetal age; namely the following:

1. Menstruation age where the age of the fetus is calculated from the first day of the last period of menstruation prior to the onset of pregnancy (Mall, 1918).

2. The mean menstruation age is similar to menstrual age but is based upon the average calculated from a large number of cases (Mall, 1918).

3. The conception age is calculated from the last day of the last menstrual period prior to the onset of pregnancy (Minot, 1892).

4. Copulation, or insemination, age is based upon trustworthy cases of known copulation time and upon calculation. It has been found to be approximately 10 days shorter than the mean menstrual age (Mall, 1918).

5. Ovulation age is calculated from the time of ovulation. However, it is difficult, at present, to determine the time of ovulation precisely (Hartman, 1936). Guyton (1979) indicates that the ovum remains viable for eight to 24 hours after it is expelled from the ovary. According to Austin (1975), the sperm remains fertile for 24 to 48 hours and motile for eight days in the human oviduct.

6. The fertilization, or true, age must be calculated from menstruation age, mean menstruation age, or copulation age (Mall, 1918). In general, present evidence seems to indicate that fertilization occurs within less than 48 hours after copulation (Carmichael, 1954).

7. "Test tube" age in which the age of the developing organism may be calculated from the time of fertilization of the egg by the sperm under laboratory conditions.

Efforts have also been made to compile tables from which ages of human fetuses can be estimated from known physical measurements. However, even if organisms of truly known ages are plentifully available, each age norm would still have to be stated in terms of some statistical average because of the many factors, such as genetic stock, specific pathology, and nourishment, which influence fetal size. Linear measurements of fetal specimens have been made on the basis of crown-rump length and crown-heel length. The former seems to be more commonly used for embryological studies (Carmichael, 1954) while crown-heel length was used by Minkowski (1928) in his extensive studies of human fetuses. Streeter (1920) prepared growth curves of the human fetus based on the relationships of weight, sitting height, foot length, head size, and menstrual age while Hooker (1944) has suggested that weight and length seem to provide a more useful index of behavior development than does age. In short, it would seem that the word "approximate" should appear before statements of human fetal age on the basis of our current diversity in methods of actual age determination.

OBSERVATIONS *IN UTERO*

Observations of human fetal behavior fall into two basic categories; namely, those that can be made through the body wall of the mother and can be felt by the mother and those observations made on fetuses which have been operatively removed for medical reasons. The mother may sometimes perceive movements, commonly referred to as "quickening of the fetus," as early as the 17th week (Feldman, 1920). As pregnancy progresses, these movements tend to increase and to fall into three general types of fetal activity. These are quick kicks, thrusts, and jerks of the extremities; slow squirming, pushing, stretching, and turning movements; and hiccups or rhythmic series of quick convulsive movements. Figure 4.1 shows the results of a study by Newbery (1941) of the amount of fetal activity from the sixth to the tenth lunar month, with the greatest increases of movement occurring in the early part of this period. It is

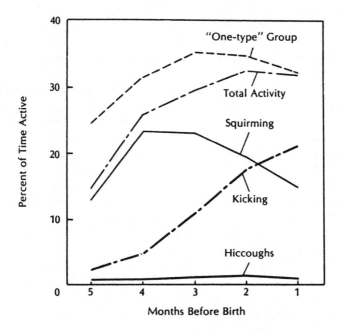

FIGURE 4.1. *Types of fetal activity. (From H. Newbery, Studies in fetal behavior. IV. The measurement of three types of fetal activity. J. Comp. Psychol., 1941, 32, 521-30. By permission of the publisher, The Williams and Wilkins Co.)*

highly likely that the general reduction in activity at the end of the prenatal period is caused by the increased restriction of the growing fetus within the limiting confines of the womb and the relatively reduced oxygen and food supply.

The activity of the mother during pregnancy would also seem to influence the activity of the fetus, according to a longitudinal study conducted at the Fels Research Institute. In this instance, fetal activity was recorded, by the mothers, under different conditions of maternal activity which included eating, exercise, smoking, reading in a quiet room, and quiet interrupted by sudden noise. It was found that fatigue and emotional stress in the mother stimulated fetal activity, as did an increase in the basal metabolism rate of the mother. If such conditions prevailed over a period of time, the resultant increases in fetal activity might result in reduced birth weight and in an irritable, hypersensitive infant with gastro-intestinal dysfunction. Smoking was also found to increase the heart rate, with this effect being more marked with advancing pregnancy (Landreth, 1958). It has previously been noted that smoking by pregnant women has been associated with reduced birth weight in the newborn child.

Additional methods of observation of the fetus through the intact body wall of the mother have involved palpation and the use of various instruments for magnifying or recording various fetal movements. The most commonly used instrument is the stethoscope but, by means of suitable amplification and recording, electrocardiographic and electromyographic recordings have also been made through the body wall of the mother when the fetus is in a favorable position. Palpations of the movements of the fetus reveal similar movements to those felt by the mother. The heart beat of the fetus can be heard and felt beginning at the 18th week of pregnancy and rhythmic contractions of the fetal thorax, often called **Ahlfeld breathing movements**, have also been felt through the mother's body wall.

Advances in electronics have resulted in the development of sonar scanning as an observational tool to examine *in utero* fetal progress (Robinson, 1973). In addition, miniaturization processes have resulted in the production of cameras which enable medical researchers to photograph the fetus *in utero*. In general, these technical developments have been used for the assessment of the physical status of the fetus in instances involving medical hazards to either the mother or child and are not employed on a continuous longitudinal basis. Therefore, the observations obtained using these techniques are similar to cross-sectional observations obtained by other methods.

Research using ultrasound to observe fetal movements between 28 and 37 weeks' gestation and habituation to a vibrating stimulus applied to the mother's abdomen indicated that habituation occurred within 40 trials for all but one of the fetuses. When the fetal responses were related to scores on the Brazelton Neonatal Behavior Assessment Scale and the Bayley Scales of Infant Development, fast prenatal habituation was associated with lower stability scores at two days after birth which may reflect a relation between prenatal habituation and postnatal reactivity. In addition, at 10 days postnatal, there was a positive association of stability with reflexes and a negative association of orientation with stability suggesting that the dimension that most clearly separates fast and slow habituators reflects some form of responsiveness to the environment (Madison et al., 1986).

Conditioning of the fetus *in utero* during the last two months of pregnancy seems to have met with some success although the permanency of establishment of such conditioning is highly questionable. Spelt (1948), using a loud noise as the unconditioned stimulus which he paired with vibrotactile stimulation over the abdominal wall, reports the establishment of conditioned responses in the fetus after 15 to 20 paired stimulations. However, similar conditioning experiments in neonates reveal that conditioning is very difficult to establish and extremely unstable during this period (Pratt, 1954). The latter observations lead one to question whether the rapidity of conditioning in the fetus *in utero* is actually fetal conditioning or whether it is just a fetal manifestation induced by hormonal responses elicited by maternal conditioning.

OBSERVATIONS OF OPERATIVELY REMOVED HUMAN FETUSES

Studies of operatively removed human fetuses often give results based upon the length of the fetus rather than age. Hooker (1944) suggests that length and weight seem to provide a better index of behavior development than age. However, the temporal connotations of age are more indicative of the progressive development of behavior, so approximate age will be used in the presentation of the following observations of prenatal human behavior development.

A cautious assessment of these observations seems to be in order in view of the fact that the administration to the mother of anesthetics which permeate the placenta will influence the behavior of the fetus. Hooker (1944) found that novocaine does not appear to affect the fetal movements and some of the fetuses studied by this investigator were operatively removed using only this type of anesthetic. Of particular interest is the report, by Fitzgerald and Windle (1942), of observations of three human fetuses, of approximately 8 weeks postinsemination age, which were not narcotized or anesthetized and continued to receive oxygenated blood from the intact placenta for a short period of time. They found, under these conditions, that excitability was high with quick trunk, arm, and leg movements being called out by pressing or tapping on the amniotic sac. These reactions occurred individually and in various combinations and did not involve a total reaction of the organism unless the stimulus was very strong. On the basis of these findings, these investigators concluded that an undamaged, unanesthetized, or unnarcotized fetus with intact blood supply has, by the end of eight weeks, developed to the extent that its neuromuscular apparatus is capable of active functioning.

Further observations of the same fetuses after severance of the umbilical cord led to the conclusion that some receptors and synapses are more easily made nonfunctional by anoxia than others. These observations revealed that arm and leg responses have been abolished in asphyxiating specimens at a time when stimulation applied to the skin of the face still elicited trunk flexion. During this same stage of asphyxiation, it was found that strong stimulation elicited mass movements involving the trunk, arms, and legs. These findings would seem to suggest that such early mass movement in operatively removed fetuses may be a function of the decrease of oxygen in the blood and concomitant stimulation of the hypersensitive fetus.

EARLY BEHAVIORAL DEVELOPMENT

The first two weeks of prenatal life are usually referred to as the germinal period. From the third to sixth week, called the embryonic period, the **medullary** groove begins to form and, within a short period of time, the primitive heart cells are laid down to begin their life-long beat in the segment which is later to to become the ventricular region (Williams, 1931). This intrinsic rhythm of the heart is determined by the metabolic process of these smooth muscle cells and not by neural innervation (Goss, 1940). During this period of rapid differentiation, the cerebral and optic vesicles become recognizable and the limb buds first appear. Muscular development also proceeds rapidly at this time but at uneven rates. The smooth musculature, which is the first to develop, is clearly formed in an embryo of 1 millimeter in length, but the striated musculature cannot be detected in fetuses less than 2.5 millimeters long.

By the sixth or seventh week of life, arms, legs, and all essential organs have been formed. The semicircular ducts, which are the balance organs of the inner ear, are well outlined at 6 weeks of prenatal life (Timiras et al., 1968). Bone cells begin to form in the long bones at 8 weeks and from this time until birth the developing organism is called a fetus. There is considerable evidence to suggest that the onset of reaction behavior in the human fetus occurs at approximately 8 weeks of age.

Tactile stimulation in the area of the mouth of fetuses 8 to 8½ weeks of age has induced responses which spread from the very localized area of the upper lip and skin around the nostrils to the whole upper lip, chin, and part of the neck (Hooker, 1944). Contraction of the long muscles of the neck may extend downward and activate body and limb girdle muscles of the upper extremities (Hooker, 1939). Quite possibly this excitation is dependent upon the deformation of the growing tips of sensory fibers (Hogg, 1941), although receptors in the underlying tissue (Carmichael, 1954) may be activated also.

Faradic, or electrical, stimulation has also been found effective in eliciting responses (Hooker, 1939). Muscular contractions including irradiation of responses to other muscles (Minkowski, 1922) can be observed in fetuses of 8 weeks of age when stimulated in this way, but no spontaneous movements have been observed at or before this time (Hooker, 1939). These observations seem to indicate that responses to stimuli at this age are either myogenic or organized neurally at the spinal level only. Previously cited studies of infrahuman mammals indicate that musculature responds to direct stimulation before the onset of true neuromuscular action.

BEHAVIOR IN FETUSES 9 TO 12 WEEKS OF AGE

Variations in the rate of behavioral development are seen to exist at the earliest stages of fetal movement. Movements of 9 to 10 week old fetuses have been described as being slow, arrhythmical, asymmetrical and uncoordinated (Minkowski, 1921), although some reports of energetic responses by even younger fetuses have been made (Woyciechowski, 1928; Bolaffio & Artom, 1924).

Spontaneous movements have been reported in fetuses of approximately 9 weeks of age (Woyciechowski, 1928; Hooker, 1939), although the origin of such movement is not fully understood. It is generally believed that even during the third month the cerebral cortex has not yet assumed any functions in relation to general bodily activity. Bolaffio and Artom (1924) did report an instance in which decerebration of an 8½ week fetus resulted in greater vividness of response, apparently indicating even at this stage some inhibition by the cortex on lower reflexes. These same investigators found that mechanical stimulation of the medulla led to respiratory movements and to a primitive form of sucking. Some immature connections between the brain and the periphery have evidently been established at this time.

The general observation is made by Hooker (1944) that during the period from 9½ to 12 weeks in fetal development a "total pattern" or response to stimuli is dominant. He found, for example, that at 11 weeks of age stimulation of the mouth area brought a response from the entire upper extremity and even the sole of the foot. Minkowski's anatomical studies (1928) show that the spinal cord and nerve trunks have no medullary sheaths before the 12th week and this may provide a partial explanation of the spread of response.

Reflex action becomes increasingly evident in the developing organism, however. Stretching of limb muscles is effective in stimulating proprioceptive organs and eliciting a response at 9½ weeks. At 11 weeks, palmar stimulation results in a quick but incomplete finger closure, apparently marking the onset of the grasping reflex. At this same period, the plantar reflex and patterned eye movements can be identified (Hooker, 1944). It was previously noted (Windle & Fitzgerald, 1937) that the spinal reflex arcs are developed by the eighth week. Specific functions can be elicited increasingly thereafter.

BEHAVIOR IN FETUSES 13 TO 16 WEEKS OF AGE

By 13 weeks, almost every joint in the body that is ever to move has gained motility (Hooker, 1944), and this fact, of course, makes it possible to observe the results of stimulation over the entire range of joint action. Strong stimulation will result in what is sometimes called a "generalized matrix of behavior," and weak stimulation of certain receptor areas leads to very specific responses. Carmichael (1951) points to the importance of vestibular and proprioceptive stimuli in establishing the postural tone of the body which in turn will affect the type of response that is elicited by any particular stimuli at any particular time. He notes that when the head is turned to one side the response may not be the same as when the head is turned to the other side. Furthermore, stimulation of the sole of the foot at this age may result in either flexion or extension of the toes depending upon the posture of the toes at the time of stimulation (Sherman & Sherman, 1925).

On the basis of our knowledge of the summation of impulses required for response at different neural levels, it is conceivable the neural mechanisms may be available at this time to allow for differentiation in response according to the strength of the stimulus and its locus. Minkowski (1922) reports that touching the tongue or lower lip of a fetus approximately 13 weeks old with a blunt probe resulted in the closure of the mouth. He also observed prominent reflexes of the trunk and extremities in this fetus but found that these were discontinued at once following **transection** of the spinal cord in the dorsal region. These results seem to prove that for this fetus at this age conduction of activation was through innervation of the spinal cord. Minkowski made the further observation that, following transection of the spinal cord, the short reflexes remained unchanged. These, however, were also abolished following total extirpation of the cord. During the course of this experiment, it was noted that destruction of the cervical cord abolished reflexes of the arms while destruction of the lumbar and sacral cord resulted in the abolition of reflexes in the legs. It would appear, then, that after the 13th week the reflex response in the human infant can, in general, no longer be considered as being on the simple two-neuron arc level but is now subject to an increasing number of modifying influences.

The development of some of the reflex responses requiring more complex neural innervation seems to be a major aspect of behavioral development during this period. Spontaneous movements have been observed at 14 weeks of age which include most body parts as well as activity of the "organism as a whole"; movements elicited by tactual stimulation have been characterized as "graceful" and "delicate." Except for the true grasping reflex, respiration, vocalization, and a few others, the fetus at this age shows most of the specific patterns of response that can be found in the neonate (Hooker, 1944). Although contralateral responses have been observed in a limited way during the ninth week (Fitzgerald & Windle, 1942), it is not until approximately 13 weeks of age that stimulation of receptor fields on one side of the body regularly leads to the response of a limb on the other side of the body (Hooker, 1944). Definite indications of reciprocal innervation during movement of a limb were noted in a fetus of about 16 weeks by Minkowski (1924), who also reports the establishment of diagonal reflexes at this time. Here, stimulation of one foot of the fetus led to movement of the arm on the opposite side. Minkowski considered these observations of diagonal reflexes as being significant in comparing the **ontogenetic** development of the human fetus with the trotting reflex noted by observers of infrahuman fetal development.

BEHAVIOR DEVELOPMENT FROM 17 WEEKS TO NORMAL BIRTH

In general, the period from 17 weeks until normal birth is marked by the increasing dominance of the central nervous system in the behavior responses of the human fetus. Direct mechanical stimulation of the motor roots of the spinal nerve in a fetus of approximately 17 weeks indicated that intersegmental spinal conduction had become well established. This particular fetus responded to mechanical stimulation of the cranial nerves at the level of the medulla by opening and closing of the mouth, presumably the result of direct stimulation of the facial nerve. Stimulation of the medulla itself resulted in changes in the Ahlfeld breathing movements but direct stimulation of the cortex did not elicit any responses (Minkowski, 1922). Mechanical stimulation of the **Rolandic**

zone of the brain of another fetus of simular age did not call forth any reaction but removal of the cerebral hemispheres did result in more vivid responses to local stimuli than had been elicited previously. In this fetus, respiratory movements in response to stimulation of the medulla were so violent that they led to elevation of the shoulder and the adduction of the arms (Bolaffio & Artom, 1924). It would appear, then, that the respiratory mechanisms seated in the medulla have achieved effective neural connections after approximately 17 weeks and that intersegmental spinal conduction of other reflexes is also well established at this level.

Rhythmic chest movements were first reported in 1890 by Ahlfeld, who noted that the responses varied from 38 to 76 per minute. This timing and the rhythmicity of the movements tend to indicate that the breathing mechanism is essentially in working order long before it is needed (Carmichael, 1954). These respiratory movements of the fetus do not normally lead to aspiration of the amniotic fluid (Windle, 1941) and some investigators have suggested that the rhythmic movements act as a sort of auxiliary pump to help the heart in its function (Carmichael, 1954). It is also considered likely that a decrease in the oxygen content of the fetal blood may be one of the causes of these movements. Richards et al. (1938) observed intact fetuses through the maternal wall during the last 20 weeks of pregnancy and, following continuous observations for five to six hours, noted a correlation of .60 between chest movements and the metabolic rate of the mother. Although at 22 weeks, some prematurely delivered fetuses are capable of briefly sustaining respiration when stimulated by air, it is not until the sixth to seventh month that the respiratory mechanism ordinarily becomes sufficiently established to permanently maintain respiration.

Response to electrical stimulation of the brain at the level of the **pons** is not reported until approximately 5 months fetal age when such stimulation resulted in synchronous responses from the muscles innervated by the facial nerve. Here, stimulation of the medulla also resulted in energetic respiratory movements, and stimulation of the cervical cord elicited energetic elevation of the shoulders together with flexion of the arms. Stimulation of the lumbar cord led to movements of the legs (Bolaffio & Artom, 1924). In fetuses of approximately 6 months of age, stimulation of the lower brain centers resulted in increased rate of respiratory movements and in shoulder, arm, and finger movements. However, stimulation of the cerebral cortex itself still produced negative results, although removal of the cortex resulted in the usual response of heightened reaction to sensory stimulation (Bolaffio & Artom, 1924). These findings, together with the known susceptibility of neural tissue to oxygen deficiency, suggest that the increases in vividness of responses to stimulation by fetuses just before death are attributable to changes in the higher brain centers.

The tracing of behavioral responses to stimulation of the sole of the foot from the time of onset of reaction to the elicitation of the adult **plantar** reflex is illustrative of the fact that the same stimuli applied to the same area may call out differing, yet quite specific, responses as the various connecting levels of the nervous system mature. Minkowski (1926) believes that the first response to stimulation of the sole of the foot is probably myogenic, produced by direct stimulation of the muscle through the thin skin, and thus does not involve any neural elements. The dorsal flexion of the toes which occurs during the third and fourth months in response to stimulation is believed to involve connections in the spinal cord. With the continuing maturation of the central nervous system and the development of effective connections to the midbrain during the midfetal period, the pattern of response changes to one of big toe extension with the other toes being flexed. Subsequent development of still higher nerve centers in later fetal life results in variable responses, one of which may be spreading of the toes. The typical Babinski reflex (big toe extension and flexion of the other toes) disappears shortly after birth with the development of cortical dominance. The adult plantar reflex (contraction of all toes) is associated with the development of cortical dominance; any reversion to, or retention of, the Babinski reflex is considered to be indicative of a lesion of the pyramidal tracts of the brain and the spinal cord (Pratt, 1954).

The trend toward increased localization of response continues as the fetus becomes older. One must, however, inject reservations into such a general statement based upon the nature and the strength of the stimuli. For example, superficial stimulation elicited localized muscular contractions in the limbs and in other specialized muscle groups in a fetus of approximately 19 weeks while strong deep stimulation of a single segment of one limb resulted in flexion of the whole contralateral limb (Bolaffio & Artom, 1924). Specificity of response tends to be more marked in the head region than in the leg region in fetuses of approximately 22 weeks (Bolaffio & Artom, 1924), with very specific activation of the muscles of the eyelid occurring in response to a single electrical stimulus (Minkowski, 1922). Vivid reaction has been obtained from all the muscles of the limbs when they are excited one at a time by percussion in a fetus of approximately 24 weeks (Bolaffio & Artom, 1924).

During the sixth month, fetuses have exhibited responses which may be classified as the first tendon reflexes rather than responses to cutaneous or muscle stimulation. Bolaffio and Artom (1924) base their recognition of the onset of true tendon reflexes at this time upon the facts that the specific responses elicited by stimuli were not observed previously and that the responses were similar to those elicited as true tendon reflexes in early infancy. Furthermore, once these responses were capable of being elicited, they continued to increase in strength during the remainder of the fetal period. During the next two months of pregnancy, muscular reflexes tend to decrease in their ascendancy over the tendon reflexes until, by the end of the ninth month, the tendon reflexes are so well established that they prevail over special muscle reflexes. With the exception of some tendon reflexes of the upper limbs which are difficult to elicit because of the small size of the limb, all tendon reflexes are found to be present during this period of life. Some of the earlier developing tendon reflexes are the biceps, triceps, and Achilles tendon reflexes and the knee jerk.

The increase in the elaboration of the types of responses together with more precise differentiation of the muscular responses during this period is indicative of the maturation of the neural mechanisms in terms of elaboration of neural connections and maturation of the various neural components. By the seventh month, certain responses have been characterized as involving synergic muscle groups (Bolaffio & Artom, 1924). Although the activity of the newborn has been classified as "mass activity" (Irwin & Weiss, 1930), the movement during such activity is not similar to the diffuse type of response noted by investigators of the early fetal period. Certainly by the end of the seventh month myelination of all the fundamental activities pathways is almost complete and the myelination of the other motor pathways is in progress (Minkowski, 1928). On the basis of these findings, it seems unlikely that one can still attribute "mass activity" to the spread of responses because of lack of medullary sheaths as may be the case prior to the fourth fetal month.

Faint sounds indicative of the onset of vocal function are reported in a fetus of approximately 22 weeks (Minkowski, 1922), and weak crying sounds were made by another fetus of about 25 weeks of age (Bolaffio & Artom, 1924). Corneal reflexes have been observed in the seventh month with direct stimulation of the cornea eliciting increasingly stronger responses as the fetus grows older (Minkowski, 1922). During the last month of pregnancy, iris reflexes have been noted, but the response of the iris is very slow and a very strong light is required before the reaction is elicited (Minkowski, 1928). Variations in the grasping reflex are reported by Bolaffio and Artom (1924). They noted that very light stimulation of the hand results in variable and inconstant responses; and strong stimulation, which because of its strength may involve the muscles or underlying tissues, uniformly elicits grasping. On the basis of such observations, these investigators concluded that the grasping reflex should not be considered as a purely cutaneous reflex in prenatal life.

It would appear, then, that all processes vital for the survival of the fetus are firmly established before the last two months of pregnancy. The heart beat, with its role in the circulatory system, and the respiratory mechanisms have been discussed. Peristaltic movements of the digestive tract, swallowing of amniotic fluid, and excretion of urine have also been developing gradually since the first half of the pregnancy period. The fetus, therefore, has achieved, by the seventh month of pregnancy, the age of viability, although some of the reflexes of later fetal life may not be functional as yet. Responses of a full-term newborn infant include the following: eyelid, pupillary, ocular, tear secretion, facial and mouth, throat, neck, head, arm, trunk, foot and leg, and the coordinate position of many of the parts of the body. Some of these responses will be discussed in greater detail in the chapter on the neonate. Suffice it to say here that the vast changes that have occurred from the original fertilized ovum to the newborn child during the short period of 280 days still stagger the human imagination—one of the ultimate products of this development.

A summary of the major structural and functional changes occurring during prenatal development is contained in table 4.1. The sequential ordering clearly indicates that the first eight weeks of pregnancy are, with the exception of the heart beat, predominantly devoted to structural development. Subsequent functional development is predetermined by such structural development. This relationship between structure and function persists during the entire life span of the individual.

Briefly, and in general, prenatal behavioral development in the human fetus may be classified as:

1. Rapid, progressive, and continuous, with variations in rate occurring between individuals.
2. Very generally, behavior development progresses from weak, diffuse, massive, relatively unorganized responses to a condition where many reactions are stronger, more specific in nature, and better organized.
3. Prenatal development of behavior appears to progress along a cephalocaudal course as does also the development of reflexogenous zones. It appears that myogenic responses precede true sensory responses and that proprioceptive mechanisms seem to be functional before the onset of function in the cutaneous system.
4. Development of essential life functions involves a long, continuous process and is completed well in advance of the time when they will be required by the newborn infant to sustain independent existence.
5. Behavior development appears first in the gross musculature and later in the fine musculature.
6. Behavior tends to develop in the limbs in a proximal to distal direction. These latter two statements must be considered broad generalizations in that it is exceedingly difficult to apply stimula-

TABLE 4.1. Summary of prenatal development

Age in Weeks	Structural Development	Functional Development*
2.5 weeks	Neural groove indicated	
3.5 weeks	Primitive blood vessels and heart; neural crest formed	Heart beat begins
4 weeks	All somites present; limb buds form; neural tube closes; optic cup and lens pit forming	
5 weeks	Premuscle masses in head, trunk, and limbs	
6 weeks	Limbs recognizable; semicircular ducts become outlined	
7 weeks	Muscles differentiate rapidly—assume final shapes and relations; cerebral hemispheres becoming large; eyelids forming	Contralateral neck flexion (7.5)
8 weeks	Digits well formed; first ossification in middle of long bones; cerebral cortex begins to get typical cells; well-represented, definitive muscles in trunk, limbs and head; olfactory nucleus appears	Contralateral neck and trunk flexion (8.5) Spontaneous movement (9.5) Mouth opening (9.5) Stretch reflex (9.5)
10 weeks	Limbs nicely modeled; ossification spreading; spinal cord attains definitive internal structure; eyelids fused	Eyelid squint (10) Ventral head flexion (10) Incomplete finger closure (10.5) Plantar flexion of all toes (11) Ipsilateral head rotation (11)
12 weeks	Sex determined by external inspection; brain attains general structural features; spinal cord shows cervical and lumbar enlargements; internal	Lip closure and swallowing (12) Dorsiflexion of big toe and toe fanning; Flexion at foot, knee, hip (12)

Age in Weeks	Structural Development	Functional Development
	ear formed; some bones well outlined; taste buds appear	Elevate angle of mouth (13)
		Complete finger closure (13)
		Contralateral responses established (13)
		Vestibular and proprioceptive influence on responses (13)
16 weeks	Face looks "human"; hair on head; most bones distinctly indicated; joint cavities appear; cerebellum assumes some prominence; general sense organs differentiating (cutaneous)	Muscular movements can be detected in utero; reciprocal innervation in movements (16)
		Diagonal responses (16)
		"Scowl" combined with head extension (16)
		Temporary diaphragm contraction (17)
		Effective but weak true grasp (18.5)
20 weeks	Myelination of cord begins; nail plate begins	Side-to-side head turning (22)
		Weak vocal sounds (22)
24 weeks	Cerebral cortex layered typically	Sucking (24)
		Sneezing (24)
		Tendon reflexes (24)
		Palpebral reflex (25)
		Permanent respiration if delivered (27)
28 weeks	Cerebral fissures and convolutions appearing rapidly; eyelids reopen	Synergic muscle action (28)
		Corneal reflexes (28)
		Audible sucking (29)
32 weeks		
36 weeks	Most general sense organs completed	Taste sense present; olfactory present
40 weeks	Myelination of brain begins	Iris reflexes

* Based mainly on data presented by T. Humphrey. Some correlations between the appearance of human fetal reflexes and the development of the nervous system. In Purpura, D. P. and J. P. Schade (Eds.), *The Growth and Maturation of the Brain*. New York: Elsevier Publishing Co., 1964.

tion to minute, specific areas of very young fetuses because of their small size.

The generalization that ontogeny recapitulates phylogeny has been noted at various times in the previous presentation. This would appear to hold for histological and **morphological** development but is questionable if an attempt is made to apply it to the development of locomotion in the human being. Although there is a general relationship in the sequence of development of behavioral capacities from fish to man and investigations have shown that the first responses in fish, amphibians, and the lower mammals involve a lateral bending of the trunk, no observations have, as yet, been made in which the first trunk movements in the human fetus are unaccompanied by arm movements. Moreover, the locomotor mechanisms of fish and amphibians require a high degree of trunk muscle integration that does not appear to be similar to the neuromotor requirements for bipedal locomotion in man. Furthermore, the great variation in the creeping behavior of infants and the lack of evidence of rhythm in the movements of the limbs of the human fetus lend little support to the generalization of ontogeny recapitulating phylogeny in the development of human locomotion.

5

The Neonate

The process of birth, which, under normal conditions, involves the contraction of the uterus so that the fetal membranes are ruptured and the developing child is expelled through the birth canal, severs the parasitic connections of the child with the mother and necessitates the autonomous functioning of the child's vegetative systems if it is to survive. As previously pointed out, all the systems required for the sustenance of life are operative about two months prior to normal birth. However, the change from a liquid environment to a gaseous one means that there has been no opportunity for the respiratory system to function normally prior to the crucial time at birth when it must function or the child will be asphyxiated. Furthermore, the agent, or agents, which initiate the act of breathing become vitally important at this time.

Studies of conditions surrounding the onset of breathing indicate that the increase in metabolites and carbon dioxide together with a decrease in the oxygen content of the blood are important factors in causing the first gasps following severance of the umbilical cord (Corey, 1931). In addition, the pressure on the chest cavity of the baby as it passed through the birth canal forces some of the fluid within the respiratory system out of the mouth and nostrils so that a partial vacuum is created in the lungs. This causes air to rush into the lungs and any remaining fluid is expelled by a cough as greater volumes of air fill the lungs with subsequent breaths (Tanner & Taylor, 1965). Other investigators show that external stimuli such as the drying of the skin and its cooling are also important factors in initiating the first breath (Barcroft & Karvonen, 1948). In this connection, a slap is sometimes effective if a baby does not start breathing upon delivery (Huggett, 1930). Barcroft et al. (1940) contend that movements of the respiratory type seem to arise from the release of an inhibitory center in the forebrain.

Prior to birth, the blood vessels of the umbilical cord, in connection with the placenta, have the function of providing nutrients and eliminating waste products from the fetal circulatory system so that the fetal lungs require only the amount of blood flow necessary for development and maintenance. In addition, the capillary bed of the fetal lungs is in a relatively compressed state and the amount of pressure the contracting fetal heart would have to exert to force all the blood through the lungs would be very great. The fetal circulation differs from that of postnatal life in that most of the blood that enters the pulmonary artery is diverted to the aorta via the **ductus arteriosus.** Within the heart, a temporary hole called the **foramen ovale** is covered by a flap which prevents blood from seeping back to the right atrium during contraction of the left atrium.

After birth, the newborn infant requires more oxygen than can be provided by the fetal circulatory system and adjustments must be made so that all the blood will pass through the lung capillary bed. The ductus arteriosus begins to constrict actively with the first breath so that it shuts down within 24 hours and then becomes a fibrous cord by the time the baby is two months old. The increased pressure required to force the blood around the circulatory system causes the flap on the foramen ovale to close down permanently, and it gradually adheres to become part of the wall between the atria. In instances where either the foramen ovale or ductus arteriosus are not sealed off so that there is a mingling of the venous and arterial bloodstreams and the baby does not receive enough oxygen, the closures can be performed surgically (Tanner & Taylor, 1965).

The birth experience itself has been considered by some psychoanalysts to be traumatic, but no evidence is available to support this claim except in the case of birth injury. Here it is probably the injury itself that must be considered responsible rather than the birth as such. In an attempt to assess the effects of the birth experience, Ruja (1948) studied the relationship between the length of labor and crying in newborn infants. Although a positive relationship was found, the results may be questioned, as crying was measured on different infants at different intervals from one to eight days after birth. Pratt et al. (1930), in a continuous study of crying in newborn infants, found that crying normally increases during the first 10 days regardless of the length of labor. This increase might be expected in the light of findings, based on electroencephalograms, that the administration of sodium seconal during labor resulted in reduced cortical activity in the infant even after all clinical signs of drowsiness had disappeared (Hughes et al., 1948). Such reduced cortical activity may well be reflected in lowered reactions, including crying, during the first days after birth. It should be noted, however, that neonatal behavior is often considered subcortical since the cortex is relatively undeveloped at birth.

On the positive side, Ashley Montagu (1962) contends that labor provides a stimulant for the autonomic systems, particularly the respiratory and urogenital. His observations of children and adults who were delivered by Ceasarean section has led him to the conclusion that these individuals are more likely to suffer respiratory and urogenital dysfunction.

Although there are some unanswered questions concerning the effects of the birth experience itself, there is certainly no doubt that the rapid transition from a protected, parasitic existence to autonomous survival in the external world is a physiological strain on the neonate. Table 5.1 briefly summarizes the main areas of transition that must be achieved by the child from prenatal to postnatal life.

The immense degree of adjustment that occurs in the vegetative functions with birth is reflected in some cases by a loss of weight during the first three days which may not be recovered until the end of the 10th day. Another indication of the physiological strain imposed upon the infant at birth is the mortality rate, which is higher during the first 10 days than at any subsequent period. Indeed, the neonatal period must be considered as a period of adjustment and perfection of the newly activated physiological and sensory functions.

A few investigators in the field of infant development have considered the neonatal period as extending to approximately the end of the first week after birth; others consider it to include the first two postnatal weeks; still others place its duration as the first month with the extreme being the first three months. Most current usage in the field of infant behavior tends to consider the neonatal period as encompassing the first postnatal month. This time period would seem to be sufficient for the adjustment and perfection of the newly activated functions and for re-

TABLE 5.1. Variables of prenatal and postnatal life*

	Prenatal	Postnatal
Physical environment	Fluid (amniotic)	Gaseous (air)
External temperature	Approximately constant	Fluctuates with external conditions
Oxygen supply	Hemotrophic; diffusion through the placenta	From lung surface to blood stream
Nutrition	Hemotrophic; dependent on nutrients in mother's blood	Based on available food and functioning of digestive tract. Indigestible wastes must be eliminated
Elimination of products of metabolism	Into maternal blood stream	Elimination by lungs, skin, and kidneys
Sensory stimulation	At minimum except for kinesthetic and vibratory	All sense modalities stimulated by a variety of stimuli

* From Catherine Landreth, *The psychology of early childhood.* New York: Alfred A. Knopf, 1958. By permission of the author.

covery from injuries such as asphyxia, obstetrical paralysis, umbilical infections, and hemorrhages incurred during birth (Pratt, 1954).

AUTONOMIC SYSTEMS

Comprehensive investigations of heart beat and pulse rate of the neonate have reported great variation under different conditions. During sleep the average pulse rate was found to be 123.5 per minute and the rate was some 94.7 beats higher during crying (Halverson, 1941). Observations through the maternal wall during the last month before birth indicate that vibratory stimuli applied to the abdomen of the mother increased the average heart rate by approximately 14.3 beats per minute. Furthermore, similar observations revealed that smoking by the mother increased the fetal heart beat approximately five beats per minute some eight to 12 minutes after smoking was started (Sontag & Wallace, 1936). Therefore, stimuli of different modalities appear to produce considerable variation in pulse rate both in the fetus and in the neonate.

Although it is sometimes assumed that the birth cry is the first respiratory response of the neonate, observations based upon high speed motion pictures indicate that gasping is the first respiratory response after birth (Schmidt, 1950; Peiper, 1951). Schmidt (1950) found that gasping lasted from 13 to 45 seconds in normal full-term infants but increased in duration to 6½ minutes in premature 8-month infants and up to 12 minutes in difficult births. Following the initial respiratory gasp, the breathing rate is, as is the heart rate, subject to a great deal of variation depending upon internal and external stimuli. There is also a marked variation from one infant to the other; the average rate during sleep prior to awakening is 32.3 breaths per minute and rises to a maximal average of 133.3 respirations per minute during crying (Halverson, 1941).

Other responses intimately associated with respiration such as yawning, coughing, and sneezing are reported to occur shortly after birth, and the birth cry itself is considered to be a concomitant of the initiation of pulmonary respiration. There is a relationship between the centers governing the respiratory, sucking, and swallowing reflexes during the sucking period of the infant so that babies are able to suck, swallow, and breathe at the same time—a facility which they will later lose for it is not possessed by adults. It is believed that the swallowing center influences the sucking center which, in turn, influences the rhythm of the breathing center (Peiper, 1939). Both Peiper (1939) and Halverson (1944) have found that swallowing occurs during the phases between breathing, and the latter investigator also reported that sucking occurs simultaneously with breathing except during strong sucking when the sucks tend to come after inspiration. Good coordination of these centers appears even in premature infants.

The transition from maternally supplied nutrient materials to independent assimilation of nutrients by means of the **alimentary** tract in the neonate may be one cause of an initial loss of weight. Other possible causes may be imperfect assimilation, or the possibility that **colostrum** does not meet the energy requirements of the newborn infant. In some cases the scantiness of the maternal milk production may be responsible. Under optimum conditions, no loss of weight may occur, although there are wide individual differences in infant adjustment.

The primacy of the feeding function is indicated by the number of motoric responses associated with this life-sustaining process. The moving of the baby's head to the midline position and the opening of its mouth when its palms are pressed back is called the *Babkin reflex*. The neonate also exhibits mouth orientation, or seeking, responses which are elicited by tactual stimulation of the lip and adjacent face areas and result in the bringing of the opened mouth to the nipple. When contact is properly established, sucking begins and the ingestion of food follows. Salivation is firmly established in the neonate and is initiated by sucking. As previously mentioned, sucking, breathing, and swallowing are coordinated so that the passage of food to the stomach presents no problem to the suckling. Arrival of the food in the stomach stimulates gastric secretion and when the stomach becomes filled the child ceases nursing. After the infant has ceased nursing and broken contact with the nipple, there is frequently some regurgitation of food which, in turn, is often followed by hiccuping.

The stomach of the neonate has been found to empty in four to five hours at the most; the intestines in seven or eight hours; and the large intestine within two to 14 hours. Carlson and Ginsburg (1915) have demonstrated, by using a balloon on the stomach of infants prior to nursing, that "hunger" contractions, similar to those found in adults, occur in the neonate. However, during the first two weeks, "hunger" contractions in normal full-term infants begin in the stomach about two hours and 50 minutes after the previous nursing period. During the period from the second to eighth week, the time duration increases until contractions start at about three hours and 40 minutes after nursing. These observations would indicate that the "hunger" contractions arise before the stomach has been emptied and cannot, therefore, be ascribed to an empty stomach.

These muscular contractions of the stomach are more vigorous in the neonate than in the adult; observations have revealed a concomitant increase in reflex excitability that was synchronous with the periods of stomach contractions. Although, in the adult, the contractions may be inhibited by introducing taste substances in the mouth, in the neonate they are only temporarily inhibited by the administration of small quantities of water or milk (Taylor, 1917). After observing 73 infants, Irwin (1932) found that general motility correlated .97 with the elapsed time between feeding periods. Bodily oscillations measured on a stabilometer during the first 15 minutes after feeding averaged 17.0 per minute, but during the last 15 minutes period prior to nursing the oscillations soared to approximately 45 per minute.

The sequence of activities in the alimentary canal is completed by **egestion** or **defecation.** The first half hour after feeding is the period during which defecation occurs most frequently with the modal number of defecations being approximately five in 24 hours (Halverson, 1940). Most defecations occur during wakefulness with the infant being active before and during the act and quiescent following the act (Pratt, 1954). The activity associated with defecation is greater than the activity prior to **micturition**, which occurs approximately 18 times during a 24-hour period. As with defecation, the greatest number of micturitions occur within the first hour after feeding and during periods of wakefulness with completion of the act resulting in quiescence (Halverson, 1940). On the basis of his own and other investigators' observations, Pratt (1954) believes it is possible that a great deal of the young infant's general motility is in some way dependent upon the alimentary processes.

SLEEP

Numerous investigators have studied the sleep of newborn infants using different criteria for defining sleep. The oldest and most widely used has been the closure of the eyes, although the criterion of decreased irritability and activity is currently being accepted as a more valid indicator. The neonate sleeps 20 hours out of 24 with the duration of each sleep period being no more than three hours and usually less (Pratt et al., 1930). Contrary to usual belief, more infants are awake during the first 15 minutes after feeding than during the last 15 minutes prior to the next nursing period, and most infants are asleep during the middle 15 minutes between nursing periods (Irwin, 1932). The depth of sleep is variable from one infant to another and it varies according to the condition and the activities of the infant prior to falling asleep. As the child grows older, the total hours of sleep decrease, but the length of each sleep period increases so that longer periods of wakefulness gradually supplant periods of sleep. In contrast with the amount of stimulation required to awaken the neonate, it has been found that weaker electrical stimuli will awaken the child as it grows older (Pratt, 1954).

Most investigation of the responses of the neonate have been carried out with quiescent infants so that the effects of experimental stimuli will not be masked by other activity. On the basis of the simple criterion of sleep being reduced motility, such responses may be considered as involving sleeping infants. Prechtl (1974) has classified the state of arousal of the infant into three categories: State 1 is non-REM or quiet sleep; State 2 is active or REM sleep; and State 3 is quiet awake. Based on these classifications, proprioceptive reflexes such as the knee and biceps jerks (muscle stretch reflexes) and Moro reflex (vestibular stimulation and neck articulation) are all increased in State 1 (quiet sleep) and are essentially absent in State 2 (active REM sleep). On the other hand, extroceptive skin reflexes and auditory orienting persist in State 2 in addition to occurring in State 3 (quiet awake) but are absent in State 1. Noninceptive reflexes, such as the Babinski reflex, appear to be independent of state of arousal as these responses occur at all levels.

Parmelee and Sigman (1983) indicate that differences in responses in each state between infants and adults are probably due to the immaturity of the state organization of the infant. A cited example of such maturational changes in reflex responses is that of the Babkin reflex (skin pressure reflex) which is not state dependent in preterm infants but becomes state dependent by term. Therefore, the behavioral responses of infants are dependent upon the state of arousal of the infant and any behavioral evaluation of the responses to sensory stimulation of newborns (both pre- and full-term) and of young infants must be based upon judgments of the state of arousal.

BODILY POSTURES

Rather well-defined resting and sleeping postures have been observed in the neonate. The arms and legs tend to be flexed and the fists clenched with even the most marked extension, such as the upper arms at right angles to the body and the forearms parallel to the head, still exhibiting some flexion. Gesell and Thompson (1938) reported that all of the infants examined in their normative survey spontaneously maintained the head predominantly rotated to one side at 4 weeks of age. All the infants also held their arms in the tonic neck reflex attitude, which involves extension of the arm on the side to which the head is turned together with flexion of the opposite arm. On the basis of these observations, these investigators concluded that the tonic neck reflex is a normal feature of neonatal infancy.

The positionings of the neonate are, in a sense, also conditioned by the previous confinement within the fetal membranes, where full extension of the limbs was impossible, and by the body proportions and muscular strength of the newborn infant. At birth, the average infant is approximately 20 inches long from the crown of the head to the heel and weighs approximately 7½ pounds. The head, with its large cranium and relatively small face, makes up one-fourth of the body length and is too heavy to be supported easily in a vertical position when the infant is placed on its back. The body, with the chest circumference approximately the same as the diameter of the head, makes up one-half of the remaining total length so that the arms and legs are relatively short in comparison with adult body proportions. The major portion of the mass of the newborn infant is, therefore, composed of the head and body so that any action of the weak limbs is ineffective with respect to motility of the body as a whole. Figure 5.1 indicates the relative proportions of the newborn in comparison with body proportions at other periods of development.

SENSORY SYSTEMS

The neonatal period marks the first time certain sensory-motor structures are activated by adequate stimuli with this stimulation in turn helping to bring about further maturation of the nervous system. The reactivity of the sensory-motor structures reveals the effects of fetal maturation but does not, in itself, induce profound developmental events or provide a basis for more than the mere beginnings of learning. The responsiveness of the neonate to internal stimuli has already been discussed in relation to the functioning of the alimentary tract. It may be

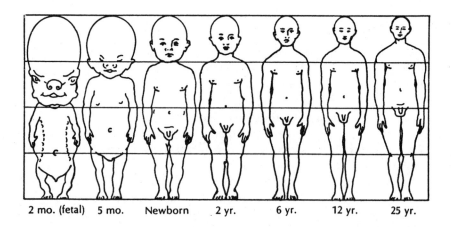

| 2 mo. (fetal) | 5 mo. | Newborn | 2 yr. | 6 yr. | 12 yr. | 25 yr. |

FIGURE 5.1. *Changes in form and proportion of the human body during fetal and postnatal life. (From C. M. Jackson, Some aspects of form and growth. In W. J. Robbins; S. Brody; A. G. Hogan; C. M. Jackson; and C. W. Green,* Growth. *New Haven: Yale University Press, 1928. By permission of the publisher.)*

recalled that the internal stimuli tend to have a rhythmic incidence and to occur over periods of fairly long duration. It is believed the transition from fetal to postnatal existence may involve a greater stepping up of internal than of external stimuli. On the basis of previously cited observations of motility in the neonate, it would appear that stimuli associated with internal processes would account for most of the infant's motility. Investigations of the role of external stimuli indicate that the responses vary according to the type, intensity, and duration of the stimulus but are always set against the background of internal stimuli and tend to add little to the total activity. Moreover, in some instances, it has been found that external stimuli will reduce total activity.

Vision

Although the optic cup which is destined to become the retina is formed by the fourth week after conception, the site of keenest vision in the retina, the macula lutea, differentiates in late fetal life continuing through early infancy (Timiras et al., 1968). Until the advent of infrared television, it was difficult to study the pupillary reflex because newborn infants tend to close their eyes even under mild illumination. However, the infrared recordings provide unmistakable evidence of substantial pupillary constriction in the light and dilation in darkness (Haith, 1978). With increased age, an increase in sensitivity of pupillary responses is shown with less intense stimuli being required to elicit responses (Sherman et al., 1936). The most invariable type of response aroused by visual stimuli is the visuopalpebral reflex, which involves the closing, tightening, or twitching of closed eyelids and is elicited by flashes of light (Pratt et al., 1930). Another response to a flash of light, the ocular-neck, involving a bending backwards of the head, is dependent upon the intensity of light (Peiper, 1926). Bright, intense flashes of light have been observed to release Moro or "startle" reflexes as well as ocular-neck, pupillary, visuopalpebral, circulatory, and respiratory responses; the incidence of the Moro or "startle" reflexes is higher during the first few days of the neonatal period (Pratt et al., 1930). Korner and Grobstein (1973) report increased alertness and active visual scanning when the newborn is placed in the soothing shoulder position.

Although the immediate responses to light changes of various intensities is excitatory and there is no apparent differentiation according to intensity, prolonged periods of illumination of the same intensity have been found to result in decreased activity (Weiss, 1934). Sudden reduction of visual stimuli, such as when the infant is subjected to darkness after having been exposed to an illumination of five foot-candles for a period of five minutes, results in an increase in activity (Irwin, 1941). However, the infant soon adapts to the dark and, once adaptation is complete, will respond with increased sensitivity to visual stimuli which would normally be inadequate to elicit responses from a light-adapted eye (Peiper, 1926).

There is little doubt that the neonate has some vision but the extent of such vision is still problematic. Coordinate compensatory eye movements have been observed as soon as 32 hours after birth (Ling, 1942). The onset of visual pursuit movements has been placed at one (Beasley, 1933) and two weeks (McGinnis, 1930) by different observers and horizontal pursuit movements tend to appear before vertical and circular pursuit movements. There are variations in the responses from one infant to another with respect to the optimum rate of movement and the distance of the moving light from the eyes (Beasley, 1933). On the basis of duration and fixation of gaze, it is generally accepted that the neonate has color vision with the gaze tending to rest longest on blue and green, shortest on yellow, while red comes in between (Stirnimann, 1944). As early as two weeks of age, newborn infants show strong predilections for gazing upon vertical or horizontal gratings rather than obliques (Leehey et al., 1975).

The early eye movements of the newborn are saccadic; that is, the child shifts his or her fixation from one stationary target to another. Smooth eye movements, which are involved when fixation is held on a moving target, gradually replace the series of saccadic pursuit movements used by the newborn to follow moving objects and smooth pursuit movements are common by 2 months. A large moving visual pattern elicits a series of smooth movements in the direction of the pattern's movements followed by saccadic fixations in the opposite direction and this type of eye movement is called optokinetic nystagmus (OKN). OKN eye movements can be elicited when the observer's head is stationary and is dependent upon certain combinations of velocity, size, and spatial frequency of the visual stimulus. In the newborn, OKN can be elicited by a moving field of vertical stripes and appears to mature before saccadic and smooth pursuit but roughly at the same time as the other motion-compensating eye movements; that is, static reflexes and statokinetic reflexes (Banks & Salapatek, 1983).

When the body and head are in motion, the eye movements that occur to compensate for the motion of the head and help to maintain fixation at a constant point in space are: 1) static reflex movements which consist of upward and downward eye movements when the head is tilted forward or backward and of counterrolling of the eyes when the head is tilted to the side; 2) statokinetic reflexes, which are elicited by angular rotations of the head and body and involve a series of smooth movements, in the opposite direction of motion, followed by saccadic fixations in the direction of motion when the rotation is fairly rapid and large in magnitude. When the head/body rotation is smaller, single smooth compensatory eye movements occur which are more accurate when the eyes are open than when the eyes are closed. These vestibular-controlled eye movements do not enable accurate fixation of a target while the head is rotated until 3 months of age. As the vestibular system is also involved in maintenance of balance, it is not surprising that infants of 12 months and older, who can stand unsupported, respond to the motion of an experimental room (whose walls and ceiling can move) by swaying or falling in the direction of the room's motion. Such experiments show that infants who are capable of upright posture use kinetic visual information to guide postural control. This visual control of posture increases in extent up to 2 years of age after which visual influence declines to adult values (Banks & Salapatek, 1983).

Observations by Dayton and Jones of 85 newborn infants, ranging in age from 8 hours to 10 days, have led them to conclude that newborn infants have the ability to see small objects quite distinctly and are able to use the eyes together (binocular vision) to a remarkable extent (*University Bulletin*, 1964). Experiments reported by Bower (1979) indicate that babies will defend themselves against a small object that approaches until it is close to them. The size of the retinal image does not appear to be a factor in this reaction because a large object that does not come near will not produce defensive reactions. In addition, infants are able to discriminate between a shadow of an object headed directly at them and of one that would be on a "miss" course. These findings indicate that infants process three-dimensional information; however, the speed of the moving objects would also seem to be a factor in such information processing as the experiments also indicate that babies cannot register visual information that is coming too fast. They appear to have a very limited information-processing rate and Bower (1979) comments that many everyday events may occur at too high a rate for babies to register all the relevant information.

Variations in response to visual stimuli may be the result of maturational differences. For example, pre-term infants may be slower to process visual information and less able to use information than full-term infants. Parmelee and Sigman (1983) reported that, at 4 months, a group of full-term infants showed significant preferences for novel stimuli that were not shown by pre-term infants of the same conceptual age. Moreover, the pre-term infants were slower to turn away from objects explored manually and visually at 8 months old. Similarly, maturational changes have been noted in visually evoked potentials (EEG's) with full-term infants having a prominent positive-negative complex almost always present. Between the first and second postnatal month, a third positive-negative complex of greater amplitude than the other two develops and all three positive-negative complexes are well formed by 3 months with the form of the visually evoked potentials becoming stable and like that of adults. Changes also occur in the latency of the visually evoked potentials with a sharp drop in latency between one and two months after full-term and then a gradual decrease in latencies until adult levels are reached by 2 to 4 years. The change in the form of the evoked potential may reflect increases in the complexity of visual material that can be processed and the change in latency with maturation may have some bearing on the speed and attentional aspect of visual information processing.

Environmental factors may also contribute to variation in visual responses with 4- to 8-month-old infants who suffered fewer birth complications showing better discrimination between novel and familiar stimuli. In addition, among pre-term infants, slow visual processing of unchanging patterns was most pronounced among infants experiencing the least social interaction at home. On the other hand, the degree of preference for novel stimuli in pre-term infants at 4 months corrected for age was positively related to social stimulation in the home measured at one month. Morever, neonatal intervention centered on tactual and vestibular modalities enhanced visual recognition memory six months later (Parmelee & Sigman, 1983). Therefore, it appears that maturational levels and environmental factors are associative and interactive in the behavioral development of visual sensitivity in infants. A very comprehensive review of the anatomical and functional development of the visual system is provided by Banks and Salapatek (1983).

Hearing

Although the main components of the middle ear and the external ear assume their final form and interrelation by midfetal life, hearing is imperfect in the newborn because of gelatinous tissue filling the **auditory** canals and impeding passage of sound waves. The progressive resorption of the gelatinous material during the first week after birth results in improved hearing (Timiras et al., 1968). The neonate responds to auditory stimuli in such ways as quivering of the eyelids, head movements, wrinkling of the forehead, crying, and awakening from sleep. Louder stimuli produce more bodily movements, increases in respiratory and heart action, and greater frequency of eyelid closure (Stubbs, 1934). However, as with visual stimuli, auditory stimuli of long durations, such as five minutes, tend to decrease bodily movements significantly in comparison with periods during which no stimuli are presented (Weiss, 1934). The most frequent reaction to auditory stimuli is the **acoustopalpebral** reflex, which is similar in nature to the **visuopalpebral** reflex (Froeschels & Beebe, 1946), and the Moro or "startle" response is elicited by sudden, loud noises. The physiological condition of the neonate has a definite effect on the responses to auditory stimuli with stimuli being most easily elicited during sleep and most difficult to activate during nursing (Pratt,

1954). The smallest percentages of responses are obtained when infants are crying and the greatest number when they are awake and inactive (Stubbs, 1934).

According to Eimas (1978), the neonate is sensitive to a wide variety of sounds including brief clicks, tuning forks, whistles, and music; continuous acoustic stimulation often results in a general quieting of the infant. A review of the literature by Eimas (1978) indicates that babies as young as a few days can discriminate sound intensity differences with the absolute threshold appearing to be significantly higher than that of the normal hearing adult. There is evidence that 5- to 7-month-old infants are sensitive to changes in tonal pattern and that infants from a few days to 5 months are capable of discriminating frequency changes. These findings indicate that the infant brings to the task of speech perception at least the auditory ability to discriminate variations in intensity, frequency, and frequency patterns (Eimas, 1978). The rapidly growing auditory competence of the full-term newborn is reflected in maturational changes in EEG characteristics of auditory evoked potentials and heart rate in responses to auditory stimuli (Parmelee & Sigman, 1983). A very comprehensive review of auditory development and speech perception is provided by Aslin, Pisoni, and Jusczyk (1983).

The ability of the neonate to localize sounds has been examined by Bower (1979) who cites experiments indicating that newborns will turn their eyes in the direction of sound. After 28 days, however, such a response may not occur; Bower comments that the infants may have lost interest in looking toward the sounds. There is some variability in the accuracy of sound location depending upon the source position in relation to the infant. Infants under 20 weeks of age were able to locate the source of sounds with considerable accuracy if the location was in the midline in relation to the body, whereas there was less accuracy in locating sound sources on the periphery. When these results were compared with sighted reaching for the same object (without sound), the results indicated the auditory location along the midline was more accurate than the visual. On the other hand, visual perpheral accuracy was much higher than auditory peripheral accuracy (Bower, 1979).

Smell and Taste

The **olfactory** epithelium becomes pseudostratified by the seventh week after pregnancy and olfactory perception is present but not well established at the eighth fetal month. The taste buds appear in the fetus during the third month and reflex responses to taste are present in premature infants of 7 months (Timiras et al., 1968).

Determination of the extent of olfactory sensitivity in the neonate is hampered by methodological difficulties in assessing purely olfactory stimulation. Although vocalization, facial responses, and general bodily movement have been observed in response to ammonia and acetic acid fumes and sucking responses have been noted in response to the fumes of valerian, it is difficult to know whether these responses should be attributed to olfactory stimulation or to irritation of the mucous membrane of the nose (Pratt et al., 1930).

Taste is considered to be highly developed in the neonate but it is uncertain whether all four taste qualities are fully differentiated. Of all **gustatory** stimuli tests, only salt solutions impaired sucking responses or caused them to cease (Jensen, 1932) whereas sucking responses are most pronounced in response to the administration of sugar solutions and are found to increase in prominence in this category with age (Pratt et al., 1930). Furthermore, the degree of satiation also affects the response, with the moderately full infant being a better discriminator of gustatory stimuli than the hungry one.

Cutaneous Sensitivity

The sense organs associated with cutaneous sensitivity (pain, deep pressure, temperature, and **tactile**) begin to differentiate between the third and fourth fetal month. There is a considerable degree of variability in the rate of development with the deep pressure **corpuscles** being completed at 8 fetal months, whereas the tactile corpuscles are not completed until a year after birth (Timiras et al., 1968).

Thermal sensitivity seems to be well developed in the neonate. Numerous investigations of various parts of the body indicate great variability from one area to another but suggest the possibility that the legs and feet are more sensitive to thermal stimulation than the head and hand areas (Pratt, 1954). It would also appear that different areas of the body have different high and low temperature thresholds where stimuli deviating from these thresholds will elicit vigorous responses. Furthermore, a definite preference for certain temperatures is indicated by the seeking movements of one foot towards the other when the latter is being subjected to a warm stimulation, whereas relatively cold stimulus will result in the withdrawal of the stimulated limb (Stirnimann, 1939). General environmental temperatures have been reported as giving rise to shivering (Blanton, 1917) and a correlation of -.205 has been obtained between environmental temperatures and general activity in the infant (Pratt, 1930). A study by Irwin and Weiss (1934) of 50 clothed and unclothed infants indicated less crying by the former with the conclusion being that clothing provides some thermal insulation from atmospheric stimuli.

Sensitivity to contact or pressure stimuli is well developed in the newborn infant but it is difficult to differentiate the effects of these stimuli from the effects of pain, thermal, or other stimuli. Although there have been no systematic investigations of the differences in tactual sensitivity of all of the cutaneous surfaces of the neonate's body, the results of numerous studies tend to suggest the face, hands, and soles of the feet as having the greatest sensitivity while the shoulders, back, breast, and abdomen have the least. In assessing cutaneous reflexes, the investigator is also faced with the problem of controlling the intensity of the stimulus so as to be sure the response elicited is purely cutaneous and does not also involve pressure sensory receptors (Pratt, 1954). Furthermore, responses to similar stimuli will change with the age of the child (Nassau, 1938). In general, the response evoked from any given body area by tactual stimuli will vary with their intensity and duration, the physiological condition of the infant, and whether the application of the stimulus involves stroking or punctiform contact. The responses elicited range from local reflexes to general body movements and include **palpebral, pupillary, Moro**, startle, **tonic neck**, withdrawal, and plantar responses.

Additional responses to tactual stimuli provide a fundamental orientation of the infant to its surroundings. Of primary importance in this regard is the mouth orientation response of the infant to contact stimulation of the cheek which was noted above in relation to sucking. Stimulation above or below the lips will result in the throwing back of the head or the dropping of the chin according to the respective area of stimulation. There are variations in the extent of these responses depending upon the locale of the area stimulated with the lips, above the lips, below the lips, and the cheek being decreasingly sensitive in the order listed. The sensitivity of the cheek area tends to decrease with age (Pratt, 1954).

Response to pain stimuli has been recorded in the neonate, but the differential sensitivity of the various areas of the body has not been fully investigated. Even for those areas investigated, there is some disagreement as to the relative sensitivity of the areas. One group of investigators has found the head areas to be more sensitive than the leg areas (Sherman et al., 1936), whereas another group noted that the head areas were least sensitive, the arms more so, and the legs most sensitive (Dockeray & Rice, 1934). The relative sensitivity of the newborn to pain in comparison with the later neonatal period is also an area in which variable observations have been recorded. In one instance, investigation of newly born infants over a period of time indicated a decrease in the average number of pin pricks required to elicit a response in both the head and the leg regions over the first few days (Sherman & Sherman, 1925) while, in another instance, no change in response was found with age during the neonatal period (Dockeray & Rice, 1934).

Children who are blind must place considerable reliance upon tactile sensory discrimination and it has been conjectured that such reliance will increase the discriminatory capacity. However, experimentation tends to show that there is no difference in tactile discrimination thresholds of the blind and sighted. In addition, the capacity and duration of the tactile storage are inferior to those of the visual system (Hatwell, 1978). But experimentation with the "tactile-vision-substitution-system" indicates that the tactile system may be more superior than previously thought. In these experiments, a sensory prosthesis transforms the visual image of an object (recorded via a TV camera) into a corresponding pattern of tactile stimulations. These tactile stimulations are transmitted to the individual's back through a cluster of 400 vibrotractors. When the individual can orient and move the camera to thus actively change the stimulation patterns, the resulting indentification of the very complex tactile pattern is possible (Hatwell, 1978).

Kinesthetic Sensitivity

The differentiation of proprioceptive nerve endings in the muscles, tendons, and about the joints tends to follow a cephalocaudal progression. Muscle spindle formation begins in the upper extremity during the 11th fetal week and by the fourth fetal month spindles have differentiated in practically all muscles. Prior to the fourth month there are only free nerve endings about the joints, but at 4½ fetal months the first mature corpuscles begin to form about the joints. At 20 weeks, spindle-type and Golgi-body type endings appear in the tendon areas of the arms and legs. In the neonate, the proprioceptive sensory endings have a finished look and three-fourths of all corpuscles about the joints are mature (Humphrey, 1964). The increasingly complex nature of the responses during prenatal functional development (table 4.1) clearly indicates the increasing influence of proprioceptive influence on responses after the 13th fetal week.

Sensitivity to movement or changes in body position are exhibited in the neonate by movements of the body as a whole or by various parts of the body. Sudden loss of support, sudden elevation of the body, and sudden jarring of the surface upon which the infant is resting result in the elicitation of the Moro or "startle" response. In these instances, the response is considered to be conditioned by static-kinesthetic sensitivity whereby the spatial movement stimulates the static receptors to elicit the response. Some investigators have expressed the opinion that the generalized responses of the newborn infant may be touched off indirectly by static-kinesthetic sensitivity to the more local responses set off directly by other stimuli (Pratt, 1954). Although the proprioceptive system may be somewhat more structurally mature at birth than some of the other sensory systems, it is highly dependent upon the structural and functional development of other bodily systems for its own functional development. The functional development of the vestibular system for the maintenance of balance is as vital as functional development of the somatosensory and proprioceptive systems for acquisition of upright loco-motion. In sighted individuals, visual input also has a major role and can, in some instances, override **vestibular, somatosensory** and propriocep-tive information. For example, when the entire visual environment moves in relation to a stationary observer, this movement is often inter-preted as movement of the individual in relation to a stationary world as this is the normal visual-proprioceptive input. Similarly, a moving audi-tory environment around a stationary blindfolded individual can elicit sensations of self-rotation and **nystagmus** in the individual (Lackner, 1978).

In instances of induced apparent self-motion by visual or auditory stimulation, the active movement of the individual's head will stimulate the vestibular system and proprioceptors in the neck. This sensory input would be different if the individual were actually moving, and the dra-matic change in vestibular and proprioceptive input is sufficient to over-ride the rotary visual or auditory stimulation. A number of investigations indicate that individuals who are actively maintaining their posture do not experience the visually induced self-motion illusion (Lackner, 1978). Postural illusions can also be evoked by vibration of a skeletal muscle. In this instance, the vibration elicits a reflex contraction of the muscle called the tonic vibration reflex. If the action of a muscle contracting under a tonic vibration reflex is resisted by restraining the controlled limb, then that limb will be experienced as moving. The direction of the apparent movement is the same as the direction of movement that would occur if the vibrated muscle were actually lengthening. Similarly, if an individu-al's Achilles tendons are vibrated, the tonic vibration reflexes will cause the individual to sway backwards. On the other hand, if the backwards motion of a blindfolded, Achilles-tendon-vibrated subject is prevented, then the stationary individual experiences a falling forward sensation (Lackner, 1978).

The force of gravity also is a contributing factor to the development of functional proprioception. During the weightlessness of orbital flight, the Russian cosmonauts felt themselves upside down when their eyes were closed. They could abolish the illusion by pushing firmly against their chairs or opening their eyes; the feeling ceased during reentry. There are also changes in the tonus of postural muscles and in eye-hand coordination during weightlessness. The ankle jerk is absent during the first 100 milliseconds of weightlessness and the balance of activity in anti-gravity muscles is disturbed, yielding inaccuracies on pointing tasks when visual feedback is restricted. In summarizing his view of sensory and pos-tural stability, Lackner (1978) comments that sensory influences on ap-parent posture and postural influences on sensory localization reflect a complex interaction of **efferent**, vestibular, and proprioceptive informa-tion about body orientation with exteroceptive information from the eyes, ears, and skin. This is an interaction that is essential to preserve the long-term stability and spatial integrity of the individual's perceptual world.

Blind children must place exclusive reliance upon the haptic sensory system for the recognition of form and shapes. The **haptic system** is the functional integration of the tactile and proprioceptive sensory mechanisms. Haptic pattern perception is slower to develop in the blind than visual perception in the sighted, but it generally follows the same lines of development. The development of the intersensory processes takes place early in life and the extent of perceptual development is greatly influenced by the number of available sense modalities. Hatwell (1978) comments that the comparison between the visual perception of the sighted and the haptic perception of the congenitally blind is always a comparison between a complete and integrated polysensorial system and an incomplete and impoverished one.

GENERAL RESPONSES

The Moro response is a general bodily response to sudden, strong light and sound as well as static-kinesthetic sensitivity. Moro, in 1918, described this response as a clasping response which consists of the symmetrical extension of the arms followed by their bowing and return to the body with the legs undergoing the same kind of movement although their involvement may not be so great (Pratt, 1954). Subsequent investigators have deemed that the Moro response is not a true clasping or embracing response as the extended arms do not hold or clasp the experimenter's arm and that it is a variation of the "startle" response, which is a purely flexion response. Both patterns of response are clearly present at 6 weeks of age but the Moro disappears after a few months, whereas the startle response persists into adult life (Landis & Hunt, 1939).

The pattern of arm movements in the Moro response is duplicated to some extent in the reaching movements observed by Bower (1976). During the first few weeks of life, infants can reach out to touch visible objects and will occasionally grasp them. However, this action disappears at about the age of 4 weeks and does not reappear again until around 20 weeks of age. Similarly, sound can activate infants to reach out and grasp objects they can hear but cannot see. This response occurs for both sighted and blind children and, as with the early visual reaching, disappears when the infant is 5 or 6 months old. A reaching response has obvious practical use for the blind infant; unfortunately, the reaching response to a sound stimulus may not reappear in the blind child.

Rotation of the body in a horizontal plane has been found to result in compensatory head movements in the same direction during rotation followed by movement in the opposite direction after cessation of rotation (McGraw, 1941b). Turning of an infant's head to the side suddenly when it is lying on its back results in the adoption of the "fencing" posture of the tonic neck reflex, and passive flexion of one leg of the infant when it is lying on its back will automatically result in the flexion of the other leg (Pratt, 1954). Responses during inversion, when the infant is suspended by the ankles, indicate a momentary backward bending of the head resulting from contraction in the cervical region (Irwin, 1936) and a flexion of the knees and of the hip resulting in an up-and-down motion of the body (McGraw, 1940b). Some investigators consider these responses to be related to early attempts at locomotion (McGraw, 1946). General body position during inverted suspension consists of the head and body being roughly aligned in the vertical plane and the arms being maintained in their usual flexed position. When on its back, the newborn exhibits flexed arms and legs, curled fingers, and some sideways inclination of the head (figure 5.2).

In general, the newborn infant is completely dominated by gravity, since it does not have the strength to hold its head or trunk upright or in alignment when suspended at the abdomen, buttocks, or at the side of the hip. It is also unable to maintain a sitting posture when placed in a sitting position, but is able, as with inverted suspension, to momentarily lift its head when placed in a prone position on a solid surface. A newborn infant will also make alternate, or "stepping," movements when held in an erect posture with its feet resting on a surface. The latter two activities have been regarded as the first indicators of future upright, **bipedal** locomotion. However, McGraw (1946), one of the earliest investigators to assign locomotory implications to these responses, believes that genuine upright ambulation is impossible in the neonate because of undeveloped equilibratory apparatus and lack of strength. Furthermore, the narrow base of steps during these stepping movements is in marked

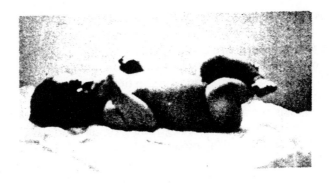

FIGURE 5.2. *Normal-term child at 4 weeks of age.*

contrast to the wide base adopted in the footwork of the beginning toddler. In the prone position, the combination of alternate arm and leg movements are classified as a swimming response (McGraw, 1946). The bilateral leg extension and flexion that also occurs in the prone position may come under this same classification in keeping with the bilateral extension and flexion during the breast stroke.

One may also speculate as to the role of the plantar reflex in such neonatal stepping movements, since tactual stimulation of the sole of the foot is involved in both these responses. Although the observations of Minkowski (1922) of the plantar reflex during the late fetal period would indicate the establishment of the adult toe flexion pattern at this time, numerous other investigators have reported widely divergent responses in the neonate. Toe extensions are reported as occurring more frequently than toe flexions (Richards & Irwin, 1934) whereas, in another instance, the nature of the response is noted as depending upon the previous posture of the toes so that a posture of flexion will result in extension and vice versa (Sherman & Sherman, 1925). A very exhaustive study of the patterning of the responses to stimulation of the sole of the foot reveals almost 200 different patterns of which the five most frequent were: foot flexion; extension of the toes and foot flexion; extension of the hallux; toes extended, fanning, and foot flexion; and hallux extension and foot flexion (Pratt, 1954).

The grasping reflex has been interpreted by some investigators, as has the Moro response, as a defensive mechanism in terms of the arboreal phylogenetic development of man and, because of its digital character, has sometimes been described as *simian*. The grasp of the neonate, which involves palm and finger flexion without thumb opposition when the infant is partially or wholly suspended, is considered to be involuntary, whereas the adult grasp, with opposing thumb, is voluntary. In terms of behavior sequence, involuntary grasping disappears at about 4 to 6 months of age, after which it is replaced by the adult form of grasping (Pratt, 1954). However, no abrupt change occurs in the grasping sequence as there is some overlapping of the two forms. Careful studies of the neonatal grasping reflex indicate two phases; namely, the closure of the fingers to light pressure upon the palm, and second, the gripping or clinging, which is considered to be a proprioceptive response to pull on the finger tendons. A discrepancy in the times of disappearnace of closure, in about 16 to 24 weeks, and of proprioceptive gripping or clinging, after 25 weeks, is accounted for by the observation that closure is a specific or limited response, whereas gripping or clinging has other movements associated with it (Halverson, 1937).

The length of time that an infant can support its own weight is often used as a measure of the strength of the grasp. The average length of suspension time with two hands has been found to be 60 seconds, and the longest time was 128 seconds (Richter, 1934). When pulled toward suspension, infants are generally able to support more than 70 percent of their body weight. During the testing of 97 infants under 24 weeks of age, Halverson (1937) found that 27 were able to support their entire weight in the process of being pulled to suspension while one infant, 4 weeks old, was able to complete the process with the right hand alone. Age would seem to be a factor, since the strength of the grasping response was not as great during the early part of the neonatal period. Furthermore, when the gripping strength of the infant was measured by means of a small, sensitive rubber capsule, it was noted that the strength of the grasp was greatest during the early part of nursing and decreased as the infant approached satiety (Halverson, 1937). The grasp of the infant is also recorded as being strongest when the infant is crying and weakest when it is asleep (Sherman et al., 1936). These results would certainly indicate that muscular tension, as it is reflected in the strength of grasp, is dependent, as are so many of the functions during the neonatal period, upon the physiological condition of the infant.

Differences have been reported in the grasping strength of the two hands; the left hand averaged 1765 grams and the right hand was found to average 1732 grams (Sherman et al., 1936). Clinging strength has also been noted as being slightly superior in the left hand (Halverson, 1937). It would appear, therefore, that the left hand is stronger than the right in the neonate, although the reverse tends to be true in the adult where right-handedness is most common. Studies of handedness in the neonate have involved attempts to assess the preferential arm motility. In some instances, no difference has been found in the preferential motility of the arms (Watson 1919), whereas in other instances a significantly greater degree of motility was observed in the right arm (Stubbs & Irwin, 1933; Valentine & Wagner, 1934). However, such motility did not appear to be related to later preferential reaching by some of the same subjects.

The movement patterns of awake newborn infants was examined by Robertson (1982) and a periodicity in spontaneous limb movements was observed which had a temporal pattern roughly similar to the interval between brief, isolated startles and transitory movements observed in sleeping newborns and raised the possibility that the temporal patterning may reflect the activity of basic timing mechanisms. Such periodicity in spontaneous movement may also be manifestation, during the waking state, of the physiological processes that control ventilation and alter the rate and depth of respiration in sleeping newborns. Although the basis for such periodicity of spontaneous movements is not established, its recognition has both social and neurobehavioral implications. In older infants, temporal patterns in behavior play an important role in the regulation of social interactions and the rhythmical fluctuations in a neonate's spontaneous movements may serve a similar function in eliciting or inhibiting adult social behavior. Variations in the temporal pattern of spontaneous movements may also be useful in the detection of subtle neurobehavioral disorganization in the neonatal period before other signs of neurological dysfunction, such as abnormal reflexes or state organization, become evident.

NEONATAL ASSESSMENT

The viability of the newborn infant is dependent upon the degree of fetal asphyxia which can occur during the terminal stages of labor and which may result in severe central nervous system depression at birth. The Apgar method of evaluating the general condition of the newborn child utilizes both physiological signs and motoric responses. The five measurement parameters together with the suggested score for variations within each item are given in table 5.2

Low Apgar scores are correlated with high infant mortality, especially at the lower gestational ages, and the flexibility, or lack of tonus, of the infant gives a good indication of gestational age. The popliteal angle (i.e., the angle of the extended knee), which is 180 degrees at 28 weeks' gestational age, is reduced to 130 degrees at 32 weeks by the increased hypertonia associated with increased gestational age and has a resultant angle of 90 degrees in the full-term newborn (Dargassies, 1966).

The popliteal angle of the full-term neonate must become modified before the child is able to extend the knee during upright locomotion. The change that occurs in the popliteal angle with increasing age after birth is probably not so much one of change of tonus as of differential growth rates of the extensors and flexors. Tonus of both the flexors and extensors is required for stability of the knee joint and a faster growth rate

TABLE 5.2. Apgar method of evaluation*

Assessed Item	0	1	2
Heart rate	Absent	Less than 100/min	More than 100/min.
Respiratory effort	Absent	Weak cry	Strong cry
Color	Blue; pale	Extremities blue, body pink	Completely pink
Muscle tone	Limp	Some flexion	Well flexed
Reflex irritability (foot stimulation)	No response	Some motion	Motion; cry

* Adapted from V. A. Apgar. A proposal for a new method of evaluation of the newborn infant. *Current Researches in Anesthesia and Analgesia*, 1960, 32, 260.

for the flexors would maintain tonus in both sets of muscles yet provide the lengthening of the flexors so the knee can be straightened.

Brazelton's Neonatal Behavioral Assessment Scale (1973) is a psychological scale designed to measure the infant's capabilities along dimensions believed to be relevant to the development of social relationships. The baby's state of consciousness is considered by Brazelton to be the single most important element of behavioral examination and the nine point scale for the various test items is concerned with noting the state of the response. The scale contains 27 test items which are generally concerned with the infant's use of a state to maintain control of reactions to environmental and internal stimuli. The examination tracks the pattern of state of change over the course of the examination and the variability of the state becomes a dimension of assessment pointing to the initial abilities of the baby for self-organization.

The test items designed to measure the infant's ability for self-quieting after aversive stimuli are a further assessment of ability for self-organization. The scale contains items designed to calm the infant and to evaluate the infant's control over interfering motor activity. The infant's response to animate (voice, face, etc.) and inanimate (bell, light, etc.) stimulation is also assessed. In addition, other items include examination of reflexes to assess neurological adequacy and give estimates of the vigor and attention of the infant. Brazelton considers the scale to be one that can be used successfully for special groups at risk and recommends repeated tests over several days in the neonatal period as being of much more value than any one assessment.

In his concern for the development of systematic efforts at relating aspects of behavior to aspects of brain function, Teuber (1978) indicates we may ask what happens to behavior after particular brain injuries and /or how the behavior in question might be acquired by young children in their early development. Such an investigation is reported by Mednick (1977) who compared maturely born infants showing one or more of a group of symptoms previously found to have a higher than normal correlation with brain damage **symptomatology** in later life and matched controls who had no neurological symptoms. The neurological symptoms were transient; that is, they disappeared by the eighth day after birth and included shivering or jitteriness, restlessness, cyanosis or respiratory distress, convulsions, frog position, and limpness.

Although the number of males having transient neurological symptoms (TNS) was 1½ times larger than the number of females, equal numbers of males and females (12) were selected from the first consecutive births beginning in January 1960. The controls were selected on the basis of match for age, sex, and social class from the 7102 maturely born infants (birth weight over 2500 grams) who had no neurological signs. The performance of both groups was assessed at the end of one year on the basis of neurological and physical examination scores and on motoric development. It was only in motoric development that there was a significant difference between the TNS children and controls; the TNS females had poorer motoric development than the males.

At 10 and 12 years of age these same individuals were tested on a designs test, role-taking test, subtests of the Wechsler IQ test, and on teacher's judgment of intellectual functioning. Significant differences between the TNS and control children were obtained for the designs test, the role-taking test, and the teacher's judgment of intellectual functioning. Item by item analysis of the teacher's judgment test indicated that only those items concerning distractibility or lack of concentration were significantly different for the TNS and control children. In both the designs test and the teacher's judgment test, the TNS females had poorer scores than the males. The TNS females in this study had scored significantly worse than the males in neonatal physical status and the poorer performance of the females on the follow-up measures may be seen as a correlate of more severe early **traumatization** (Mednick, 1977).

Although the neonate's movement capabilities are limited in comparison with the movement capabilities of an adult, the degree of functional capability is an indicator of the structural and functional maturation of physiological and neurological processes. Table 5.3 summarizes the motor and sensory characteristics of the full-term, well-nourished newborn. With the successful transition from the relatively sheltered prenatal environment, the newborn infant has the physiological and neurological endowment for continued interaction with the environment for the optimal structural and functional development of the individual.

TABLE 5.3. Summary of motor and sensory characteristics of the neonate

Motor Characteristics	Sensory Characteristics
Respiratory associated: sneezing, crying, hiccups, coughing, yawning, burping	*Visual:* pupillary; visuopalpebral; ocular-neck; binocular vision; coordinated, compensatory eye movements; color & line discrimination; limited information-processing rate
Feeding associated: sucking, Babkin reflex, mouth orientation or seeking, swallowing, regurgitation	*Auditory:* acustopalpebral, intensity, tone, frequency, frequency patterns, sound localization
Resting or sleeping posture: flexed arms, legs, hand; tonic neck reflex	*Taste:* depends upon hunger level; sugar increases sucking; salt impairs sucking
General: "Moro" or startle; Babinski reflex (plantar); swimming; trotting; grasping, seeking; withdrawal; shivering; compensatory head movements during rotation; momentary head elevation in prone position; facial movements, frowning, wrinkle forehead, etc.; general arm and leg movements	*Smell:* vocalization, facial and bodily movements to sharp odors; sucking for pleasant odors
	Cutaneous: unpleasant stimuli—withdrawal and survival responses; pleasant—seeking and quieting; pain; pressure; temperature; tactile
	Kinesthetic: muscle, tendon and joint position and movement; vibratory; gravity

6

Motor
Behavior
of Infants

Once the infant has successfully established the physiological transitions after birth necessary in its adaption to the new environment, the processes of growth and maturation proceed apace in the development of behavior necessary for the continued successful functioning of the organism. The term *growth* is usually assigned to measurable physical and biological changes in the development of the individual but the definition of maturation leads to a greater divergence of opinion among investigators in the field of child development. Gesell (1933) considers maturation to be the intrinsic regulatory mechanism which preserves the balance and direction of the total pattern of growth. Krogman (1950) defines maturation as a time-linked phase, or process, leading to the ultimate status of maturity of each different structure.

MATURATION AND LEARNING

Although no exact definition of *maturation* has been universally accepted, the term is most frequently used to describe changes which develop in an orderly fashion without direct influence of known external stimuli but which are almost certainly, in part at least, a product of the interaction of the organism and its environment. With respect to higher organisms it is certainly true that no adaptive function is at its optimum of perfection from the moment of its inception. For example, at a certain stage in development it becomes possible for the child to attempt to walk. Our common expression, "learning to walk," recognizes the need for practice to perfect this function.

Investigators in the field of development are frequently confronted with the problem of distinguishing between changes in behavior resulting from the processes of maturation and of learning on the part of the individual. Essential characteristics of maturation are usually listed as:

1. The sudden appearance of new patterns of growth or behavior
2. The appearance of particular abilities without benefit of previous practice
3. The consistency of these patterns in different subjects of the same species
4. The orderly sequence in the manifestation of different patterns.
5. The gradual course of physical and biological growth toward the attainment of mature status

A number of studies on lower animals have demonstrated the importance of interaction between the organism and its environment. The technique of restricting function beyond the normal period of inception of a particular behavior characteristic has been employed in a number of these investigations. Spalding (1873) hooded young chicks and kept them from the hen for varying periods of time. Those chicks that had been hooded and kept from the hen for only a day or two would, upon release, run to the hen in response to her call, whereas chicks that had been kept from the hen for a period of 10 days or more did not respond to the calls of the hen. These results led Spalding to surmise that the moment of "ripeness" during which the chick can be induced to respond to and follow the hen had been exceeded in the latter instance. Similarly, restraining young swallows beyond the time when they would ordinarily begin to fly indicated varying degrees of efficiency among the birds during their first flight although all were able to fly (Spalding, 1875). Moreover, 10 weeks of confinement of young buzzards starting just as they were beginning to feather resulted in a high degree of impairment of flight and balancing ability on the part of the confined birds in comparison with their unrestrained nest mates who were soaring with adult skill by this time. Subsequent observations over a period of several weeks revealed a continued impairment in the flight of the experimental birds which was attributed to their prolonged confinement (Dennis, 1941).

Similar results have been obtained by investigators working with mammals. Introduction of mice into the cages of kittens who have previously never seen a mouse produces remarkably different results with increasing age. If the mouse is introduced for the first time when the kitten is in its second month, the change in behavior of the kitten is so marked that kittens may be conceived to kill mice instinctively. This behavior is increasingly difficult to evoke if the mouse is introduced for the first time at a later age of the kitten (Yerkes & Bloomfield, 1910). More recent experimentation with chimpanzees has carried the period of restriction still further, in some cases completely depriving the animal of any opportunity for the exercise of certain functions over periods of time as long as one year. Permanent impairment results from such experimental deprivation.

Studies involving restriction of activity in humans do not, in general, reveal such dramatic results as those with animals. Moral considerations prevent investigators from carrying experiments to the extent where serious malfunctioning or **atypical** behavior will result. Some restriction was involved in a study by Dennis (1935, 1938) in which twin girls were reared from the age of 1 month to 14 months under nursery conditions with a minimal amount of motor and social stimulation. When the development of these infants was compared to standard norms, it was found that they were retarded in certain motor achievements beyond the age range for the appearance of these items in normal infants. Social development, however, showed no appreciable difference between the ratings of the twins and standard norms so that customary social stimulation does not appear to be indispensable for normal social behavioral development at this age.

Various cultures often impose restrictions upon the motor activity of infants and these provide a fertile area of exploration without infringing upon the mores of the culture. Such physical restrictions were placed upon infants in the Albanian culture, where babies were bound to small wooden cradles during the first year and released only for purposes of cleaning. An investigation which rated the Albanian children on the basis of the Viennese infant tests indicated some retardation in motor development on the part of these children, particularly during the third year. Social development, however, was found to be normal in the Albanian children, as could logically be expected since they received the greatest amount of stimulation in this area (Danzinger & Frankl, 1934).

Similar studies of the influences of cradle binding as employed by the Hopi Indians, however, revealed no appreciable degree of difference in motor development in comparison with the norms for American infants (Dennis, 1940). In this instance, as opposed to the more stringent binding restrictions of the Albanians, the Indian infants were allowed varying amounts of freedom from the confines of the cradle. During the first three months of cradle binding, the Hopi child was, except for approximately one hour daily, constantly bound to the cradle. After three months, the number and time duration of the periods of freedom were increased. More Hopi children are being reared with complete freedom of movement, and a comparison of 43 of these with 63 Hopi infants who had been reared on cradle boards indicated that the median age of walking for the latter group was 14.98 months while that of the free group was 14.5 months (Dennis & Dennis, 1940). These results were, however, based upon the recollection of parents whose children were from 2 to 6 years of age at the time of this study and there may, therefore, be some question as to the reliability of this information. In general, the results of these studies indicate that the physical restrictions imposed by the Hopi Indians on their infants by cradle binding were within the range that can be tolerated by humans and still result in normal progress. In comparison with the Albanian cradle binding, the results also tend to indicate that the amount of motor activity required by the infant for normal development increases throughout the first year.

EFFECTS OF ADDITIONAL PRACTICE ON DEVELOPMENT

Rather than attempting to assess learning by the technique of restricting practice, most investigators in human behavior development have tended to augment normal opportunities by additional practice as a more culturally acceptable method of approaching the problem of differentiating maturation and learning. A very careful study by Gesell and Thompson (1929), using identical twins, of the effects of practice at the threshold age for climbing and cube-combining indicated to these investigators that learning appears to be profoundly conditioned by maturation. Starting at 46 weeks of age, Twin T was given 10 minutes of practice and encouragement for six days a week in climbing a four-tread staircase and in manipulating cubes. The training continued for six weeks and was directed towards an expansion of the activities, not just their initiation. During this first training period, Twin C, the control twin, was deprived of stairs and cubes but not restricted in any other way. At the end of the six weeks of training, or at 52 weeks of age, experimental twin T was able to climb the stairs in 10 to 18 seconds. At the same age but with no previous training, control twin C was able to climb the stairs in 40 seconds. However, two weeks of training started at 53 weeks and similar to that given to Twin T lowered C's time to 10 to 18 seconds by the end of this particular training period. Neither twin was then trained nor tested until one week later at 56 weeks when the retest results were:

1st Trial	Twin T	11.3 seconds
1st Trial	Twin C	14.8 seconds
2nd Trial	Twin T	13.8 seconds
2nd Trial	Twin C	13.9 seconds

On the basis of these results Gesell and Thompson concluded that training does not transcend maturation but that maturation does tend to modify or supplant the results of training.

Furthermore, Gesell and Thompson noted that, although the times for the completion of stair climbing were similar at the end of the experiment, Twin T was admittedly more skillful prior to the inception of Twin

C's training period and tended to remain more skillful 10 weeks later. Sixteen weeks after the beginning of Twin C's training period, Twin T was still reported as being more agile, less afraid of falling, and walking faster. Twenty-six weeks later Twin T was noted to traverse more ground during play and to be more mobile. McGraw (1946) expresses the opinion that the real issue in the Gesell and Thompson study is not whether practice had any effect on the emergence of the climbing or cube building activities but involves a consideration of the relative effects of practice as associated with the time of introduction of the practice period. Certainly it would appear that the practice sessions were much more effective at the later period when the infant had presumably achieved the degree of maturity necessary for rapid improvement to accrue from such practice.

Similarly, an experimental study of young children trained in cutting with scissors, buttoning, and climbing a ladder showed that, although the experimentally trained group exceeded the nonpractice control group in all tests after 12 weeks of practice, the control group was able at a later date with only one week of practice to achieve the same level of performance as the experimental group (Hilgard, 1932). The greater profit from training within a shorter period of time shown by the control youngsters at a slightly older age led this investigator to conclude that factors other than training contributed to the development of the three skills used in the study. Maturation and practice in related skills were cited as each making partial contributions to the more effective later practice period. It would appear, therefore, that for short-term training the period in the maturation of the child at which training is undertaken must receive serious consideration for the achievement of the most effective results from the least amount of practice.

A longitudinal study of fraternal twin boys was undertaken by McGraw (1935) to determine the age at which children will show improvement in various motor activities from practice. The experimental twin, Johnny, was trained in activities in which he was somewhat capable from the time he was 21 days old until the age of 22 months, while the control twin, Jimmy, was kept in a crib so that his activities were comparatively restricted. Additional items were added to Johnny's practice repertory as he grew older and was more capable of performing the new activities. During the course of the experiment, the behavior development of the twins was compared to that of a group of 68 children who were also being observed in these same activities. Johnny was advanced in those events in which he had received training while Jimmy fell within the developmental norm range. On the basis of her observations, McGraw concludes that there are critical periods for any given activity when it is most susceptible to modification through repetition of performance. She also points out that phylogenetic activities, those which every child must acquire in order to function biologically as a human being, are maturationally fixed and less subject to modification through repetition of performance than are the ontogenetic activities, namely those which an individual may or may not acquire.

One of the basic motor skills that is influenced to some degree by practice is throwing, but the effectiveness of the training program is also dependent upon the age of the child. Dusenberry (1952) trained 14 boys and 14 girls in overhand ball-throwing techniques for six instruction periods at one week intervals. The trained children were compared with a control group who had been equated on the basis of age, sex, race, and the average distance of the five throws given during the pretraining testing. Table 6.1 shows that the training was much more effective for 5- to 6-year-olds than it was for 3- to 4-year-olds. Although significant gains were registered for both sexes at 5 to 6 years of age, the gain for the trained boys from initial to final test was much greater than for the trained girls. Moreover, the amount of gain by the trained girls at either of the age groupings was not great enough to overcome the sex difference in throwing performance, and the score for the trained girls did not reach the score for the control boys at the same age level. For the trained boys, the amount of gain tended to be greater for boys who threw well on the initial test; the correlation between these variables was .46. Dusenberry noted that the boys evidenced better use of their bodies and had more advanced arm and hand movements than did the girls.

There is, then, considerable variability in the relative influence of maturation and learning which is dependent upon the age of the individual and the nature of the activity. Klissouras and Marisi (1976) have surveyed the genetic basis of various physical performance tasks and report mean heritability coefficients of .68 for motor ability; .79 and .60 for

TABLE 6.1. Training effects in ball throwing at various ages*

	Age in Years	Initial Throw (Ft.)	Final Throw (Ft.)	Difference
Boys				
Control	3-4	18.90	22.20	3.30
Trained	3-4	18.05	22.60	4.55
Control	5-6	34.95	36.65	1.70
Trained	5-6	32.75	43.80	11.05
Girls				
Control	3-4	12.85	13.90	1.05
Trained	3-4	13.55	14.35	0.80
Control	5-6	21.00	20.15	−0.85
Trained	5-6	21.65	26.25	4.60

* Adapted from data by L. Dusenberry, A study of the effects of training in ball throwing by children ages three to seven *Res. Quart.*, 1952, 23, 9–14.

initial and final pursuit motor scores, respectively; .88 for physical dexterity; and .53 for tapping ability. They indicate that phylogenetic activities, such as walking, and simple motor activities are more conditioned by heredity than complicated and ontogenetic activities, such as throwing and balancing. The strength of genetic control is considered as diminishing systematically throughout the course of practice. Familial patterns in activity level, according to Willerman and Plomin (1973), also tend to occur. These investigators report mother-child and father-child correlations of .48 and .42 respectively for activity level. In addition, their survey of child-rearing indicated that mothers and fathers of active boys tended to be less protective and indulgent.

In summary, numerous investigators have stressed the consistency of the sequential order of development of locomotion in infancy (Gesell, 1928; Shirley, 1931, 1933; Bayley, 1935; McGraw, 1940a). There would appear to be little modification of the development of bipedal locomotion through practice, nor is there evidence that practice will have much influence on the subsequent development of running and jumping. Throwing, particularly the overhand throw, seems to be influenced to some extent by practice.

With ontogenetic, or culturally influenced, activities such as bicycle riding or roller skating, however, the availability of equipment and the opportunity for practice have a marked influence upon the acquisition of these skills. The observations of McGraw (1939b) on the twins, Johnny and Jimmy, illustrate this point. With training, Johnny was able to roller skate soon after he was able to walk, whereas some individuals never achieve this skill throughout their entire lives. Early training does, moreover, seem to have a very definite effect upon the individual's general "rapport" or "feeling" for motor activities. Although later observations of Johnny and Jimmy revealed, on the basis of objective tests, that both were of somewhat equal skill level, Johnny, who had been given the greater opportunity for motor activity during his first two years, still exhibited superior motor coordination and also more assurance in his movements many years after the termination of the experiment than was shown by the previously less active Jimmy (McGraw, 1939b).

PHYSICAL GROWTH

The physical growth of the infant with its developmental changes in body proportion has a very definite influence in the motor behavior possibilities available to the infant. For example, the mode of prehension of the infant will be influenced by the size of the child's hand in relation to the size and mobility of the object to be seized. Aside from the problems of strength, it would also seem logical that the large head and small limbs present problems of both balance and motive power in the achievement of upright locomotion.

At birth, one-fourth of the body length is taken up by the head with the ratio of trunk length to lower limb length being approximately 4:3 in the remaining three-fourths of the total body length. During the first half year the rapid growth is mainly a process of filling out and broadening with only relatively slight changes in body proportion. While growth continues to be rapid during the remaining period of infancy, this subsequent growth is marked by increasing changes in body proportion. The period after the first six months up until puberty is noted for slow head growth, rapid limb growth, and an intermediate rate of growth in trunk length so that by the end of 2 years of age the lower limbs and trunk of the child are approximately equal in length (see chapter 5, figure 5.1).

Although the weight of the male exceeds that of the female by 4 percent and the height excess is 2 percent over the female at birth, the greater maturity of the female is reflected even at the early age of 8 weeks in the relatively longer lower limbs. The percentage rate of growth does not differ significantly between the sexes even though the growth increment tends to be larger for the male. Therefore, it is entirely possible that the slightly longer lower limbs together with the lesser weight of the female may be a factor, in addition to greater maturity, in the tendency for females to acquire skill in upright locomotion before males.

The variables affecting physical growth have been reviewed and investigated by Tanner (1978) who categorizes these into nine general factors. These are outlined briefly in the following discussion but should be kept in mind as factors influencing physical growth during the entire life span of the individual.

1. The Genetic Aspects of Size, Shape, and Tempo of Growth

The role of heredity in the development of the individual was stressed in the chapter dealing with heredity. The familial similarity in body size and shape is illustrated by Susanne's investigation (1975) of the relationship between parents and children and among children in 125 families. All possible combinations of familial relationships were examined with respect to the bodily measurements and those for height varied from .47 to .57. This fairly substantial relationship is in keeping with previously reported observations by Malina et al. (1970) that children tend to be tall when both parents are tall. Similarly, short parents tend to have short children. The relationship between parent size and children's size holds for both sexes and for both whites and blacks. In a subsequent study, Malina et al. (1976) reported that heritabilities of stature, as given by the mid-parent child regression, were 37 percent for blacks and 49 percent for whites, thus indicating more dissimilarity of black parents and their children.

The correlations reported by Susanne (1975) for other bodily measurements were not as high as those for height but were mainly in the .3 to .4 range. The size of those correlations more closely resembles the relationship between mothers and daughters for the age of onset of **menarche**. This aspect of physical growth is discussed more fully in chapter 9 on adolescence. Tanner (1978) illustrates the genetical control of the tempo of growth with the coincidence of growth curves, equated for developmental age, of three sisters.

2. The Effects of Nutrition on Physical Growth and Tempo of Growth

Nutritional effects on physical growth are disussed in chapter 2 dealing with prenatal maternal influences. Similar results are noted for children, but here the effect on structural development may not be as great as it is during the periods of structural differentiation. Tanner (1978) distinguishes between nutrition effects on tempo of growth, on final size, on shape, and on tissue composition. The first to be affected appears to be tempo with the undernourished child slowing down in growth to wait for better times. He points out that children who are subjected to an episode of acute starvation recover more or less completely provided that the adverse conditions were not too severe nor did not last too long. Chronic malnutrition during most or all of childhood will result in smaller adults. However, undernutrition does not appear to alter shape significantly.

Since **ponderal** growth in infancy follows the general course of growth in height, pediatricians rely on weight gain as evidence of adequate nutrition. Indications are that infants from poorer homes are shorter and weigh less than those from economically adequate homes (Bakwin & Bakwin, 1931), while the retardation in bodily dimensions which accompanies retardation in weight is greater for the transverse than for the vertical dimensions. This results in the youngsters from poorer homes being comparatively more linear than those from economically adequate homes. In instances where proper care is given to infants from poorer homes in a clinic, the height and weight are raised and a change also occurs in the relative body proportions so as to conform with the norms of a control group (Bakwin & Bakwin, 1936). Studies indicate that there is no difference in size between black and white infants in similar economic circumstances (Bakwin & Patrick, 1944).

3. Differences Between Races

Racial characteristics are inherited from parents and are considered to have developed through a complicated interaction between genetical and environmental factors. These processes continue to contribute to population differences in average adult size, the tempo of growth, and bodily shape. An extensive investigation of the height curves of the major population groups—European, African, and Asiatic—was completed by Eveleth and Tanner (1976). This shows similar heights for Europeans (London children) and Afro-Americans for males but the Afro-American girls tend to be slightly taller than European girls. This differential appears to be partly due to the faster growth tempo of the Afro-American girls who achieve menarche about .3 years earlier than European girls. For both sexes, the Asiatic group (Hong Kong) is distinctly smaller than the other two groups. The difference here appears to be mainly the gene pool as the Asiatic girls tend to achieve menarche .5 of a year sooner than the Europeans.

When all racial groups grow up in good environments, the greatest differences between the races are those of body shape. The body shapes of children tend to be very similar for all racial groups, but after adolescence, differences become pronounced. Asiatics have the shortest leg length in comparison with body height and the Africans (Nigeria) the longest leg length, with the Europeans holding an intermediate position. The hip-shoulder ratios of Europeans and Asiatics tends to be similar, whereas Africans of both sexes have slimmer hips for a given shoulder width. In addition, African males have more muscle and heavier bones per unit of body weight and proportionately less fat in the limbs than the other groups (Tanner, 1978).

The tempo of growth is faster for the African as the newborn is ahead of the European newborn in skeletal maturity and motor development. In areas where there are no nutritional disadvantages, the African stays in advance in dental maturity and bone age. Tanner (1978) indicates that a nationwide survey of the United States resulted in mean ages of menarche of 12.5 years for Afro-Americans and 12.8 years for the European-descended. Asiatics tend to have as fast a growth tempo as the Africans, especially in later childhood.

4. Seasonal and Climatic Effects on Growth

The mean growth rates of children are reported by Marshall (1975) as reaching a maxima in mid-winter and a minima in mid-summer for 300 children in the Orkney Islands. Since the difference between the maximum and minimum growth rates for the boys was 5.26 cm/year and for the girls 5.46 cm/year, the seasonal variations in temperate zones is appreciable. In tropical countries the seasonal variations tend to be governed by the rainy and dry periods together with the food supply and frequency of infections.

The climate appears to be one of the long-term environmental factors contributing to racial differences. The long limbs of the African allow for greater heat dissipation, whereas the stockier build of the peoples of the temperate and polar regions tends to retain heat. These changes in body shape have been a result of changes over many generations and do not have an immediate effect on individual children. One geographic variable that does have an immediate effect on growth is that of altitude. Tanner (1978) reports that the high altitude of the Peruvian mountain areas induces a larger chest circumference and bigger lungs in Quechua children growing up there than occurs in sea coast-raised Quechua children. Other climatic and seasonal growth effects are associated with the adolescent growth spurt and are discussed in chapter 9.

5. Effects of diseases

Minor diseases have a minimal effect on the growth of well-nourished children. Major diseases and chronic occurrence of minor diseases may slow down growth, generally followed by catch-up growth when the condition is cured. When continual minor diseases are also associated with undernutrition, there is a tendency for these children to be smaller (Tanner, 1978).

6. Psychosocial stress

Tanner (1978) points out that fairly severe stress is required before there is a slowing in the growth rate when there is sufficient food. In such instances it appears to be an inhibition of the growth hormone that causes failure to grow. When the stress is removed the growth hormone is secreted again and catch-up growth occurs. Although most psychosocial stress situations have been recorded as occurring in institutions, adverse home conditions may also produce psychosocial stress.

7. Urbanization

A survey of a number of studies indicates that urban children are taller and mature earlier than do their counterparts in villages or rural areas. Tanner (1978) attributes such differences primarily to nutritional factors—the rural children expend more energy in physical activities than do urban children, whereas the total caloric intake is approximately the same and frequently less for the rural children. Davies et al. (1974), using data from children aged 7–15 years attending urban and rural schools in Tanzania, reported no significant differences between the two groups in height, weight, skinfold thickness, and arm circumference. In a comparison with European children, the East African children were noted as being smaller and lighter. However, the comparative groups were approximately the same in ages at which peak height and weight increases occurred and in their shape, that is, weight for height.

8. Effects of Numbers in the Family and of Socioeconomic Status

There is a decreasing growth rate as the number of children increases in the family so that the first born children are somewhat taller at each age level than later born children. Tanner (1978) comments that the more mouths to feed or children to look after, the more slowly the children grow. However, the effect is one of growth rate and not of ultimate stature as the adult height of children in a family does not differ systematically on the basis of birth order. This slowed tempo of growth for the increasing numbers of children in a family is a trend that occurs regardless of socioeconomic status. Most studies tend to indicate that the children reared in higher socioeconomic levels tend to be taller at all age levels and as adults. They also tend to have a faster tempo of growth than do children reared under less favorable socioeconomic conditions. However, an investigation of height, weight, and menarche in Swedish urban school children conducted by Lindgren (1976) indicates no difference in height and age at menarche according to father's occupation. This would seem to indicate that even the lowest socioeconomic levels in Sweden are able to provide a standard of living which is conducive to optimal growth in the child.

9. Secular Trend

Data that have been collected for approximately the last one hundred years in industrialized countries show that children have been getting bigger and growing to maturity faster. This secular trend in growth is illustrated by a number of figures in chapter 9 on adolescence. It is a trend that appears in the height and weight of children even at birth, but averages are masked here to some extent by the increasing survival rates of low-birth-weight children. The secular trend appears to be most marked in the late childhood and adolescent years with Tanner (1978) reporting that the trend is much smaller in adults than in children. He concludes that much of the secular trend in children's heights is due to their earlier maturing.

The secular trend in onset of menarche (see chapter 9) mirrors that for physical growth. The onset of menarche has been occurring at an earlier chronological age over the last hundred years. This means that the tempo of growth has increased considerably as children have been growing bigger over a shorter period of time. There may be some slowing down of this secular trend in growth for Tanner (1978) reports the age of onset of menarche as leveling off in Norway from 1950 to 1970 and markedly slowed down in London after 1960.

When one considers the many factors that influence the growth of the individual it is not surprising that there is a great deal of variability in development among individuals. Moreover, all of these factors tend to contribute to increased differences among individuals as they become older. Therefore, any student of human growth and development must have a keen appreciation for the uniqueness of each individual.

DEVELOPMENT OF UPRIGHT LOCOMOTION

During the first two years of postnatal life, striking progress is made by the comparatively helpless newborn infant in its development. Within this short period of time, the infant becomes a young child who has assumed an erect posture and is capable of bipedal locomotion. At the same time, the upper extremities have also been undergoing rapid developmental changes so that by the end of this period the child has attained manual dexterity in reaching, grasping, and fine manipulation. While, for purposes of discussion, it is more convenient to treat locomotor and prehensive development separately, it should be remembered that these developmental processes are occurring simultaneously although there may be variations within any individual with respect to either as compared to developmental norms.

Studies of the development of erect posture and bipedal locomotion in the human infant have centered around the identification of phases, the order of appearance of phases, and the factors associated with the time of onset of these phases. As different investigators have, in some instances, identified different phases, there are naturally some slight discrepancies in time sequences. Moreover, observations tend to be based upon averages of performance of a number of children so that it is also possible that all phases do not occur in all children nor that their duration is the same for all children. The classical studies of Shirley, of Gesell, and of McGraw are illustrative of the approaches that have been taken in investigations of the acquisition of upright locomotion and form the bases for test item selection for most normative scales.

Descriptive Approach

Although listing a greater number of activities as indicative of locomotor development, Shirley (1931) combines them into five main stages which are descriptive of the progressive phases necessary for the achievement of upright posture, of walking, and of a temporary means of locomotion, usually creeping, until bipedal locomotion is established. These stages, together with their inclusive activities, are listed in table 6.2 and pictured in figure 6.1, and may be considered as descriptive of the

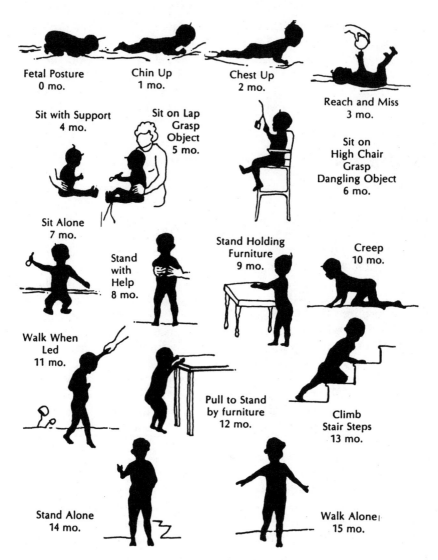

FIGURE 6.1. *Developmental sequence in bipedal locomotion. (From M. M. Shirley,* The first two years. A study of twenty-five babies. Volume II. Intellectual development. *Minneapolis: University of Minnesota Press, 1933. By permission of the publisher.)*

motoric activity of the child at particular phases in the acquisition of upright locomotion.

In table 6.2, the activities with an asterisk (*) indicate those which Shirley believes mark progression in the development of upright posture; those with an accent mark (') are indicative of progression in the

TABLE 6.2 Development of locomotion†

Stage	Time of Onset	Activity
1. Postural control of upper body	Before 20 weeks	Chin up* Chest up* Stepping' Sit on lap*
2. Postural control of entire trunk and undirected activity	25 to 31 weeks	Sit alone momentarily* Knee push or swim Rolling Stand with help' Sit alone 1 minute
3. Active efforts at locomotion	37 to 39.5 weeks	Some progress on stomach Scoot backward
4. Locomotion by creeping	42 to 47 weeks	Stand holding to furniture* Creep Walk when led' Pull to stand*
5. Postural control and coordination for walking	62 to 64 weeks	Stand alone' Walk alone'

† Adapted from M. M. Shirley, *The First Two Years. A Study of Twenty-five Babies. Volume 1. Postural and Locomotor Development.* Minneapolis: University of Minnesota Press, 1931. By permission of the publisher.

attainment of bipedal locomotion. According to this investigator, the unmarked activities are those employed by the child to provide a temporary means of locomotion. These activities merely overlap the other two categories without adding to their development other than by the incidental resulting increase in strength.

Kinesiological Approach

A listing of 23 stages in the development of behavior eventuating in standing and walking has been divided into activities which are considered to be either **flexor-** or **extensor-**dominated by Gesell and Ames (1940). Here all stages are believed to exhibit the slow but sure sequence of postural transformations necessary for the final achievement of upright posture and locomotion, with none of the stages being considered as capable of dismissal on the basis of their possible recapitulatory or vestigial nature. Compression of these 23 stages into four cycles, each comprised of what is considered to be a "continuum of closely related stages," illustrates, to some extent, the fluctuations in dominance between extensors and flexors as well as the integration of unilateral, bilateral, and crossed lateral movements into more complex movements. In

general, upright locomotion eventually involves a permanent preponderance of extensor action, and the most mature expression of flexor
dominance occurs in creeping (figure 6.2). The emphasis placed by Gesell on flexion and extension and on unilateral, bilateral, and alternate
limb action in the analysis of growth cycles relative to the patterning of
locomotion indicates a kinesiological approach to the development of
upright locomotion.

Gesell's four cycles have been summarized by Rarick as follows:

1. In the first cycle (stages 1–10, covering the first 29 weeks of life)
   the dominant pattern of bilateral flexion of arms and legs which is
   present at birth gradually gives way to more mature unilateral
   flexion of the extremities. During this cycle the trunk remains in
   contact with the supporting surface, although the extremities are
   used with limited success for circular locomotion.

2. During the second cycle (stages 11–19, the 30th through the 42nd
   week) the infant is able to elevate the trunk above the table surface. This requires a temporary reversion of the arms to the more
   elemental position of bilateral flexion. The predominate motor
   patterns of this cycle include bilateral extension of arms and bilateral extension and flexion of the legs as observed in the backward
   crawl, the low creep, the high creep and rocking. In Stage 19 the
   creep involves a high level of movement with rather involved
   coordinations, for not only is there alternate extension of the arms
   and alternate flexion of the legs, but these movements occur with
   the members of the opposite side moving alternately.

3. The third cycle (stages 21a and 21b, the 49th through the 56th
   week) entails a temporary reversion to an immobile bilateral extension in maintaining the plantigrade stance. Shortly thereafter,
   arms and legs extend forward alternately in plantigrade progression, the right arm and leg moving simultaneously.

4. The fourth cycle (stages 22 and 23, the 50th through the 60th
   week) finds the infant capable of full trunk extension and assum-
   ing an upright posture. Walking follows as the arms and legs extend bilaterally, but with the movements occurring alternately.*

From the foregoing excerpt and from figure 6.2, partial reversion at
intervals to a less mature pattern is indicated, so that total progression
towards a more mature state is of a spiral nature (Gesell, 1954). Such an
interpretation is not forthcoming from other investigators, however, and
seeming "delays" or "reversions" are explained in terms of the development of functional equilibrium. The infant must be able to control its

---

* From G. L. Rarick, *Motor Development During Infancy and Childhood*. Madison Wis.: University of
Wisconsin, 1954. By permission of the author.

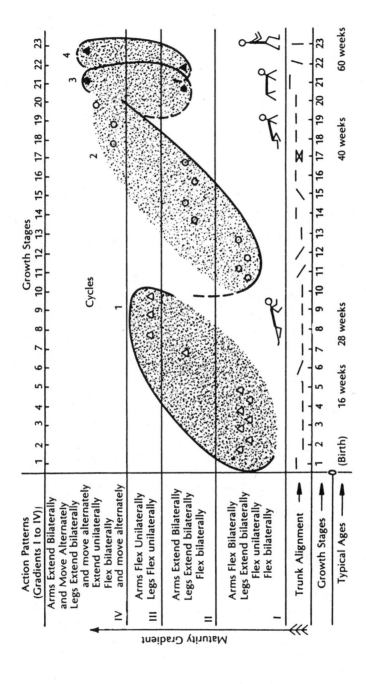

FIGURE 6.2. *Growth cycles in patterning of prone behavior. (From A. Gesell and L. B. Ames, The ontogenetic organization of prone behavior in human infancy. J. Genet. Psychol., 1940, 56, 247–63. By permission of the publisher, The Journal Press.)*

113

body in any new postural alignments in a static position before it can undertake the shifting postural sets which accompany a new skill (Shirley, 1931). In short, mastery of upright posture and locomotion depends upon the functional development of equilibrium, which has a **cephalic** status in the vestibular apparatus and a **caudal** status with the foot as the final fulcrum of locomotion. With each new postural alignment, then, cerebral adjustments involving both equilibrium and neuromuscular responses would be required in a static posture before control could be expected in more complicated dynamic movements.

Neuromuscular Approach

The neuromuscular approach to the acquisition of upright locomotion is stressed by McGraw (1945) who analyzes prone progression and erect locomotion separately. The nine phases in the development of prone progress range from newborn to beginning and advanced spinal extension; propulsion in the superior region and inferior region; assumption of creeping posture; deliberate but unorganized progression; organized progression; and finally integrated progression. McGraw associates the movement of the legs in the newborn phase with subcortical innervation, whereas the lesser activity of the **cervical** spine and upper extremities is considered indicative of **cortical** inhibition prior to the onset of cortical control. The beginning and advanced spinal extension and propulsion in the superior and inferior regions are indicative of the cephalocaudal progression in the development of cortical control of muscular functioning.

Of the following seven phases considered by McGraw (1945) to be characteristic of the development of erect locomotion, the first four require that the child receive support in the erect position (figure 6.3).

1. *Newborn or reflex stepping,* which occurs before 15 weeks, is a phase in which the flexed leg, feet together, reflexive stepping is not in functional relationship with the head or upper body where there is little volitional support on the part of the child. These muscular responses of the child during this phase are considered by McGraw to be indicative of functional innervation at the subcortical level.

2. *Inhibition or static phase* is modal from 15 to 20 weeks and involves equilibratory control of the head by the child, but a diminution of the stepping response is indicative of the inhibition of subcortial innervation as a precursor to the development of functional cortical innervation.

3. *Transition phase,* which includes bouncing up and down with both feet, stepping movements, or stamping one foot in addition

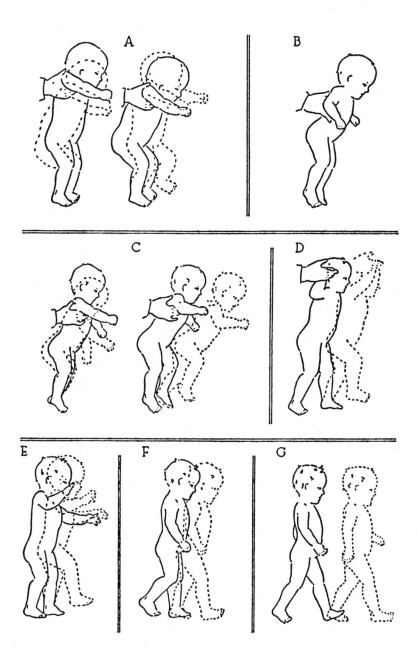

FIGURE 6.3. *Seven phases of erect locomotion. (From McGraw, M. B. The Neuromuscular Maturation of the Human Infant. New York: Hafner Publishing Company. Reprint Edition 1963–1966. Copyright © 1943 Columbia University Press. By permission.)*

to greater muscular control of the trunk and head when the child is held in an upright position, occurs from approximately 20 to 30 weeks. It is considered by McGraw to be indicative of more advanced cortical development with functional innervation becoming manifested in the inferior regions for the cephalocaudal sweep of cortical control.

4. *Deliberate stepping* occurs when the child is led, and the child's observation of foot action as steps are taken is considered to be indicative of cortical involvement and control by the child in the muscular actions being performed. This type of volitional walking pattern is modal from 30 to 35 weeks.

5. *Independent stepping*, which is modal from 35 to 60 weeks, marks the onset of the child walking alone with arms extended, knees high, spacing between the feet, use of the entire sole of the foot, and foot movements which are staccato and isolated. During the initial stages of this phase, cortical attention is necessary for the maintenance of balance and, to some extent, for the placement of the feet, but with increased control these aspects become more automatic.

6. *Heel-toe progression* is indicative of better neuromuscular coordination so that there is a smooth transfer of weight from reception at the heel to the propulsion at the toe. In addition, the length of step and the time interval between steps becomes more consistent with the child giving less and less conscious attention to erect locomotion after 18 months.

7. *Integration or maturity of erect locomotion*, which occurs at approximately 2 1/2 years, is marked by the synchronous swinging of the arm with the opposite lower extremity, more refinement of coordination and integration of movement. Thus the child moves confidently and needs pay little or no attention to erect locomotion in the course of motoric activities.

General Comments

The crucial role that locomotion plays in the functioning of animals has led to extensive investigations of the limb movement and of neuromuscular innervation and integration (Pearson, 1976). For humans, the pictorial and descriptive recordings of fundamental movement patterns (Wickstrom, 1970; Shirley, 1931) and the kinesiological analysis of limb action (Gesell & Ames, 1940; Cooper & Glassow, 1963) form the major thrust of research on erect locomotion as may be expected due to moral constraints on research with humans. Pearson (1976), in an examination of the neural control of walking in adult vertebrate and invertebrate animals, reports that centrally generated patterns are responsible for determining the order in which different muscles are activated. The neuromuscular hypothesis proposed by McGraw (1945) for the development of motoric activities in humans, which was based upon the anatomical development of the nervous system by Conel (1939, 1941), would seem to have considerable merit in the light of Pearson's observations.

Using McGraw's neuromuscular hypothesis, the seeming "delays" or "reversions" in Gesell's kinesiological approach might be explained in terms of periods in which neuromuscular patterns are being consciously developed by the child in its progress towards upright locomotion through a series of bodily activities that have a decreasing base of support and an increasingly higher center of gravity. Cyclic increments might then be interpreted as indicative of increasing integration of balance and centrally generated patterns to achieve coordinated movement which is mediated at a subconscious level.

Zelazo (1983) has proposed a theory that the individual components of walking (stepping, standing, and placing) are present at birth, can be maintained with practice and consistent use, and can produce an earlier onset of walking. The fact that independent erect locomotion rarely occurs before 9 months in most societies is considered to be a maturational limitation that may be cognitive in part. On the other hand, Thelen (1983) argues that cognitive assumptions are unnecessary and explains the disappearance of the neo-natal stepping to be the result of increasing leg mass and the retention of this reflex as simply an exercise effect. According to Thelen, learning to walk is a complex, gradual process of maturation of motivation; the integration of subcortical pattern-generating centers of neural substrate for control of posture and balance; and important changes in body proportions and bone and muscle strength. Kinematic analysis of stepping patterns indicate that when infants begin to walk independently their step patterns are different from newborn stepping and supine kicking and are more similar to adult-like steps (Thelen, 1986). Thelen (1983) considers that the control of walking is likely the province of mechanisms phylogenetically more primitive than the human cerebral cortex.

In general, the developmental trends in the acquisition of upright locomotion are as follows:

1. There is a transition from flexor to extensor dominated limb action.

2. The transition from early locomotion on the stomach through creeping to upright locomotion involves decreases in the size of the base of support.

3. The decreases in the size of the base of support are associated with increasingly higher levels of the center of gravity.

4. Each higher level of center of gravity and/or decrease in the size of the base of support is accomplished first in a stationary position prior to movement.
5. Decreases in the size of base of support, increases in height of the center of gravity, and transition from stationary position to dynamic movement all place increasing demands upon higher levels of balance.
6. A change from bilateral to alternate limb action accompanies the change from stationary to moving position.
7. The transition from bilateral to unilateral limb action requires development of muscle strength and bone mass to support the body unilaterally.
8. Control and coordination is established in a cephalocaudal progression.

Variations in the time of onset of various phases of locomotion are most clearly indicated in a comparison of the median ages at which both Shirley and Bayley observed such motor activity in 25 and 61 infants, respectively (Bayley, 1935). As well as pointing up variations in performance ages, figure 6.4 indicates that the development of children in California, the site of Bayley's study, tends to be generally more advanced than that of the children of Minnesota where Shirley's records were obtained.

The study of 25 children from birth to 2 years of age by Shirley (1931) also revealed additional trends in locomotor behavior other than the sequential developmental phases which are considered to be typical of locomotor behavior in the attainment of upright posture and walking. As soon as walking alone occurs the child is able to increase speed rapidly and, in the process of doing so, also increases the length of step, decreases the width of the step, and gradually reduces the angle at which the leg is raised. Increasing ability of the child to maintain balance during upright locomotion is reflected by decreased use of the arms for balance and the reduction of the base of support involved in the decrease in the width of the step together with a reduction in the degree of toeing out of the foot.

Although Shirley did not find any definite relationship between her measures of motor development and anatomical and physiological measurements of the child, Norval (1947) noted that, for newborn infants of the same weight, a difference of one inch in length tends to indicate that the longer child will, on the average, walk 22 days earlier than the shorter child. Sex difference is commonly noted to favor females in the earlier onset of walking, but Nicolson and Hanley (1953) report the mean age for walking of 114 boys to be 13.4 months while that for 123 girls was 13.6 months. Certainly physique, heredity and environment play a definite part in the time of onset of upright posture and walking. Small boned and

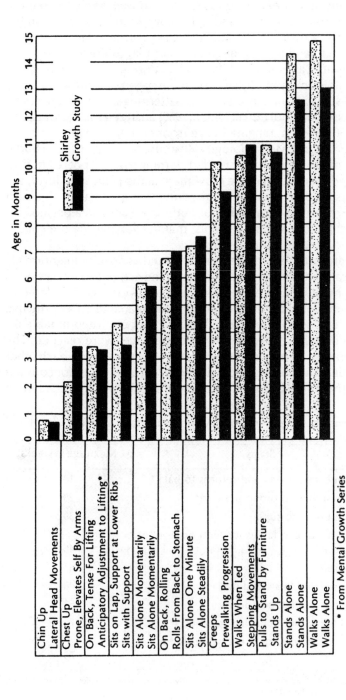

FIGURE 6.4. *Comparison of data from Shirley and from California Infant Growth Study on median age of first passing certain motor items. (From Nancy Bayley, The development of motor abilities during the first three years. Monogr. Soc. Res. Child Develpm., 1935, 1 (1), 1–26. By permission of the author and publisher.)*

muscular infants have been noted as tending to walk earlier than those who are short, rotund, and exceedingly heavy while an association has also been made between early skill in walking and such factors as good muscular strength and interest in gross motor play (Shirley, 1931).

The amount of attention a child receives during the course of learning motor skills is undoubtedly a factor in the speed of acquisition of the skill. It may also have some influence on patterning of movement at various skill levels of the individual. Pikler (1968) analyzed the motor development of 736 children, ranging in age from birth to 3 years, who were reared at the National Methodological Institute for Infant Care in Budapest. The conditions of rearing included clothing that was not restrictive; a suitably sized space to facilitate movement at the child's age level; appropriate toys; and no "teaching" by adults. The no "teaching" aspect involved the refraining by an adult of putting the child in a position, or causing the child to make movements, that in everyday life the child is not yet able to execute without help.

The children at the institute were reported as developing normally both **somatically** and behaviorally and as being active and interested in their environment. Their development and behavior was considered to be similar to that of children brought up within a family. The principal stages of motor development reported by Pikler are listed in table 6.3 which also shows the average ages when the stages were reached. The stages marked with an asterisk (*) were found to always follow each other in regular order. The sequence of stages c, d, e, f, and g was not constant but each of the stages occurred after c and preceded stage i. Standing

TABLE 6.3. Principal stages of motor development in self-taught children†

	Stage	Mean age in weeks
a.	Turns from back on side and returns to back*	18
b.	Turns from supine to prone position*	25
c.	Turns from prone to supine*	30
d.	Creeps on hands and knees (or feet) on level or rising terrain	46
e.	Sits up by self	47
f.	Kneels by self and lets self down	48
g.	Stands by self and lets self down	51
h.	Starts walking without clinging to objects*	70
i.	Walks well; uses walking in everyday life for locomotion*	75

† Adapted from E. Pikler, Some contributions to the study of gross motor development in children. *Journal of Genet. Psychol.*, 1968, *113*, 27–39.

preceded starting to walk in 90 percent of the children. The age of mastery of the various stages appears to be somewhat later than that of comparable age groups where there is more help from adults. However, a survey of the findings of six other investigators leads Pikler to the conclusion that the gross motor abilities of the children at the institute were not appreciably delayed in comparison with instructed children. In addition, long years of experience led to the conviction that the children who sat and walked on their own initiative and through their own independent efforts tended to move more steadily, less spasmodically, and with more harmony and adroitness than do other children. Pikler also believes that self-taught children are less prone to accidents under normal circumstances. She cites the fact that from among the 1400 children whose motor development took place at the institute since its founding 20 years previously, there was no case of fracture either at the institute or later.

The interest of parents in the motoric performance capabilities of their children tends to preclude the use of the self-taught approach reported by Pikler. However, this study does point out the fact that certain aspects of functional motoric development appear regularly and in invariable sequences in the human infant.

PREHENSION DEVELOPMENT

Although the newborn infant will grasp an object of appropriate size that is placed in the palm, prehensive activity involving eye-hand coordination must await the attainment of control of the oculomotor muscles. Infants will take little notice of a cube or similar sized object placed within reach nor make any effort to reach them before 16 weeks of age. After this time, the sight of objects will result in arm activation but not reaching as such. By the time the youngster is 20 weeks old, the "corralling" action of both arms and hands working together has developed to the extent that the infant begins to consistently attain the object rather than pushing it out of reach through lack of control when contact is made. After the object has been corralled, it is often picked up in one hand by a palm grasp in which the thumb and fingers retain the object against the palm of the hand. Four weeks later, prehension involves the approaching and grasping of an object with one hand; however, such reaching is composed of the distinct movements of raising the hand, a circuitous thrusting forward of the hand, and then a final lowering of the hand to grasp the object. By approximately the 40th week, reaching and grasping have become coordinated into a single, continuous movement (Halverson, 1931; Gesell & Ilg, 1946).

The use of the hand in grasping objects undergoes a change from the thumb and finger palm grasp of early prehension to the mature pincer-like movement of the thumb against the forefinger. This development involves an **ulnar-radial** shift in the positioning of the grasped object that is closely associated with the increased use of thumb opposition. While the crude palmar grasp which tends to favor the ulnar aspect of the palm is evident at 20 weeks, there is a definite trend towards preference for the radial area of the palm for grasping and manipulating objects by 28 weeks. With the development of the thumb-index finger approach to objects which require precise prehension by the end of the first year, the ulnar-radial shift becomes complete. Figure 6.5, based upon **cinematographic** records, illustrates this progressive development of grasping.

The complexity of the processes inherent in the developmental progression of voluntary reaching and grasping is indicated by the six component coordinate acts that Landreth (1958) believes to be involved in the development of prehension. These acts involve transitions and include:

1. The transition from visually locating an object to attempting to reach for the object.
2. Simple eye-hand coordination, to progressive independence of visual effort with its ultimate expression in activities such as piano playing and typing.
3. Initial maximal involvement of body musculature to a minimum involvement and greater economy of effort.
4. Proximal large muscle activity of the arms and shoulders to distal fine muscle activity of the fingers.
5. Early crude raking movements in manipulating objects with the hands to the later pincer-like precision of control with the opposing thumb and forefinger.

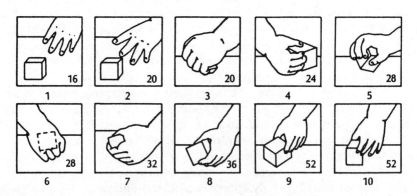

FIGURE 6.5. *Developmental progression in grasping. (From H. M. Halverson, An experimental study of prehension in infants by means of systematic cinema records. Genet. Psychol. Monogr., 1931 10, 107–286. By permission of the publisher, The Journal Press.)*

6. Initial bilateral reaching and manipulation to ultimate use of the preferred hand.

Neural development undoubtedly plays a primary role in the acquisition and development of all motor skills, including prehension, and, in the case of those activities which are not reflex in nature, it would appear to precede such motor development by a considerable period of time. The greatest cortical development of the newborn infant has been found to be in the area of the anterior central gyrus which mediates movements of the neck and shoulders while the greatest change that occurs by the time the infant is one month old is noted to be in the region of the hand of the motor area of the **gyrus centralis** (Conel, 1939, 1941).

In addition to the increasing evidences of coordination and of precision of movement which reflect improvements in neuromuscular functioning, the number of objects which the infant handles adds a further measure to the complexity of manual dexterity and as such provides an overt indicator of neuromuscular functioning and maturation. A study of 178 infants in which such objects as a block, rattle, ball, steel tape measure, metal tube, and tongue depressor were handed to the children indicated that approximately 80 percent of infants would accept and hold one object at 5 months, two objects at 8 months, and three objects at 11½ months (Lippman, 1927). Although this study indicates increased complexity of manual dexterity as measured by the number of objects handled, it is quite obvious that the items differ in size and shape. Therefore, caution should be exercised in accepting the figures as being exact with respect to both the number of objects and the age placement. Such caution is based upon the factors of the size of the child's hand and the size, shape, and texture of the objects, which will affect the child's mode of prehension and the number of objects successfully handled (McGraw, 1946).

PREFERENTIAL HANDEDNESS

The development of preferred handedness has been of concern to numerous investigators on a purely developmental basis, both as it is related to cultural influences, and as a possible factor in the development of speech or reading problems. The earliest postnatal manifestation of hand preference is believed, by some investigators, to be the tonic neck reflex. However, it has been noted that, during the first three months, one-third of infants consistently assume a right tonic neck reflex while an equal number adopt the left tonic neck reflex with the remaining third using either a right or left posture in a somewhat ambivalent manner. These ratios provide somewhat different values than are actually reported for right and left handed preference so that some investigators are reluctant to accept handedness as an index of physiologic unilaterality. It has, however, been found that a strong infantile left tonic neck reflex is correlated with emphatic constitutional left handedness (Gesell, 1954).

More recently, head orientation position during birth and in the infant neonatal period has been examined in terms of hand preference at 19 weeks of age (Goodwin & Michel, 1981). Infants who were delivered from a head turned to the right position exhibited a neonatal right supine head orientation and a right-hand preference in visually guided reaching tasks at 19 weeks. Contrary to prediction, infants who were delivered from a head turned to the left position did not exhibit a left-sided preference in either neonatal head position or hand preference. Their results led Goodwin and Michel to conclude that further investigation was needed into the relationship between prenatal and postnatal postural asymmetries and the continuing development of laterality.

During infancy and well into childhood, there is a considerable interchanging of the use of either hand and of both hands until unilateral dominance is eventually achieved or, as in some instances, the individual has developed a higher degree of ambidexterity than is usually attained by individuals who are classified as unilaterally dominant. In one study of the development of handedness, contact with the object by the infant of 16 to 20 weeks was found to be unilateral and with the left hand. At 24 weeks, contact was bilateral, and four weeks later it was unilateral with contact usually being made with the right hand. By 32 weeks, it was again bilateral after which time unilateral dominance alternated from right to left hand for the remainder of the first year. The right hand again dominated between the 52nd and 56th weeks followed by considerable interchangeability by 80 weeks. At two years, the right hand was in ascendency but there was again bilaterality between 2½ and 4 years. Following this, the right hand continued to become increasingly dominant (Gesell & Ames, 1947). Clearly there is a great deal of interchangeability of hand preference in most infants but great individual differences exist in the amount of such interchangeability and in its patterning. For example, another study indicates that infants will accept objects in the right hand 50 percent of the time at 4½ months, whereas the previously cited observations of Gesell and Ames indicate that this is a period in which the left hand is preferred (Lippman, 1927).

The nature of the task and the age of the infant both appear to be factors affecting the hand preference of children. For example, in a study by Ramsay and Weber (1986) in which children were tested for hand preference in removing toys from a box with a clear Plexiglas door, 12- to 13-month-olds showed a hand preference for incompletely differentiated bimanual attempts, preferring to open the door with both hands and to remove the toys with the right hand. The older 17- to 19-month-olds showed a hand preference for the strategy involving completely differentiated bimanual attempts, preferring to open the door with the right hand and to remove the toys with the left hand. In a study of 40 nursery school children who were tested on hand preference in spinning a top, spooning sand, shaking a rattle, and hammering a block, Updegraff (1932) placed 35 in a right hand preference category while the remaining five were considered to be predominantly left handed. Examination of these unilateral dominance classifications, however, revealed that use was made of the right hand between 50 to 97 percent of the time by those placed in the right handed category while the percentage use of the left hand by the children considered to be left handed was 55 to 85. Similar studies of 44 nursery school children by Hildreth (1948, 1949) revealed that children tend to be more right handed and more consistent in their use of this hand in taught activities such as drawing with a crayon, eating with implements, and throwing a ball than they are in the untaught activities such as eating with their fingers. Such results certainly support the position that children of this age are not exclusively right or left handed.

Right handedness is not only found to be more common in learned activities but also increases with age in our culture. Eighty to 90 percent of nursery school and kindergarten children are right handed, while among adults the percentage ranges from 95 to 97 (Landreth, 1958). However, boys, who tend to be less responsive to and/or less subjected to as much social training as girls, are more often left handed than the opposite sex. Moreover, retarded children and mental defectives, who are also less responsive to social training, have twice as great an incidence of left handedness as normal children. The changing mores of our culture and increase in knowledge are creating a greater leniency on the part of the public to left hand preference, resulting in a current increase in the proportion of left handed children. Whether this increase will ever approach the approximate 50–50 percentage base that is found in eyedness is questionable, however. Even in primitive societies where little attention is given to handedness, the proportion still favors right handedness while exposure to a classroom situation markedly tips the scales in favor of the right hand. For example, 1047 African primary school children, aged 6 to 13 years, were tested with three tests of handedness, namely, unscrewing the cap on a bottle, cutting out a paper circle with scissors, and erasing a word, and only .5 percent of the children were found to be left handed (Verhaegen & Ntumba, 1964).

It would appear, therefore, that hand preference is, to a great extent, culturally conditioned and would seem to have been so historically. A left handed person would have been at a considerable disadvantage in the not too distant past when swords were worn on the left side. There is still a holdover of this custom in the European positioning of the woman in relation to her male escort. Regardless of the position of the gutter, which has affected such social niceties in other areas, the female is always to the right of the male. This was to prevent the man's sword from becoming entangled in the voluminous female skirts.

Since our culture is oriented to favor right handedness, some pressure is usually exerted upon children to change from preferential use of the left hand to that of the right. Six prognostic indicators for a favorable transfer of handedness have been suggested by Hildreth (1950). These should be considered so as to avoid the possibility of conflict with any innate disposition toward hand preference. They are as follows: (1) the child should be under 6 years of age and (2) use both hands interchangeably with (3) the handedness index being bilateral. In addition, the child must be (4) above average in intelligence and (5) be agreeable to the change with the (6) resulting trial period showing no difficulty in transition from the left hand to the right.

The period of late infancy and early childhood is the time in which mental integration, manual lateral dominance, and speech are all in a period of rapid development. Thus it is entirely possible that a feeling of insecurity with respect to manual dexterity may transfer to speech (Landreth, 1958). Whether there is actually a cause and effect relationship here is not clear, however. It has been observed that some left handed children have begun to stutter when attempts were made to change their hand preference. There are more stutterers among left handed children and children who are inconsistent in their handedness than among right handed children. There is also a greater incidence of stuttering among boys than among girls. However, stutterers frequently exhibit other behavior difficulties, not necessarily inconsistent handedness. It is quite possible that both types of problems stem from some more deep-seated cause and that the apparent relationship between them is due to their simultaneous occurrence.

GENERAL TRENDS

It is very obvious from the foregoing that all aspects of the development of the child are interrelated and cannot be broken into separate entities. Furthermore, there is a patterning to this whole development that is reflected in the separate facets that have been outlined. McGraw (1939a) holds that there are four outstanding periods which may be classified roughly in terms of the type of development taking place during the first two years. The first period, of approximately four months, is identified by a marked diminution of the rhythmical and atavistic reflexes which are characteristic of the newborn. The next four to nine months, or second period, is typified by the development of voluntary movements in the superior spinal region and the comparative reduction of activity in the region of the pelvic girdle and lower extremities. The third period, which extends through the 14th month, is marked by the increasing control of activities in the lower spinal region. The fourth period, which covers the remaining 10 months, is characterized by the rapid development of conditional and symbolic associational processes including language.

Other investigators have identified slightly different aspects and placed slightly different emphases on them but the general trends observed in behavior development tend to be very similar. Gesell makes this statement:

> In the first quarter (4–16 weeks) of the first year the infant gains control of his twelve oculomotor muscles.
>
> In the second quarter (16–28 weeks) he comes in command of the muscles which support his head and move his arms. He reaches for things.
>
> In the third quarter (28–40 weeks) he gains command of his trunk and hands. He sits. He grasps, transfers, and manipulates objects.
>
> In the fourth quarter (40–52 weeks) he extends command to his legs and feet; to his forefinger and thumb. He pokes and plucks. He stands upright.
>
> In the second year he walks and runs; articulates words and phrases; acquires bowel and bladder control; attains a rudimentary sense of personal identity and of personal possession.*

Behavior development during infancy can be correlated fairly well with neurological development. The prominence of the atavistic Moro, grasping, and swimming reflexes indicates that subcortical control of movements is at its maximum toward the end of the first month. After this time there is a progressive decline in these subcortical movements attributed to the onset of cortical inhibition. Later cortical control is first observed in the muscles of the upper body before it appears in the region of the pelvis and lower extremities and typifies the cephalocaudal principle of developmental direction. The inception of cortical control in a given activity is believed to be marked by staccato and poorly coordinated movements, while further neuromuscular development and cortical control is reflected by an increasing integration of movements rather than actual changes in motor pattern (McGraw, 1941a). The principle of developmental direction explains the cyclic, or spiral, nature of the development of upright progression in terms of successive cephalocaudal sweeps of development in response to the ascending levels of neural organization appropriate to a certain period (Gesell, 1954).

In addition to the principle of developmental direction, both cephalocaudal and proximo-distal, which has been a recurring feature of this presentation, other developmental principles have been stated as vital to the functional unity of the human organism. Though the primitive modes of locomotion—such as pivoting, rolling, forward and backward crawl,

---

* From A. Gesell, The ontogenesis of infant behavior. In L. Carmichael (Ed.), Manual of child psychology. New York: John Wiley & Sons, Inc. 1954. By permission of the publisher.

rocking, creep-crawl, creeping, and cruising—may suggest recapitulation, they should, according to Gesell (1954), be mainly regarded as functional expressions of necessary, though transient, stages in the organization of the neuromotor system. Such organization involves the most fundamental component of muscular movement; namely, the functional relationship between flexion and extension in the counteraction of antagonistic muscles. Gesell, therefore, believes that a principle of reciprocal interweaving is one of the biological determinants of development. Neurologically, it involves the intricate interweaving of the neural mechanisms of opposing muscle systems into a reciprocal and increasingly mature relationship.

From the discussion of hand preference, it would seem that inconsistency and instability of manual lateral dominance may be reflected in other behavioral areas. To Gesell (1954), hand preference is only one aspect of the principle of functional asymmetry which, in itself, is a special inflection of the principle of reciprocal interweaving. He believes that an asymmetrical focalization of motor set is essential to effective attentional adjustments and that unidexterity of eye, hand, or foot is not so much a representation of absolute skill difference as it is a predilection for stabilized psychomotor orientations.

Additional principles, namely, individuating maturation and self-regulatory fluctuation, are also believed to define vital aspects of growth and behavior. The principle of individuating maturation encompasses the mechanism by which the behavioral organism achieves its species characteristicness, and at the same time makes specific adaptations to its environmental field. For example, the sequential patterning of the behavioral activities terminating in the acquisition of upright locomotion is determined by intrinsic factors and, as such, is species characteristic. However, the minor deviations in technique in the sequential patterning may be accounted for by varying hereditary backgrounds and the interaction of the child's particular intrinsic genetic inheritance with the particular environment and, as such, are a manifestation of the individuating aspects of maturation (Gesell, 1954).

The principle of self-regulatory fluctuation is indicative of the tendency of some behavioral traits to oscillate between two self-limiting poles during their progressive movement toward maturity and stability. It may be recalled that the heart and respiratory rate in the neonate are higher at the resting level and greater in range than in the adult, with progress towards the mature state being marked by a decrease in both the resting frequency and the range during maximal and minimal effort and excitation. Gesell (1954) cites the fluctuating reduction from 19 hours sleep required by the infant during the fourth week to 13 hours in the 40th week as being indicative of such self-regulatory fluctuation (figure 6.6). Certainly the modern emphasis in physiology on the importance of

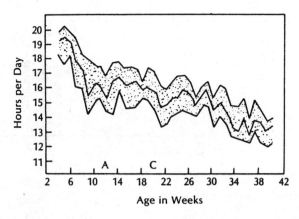

FIGURE 6.6. *Child J. Sleep chart from 4 to 40 weeks. (From A. Gesell and F. L. Ilg, The feeding behavior of infants: A pediatric approach to the mental hygiene of early life. Philadelphia: J. B. Lippincott Co., 1937. By permission of the publisher.)*

homeostasis would support the importance of this principle in the functioning of human beings.

The changes that occur in degree of myelination for various parts of the nervous system are summarized in table 6.4 in association with various aspects of manual and locomotor development. The summarizations encompass the period from birth to completion of myelination of the cerebral cortex to illustrate the continuity of the process of structural completion and the resultant motoric functional capacity. In general, the summary indicates the cephalocaudal and proximal-distal directions in the early development of locomotor and manipulative skills. It also illustrates the increasing complexity of movements following myelination of the cerebellum. The myelination of the corpus callosum, which joins the two hemispheres of the brain, is a precursor to the development of optimal alternate arm-leg action in such things as the throw and the kick. Although the pattern development of the various motoric activities is discussed in greater detail in the following chapter, the myelination will not be covered. However, the age designation for the various phases of myelination allows for comparative assessment of motoric activities subsequently mentioned but not listed in the summary.

SUGGESTED DEVELOPMENTAL ACTIVITIES

1. Crib mobiles and/or other objects which are interesting and/or colorful, but not potentially harmful, and that can be hung securely from the crib or playpen provide opportunities for very early visual exploration and later also tactual exploration of objects.

TABLE 6.4. Summary of postnatal development

Age	Degree of Myelination*	Manual Development	Locomotor Development
Birth	Motor roots ++ Sensory roots + Optic tract + Superior cerebellar peduncle +	Grasp reflex	Trotting and swimming reflex
4 months	Sensory roots ++ Optic tract ++	Crude reaching; palmar grasp	Sit with support
6 months	Superior cerebellar peduncle ++ Middle cerebellar peduncle + Pyramidal tract +	Reaching smoother; radial shift in grasp; more manipulation of object	Sit alone momentarily Rolling over
9 months	Striatum +	Reaching well coordinated; radial grasp and manipulation	Creeps Walks when led Pulls to stand
12 months	Pyramidal tracts ++ Striatum ++	Pincher grasp and manipulation; controlled release of objects	Stands alone Walks alone
2 years	Corpus callosum +	Increased control of manipulation; force may be applied to released objects; arm outstretched in catching	Rocker action of foot; run becoming smoother 2-foot hopping; mark-time stair climbing
3 years	Middle cerebellar peduncle ++	Anterio-posterior throwing action; arm scooping in catching; can strike stationary object with paddle	Well-coordinated walk; more control in run; 1-foot hopping; alternate foot stair climbing

Age			
4 years	Reticular formation +	Horizontal arm action in throw; elbows in front, vise grip in catching	Galloping Adjust to ball in kick and catching
5 years	Corpus callosum ++ Intracortical neuropil and association areas +	Ipsilateral step forward in throw; elbows at side, hands cupped in catching; can strike thrown object underhand	Turn and stop in run Skipping Use entire leg in kick
6 years		Alternate arm-step forward action in throw; one hand catching	Alternate foot-arm action in kick; good control of locomotor actions
15-20 years	Intercortical neuropil and association areas ++	Adult movement patterns	Adult movement patterns

* Based mainly on P. R. Dodge; A. L. Prensky; and R. D. Feigin, *Nutrition and the developing nervous system.* St. Louis: C. V. Mosby Co., 1975.
+ = moderate amount; ++ = heavy amount

2. During early infancy, object manipulation is vital in object concept development and is enhanced by exposure to a wide variety of various types of objects such as rubber squeeze toys, rattles, soft cuddly animals, and teething toys.

3. Common household objects of various sorts that will not be potentially dangerous (e.g., plastic buckets, utensils, discarded junk mail, etc.) and can be manipulated (and banged) without damage provide visual, tactile, kinesthetic, and/or auditory input.

4. Various shaped sponges for bath play encourage exploration and a feeling of confidence in water.

5. Music boxes provide variations in temporal sequencing of auditory input and encourage young children to move rhythmically in response to such temporal sequencings.

6. Baby walkers or horses can stimulate alternate leg action before the child has developed sufficient balance and stength for independent upright locomotion.

7. Larger-sized push toys can encourage locomotion during early phases and can be used as pull toys during later upright locomotion.

8. Cardboard boxes of various sizes provide creative opportunities such as stacking, storing other toys, constructions of various sorts; and larger ones can be used as a playhouse.

9. In later infancy, provision should be made for creative activities such as sandbox play and water play outdoors.

10. Opportunities and toys for imitative play should be made available for such activities as playing house, doctor, policeman, fireman, cooking, and grocery shopping.

7

Perceptual-Motor Integration

Although researchers are finding that the sensory capabilities of newborn and very young infants are much better than previously supposed, these must still undergo a considerable amount of maturation before adult levels of sensory capabilities are achieved. In addition to the maturation of each separate sensory system, the various systems must be integrated to enable each individual to optimize information input. These processes can be illustrated with reference to the development and operations of the computer.

Developers of the computer used their knowledge of the similarities between electrical impulse and neural functioning to build the first computers. These computers had a single input system (keyboard), one mode of operation (usually mathematical calculations), and were much slower, less precise and capable of only relatively simple functioning within one mode in comparison with modern computers. The early level of computer development can be compared with sensory capabilities for each of the sensory systems of the newborn, whereas the faster, more precise modern computer with its increased functional capacity is more indicative of the mature sensory input system.

Although computers are used extensively in neurological research and computer developers use neurological findings to build increasingly complex computers, these are still relatively simple in comparison with the complexity of functioning of the brain. One of the main aspects associated with complexity of functioning is the number of input modalities and the integration of these inputs. Whereas some of the instrumentation available to provide input modalities to computers may have a much wider range of sensitivity than do human input sensory systems, the number of different input modalities that can be processed simultaneously by present-day computers is small in comparison with the number of sensory inputs that are processed by the human brain. The reason for this is that each additional input that is added greatly increases the complexity of the circuitry if that input is to be effectively integrated with the other input modalities. Even with present-day miniaturization (computer chips), the size of the computer that would be required to handle the complex of input modalities that would be required to duplicate all the sensory inputs to the brain would vastly exceed the size of the human brain and may well be prohibitive.

Of even greater importance is our current lack of knowledge of exactly how these various sensory inputs are integrated in the brain to provide an "understanding" of these sensory inputs. In addition, the brain has the ability to build on, unite and/or integrate these "understandings" to produce new and/or modified "understandings." Such integrative flexibility, which is a prime feature of human intelligence, is one of the goals of computer research and is exemplified to a limited degree in the "supercomputers." This integrative flexibility is also of prime concern to researchers in the area of child development as is the quest for increasingly better understanding of the developmental aspects of sensory inputs.

SENSORY INPUTS

The sensory input capabilities of the newborn and very young infants have been discussed in a previous chapter and should be kept in mind during the following discussion which is concerned with developmental changes in information processing. How an individual processes sensory input is called perception and when such perception involves sensory input from the motor system and/or results in action of the motor system, such information-processing is termed *perceptual-motor*. In all instances, the information-processing is influenced by the sensory input itself (preperceptual) as well as the interpretation of the sensory input (perception). As indicated in the introduction, the preperceptual aspects of sensory input involve the speed with which the sensory stimulation reaches the brain and the precision (i.e., strength, duration, etc.) with which the sensory end organ records and transmits the stimulus. An additional aspect of preperception is how long this sensory input persists in the brain as a "memory trace" or "storage." If this latency period is long, a longer period of time is available to process the information. However, this also means that the perceptual process would be slowed down as it would take longer to "clear the circuitry" to make it available to process new information. In brief, the most efficient information-processing involves fast preperceptual and perceptual phases.

The speed of preperceptual processing has been investigated by using a masking procedure which involves the presentation of two brief stimuli of the same sensory modality in rapid succession and the subject must identify the first stimulus (in backward masking) or the second stimulus (in forward masking) in a forced choice. Because the second stimulus of a pair interferes with the storage of the first stimulus at relatively short stimulus onset asynchronies, performance is generally better with forward than with backward masking. For adult subjects using auditory stimuli, interference with performance in backward masking decreases to an asymptotic level at stimulus onset asynchronies of about 250 milliseconds and Mazzaro (1972, 1973) concluded that this may be the period for which storage is useful in the auditory recognition process. Masking studies using the visual modality have also reported a 250 millisecond duration for adults in preperceptual visual processing (Lasky & Spiro, 1980). This similarity of duration of preperceptual processing for auditory and visual stimuli may have implications for the integrative process of these two sensory input systems especially as they relate to language development which will be discussed later. At this point in the discussion, however, consideration must also be given to the question of whether changes occur in the preperceptual processing duration during the maturation process.

Although masking procedural techniques appear to be appropriate for assessing preperceptual processing duration, modification of the adult testing procedures are necessary when testing very young infants. Cowan, Suomi and Morse (1982) used a non-nutritive sucking discrimination procedure to investigate preperceptual auditory storage in 8- to 9-week-old infants. In a series of three experiments, these investigators established the validity of the non-nutritive sucking procedure and administered forward and backward masking auditory pairs. As with adults, forward masking was better than backward masking but discrimination occurred in the backward masking condition with a stimulus onset asynchrony of 400 milliseconds but not at 250 milliseconds as occurs with adults. To these investigators, their results suggested that preperceptual auditory storage contributes to auditory perception in infants in a manner similar to that of adults. However, the useful lifetime of an auditory trace may last longer in the infant in terms of either the duration of the trace or its participation in the recognition process. Similar results of increased preperceptual processing duration for 5-month-old infants has been reported in a visual modality study using tachistoscopically-presented visual stimuli (Lasky & Spiro, 1980).

The longer duration of the preperceptual stimulus trace in the very young infant provides more time for the analysis of any one stimulus. However, it also means that the preperceptual storage mechanism would be freed for information intake less frequently so that rapid sequences of stimuli that exceed the duration of a single preperceptual stimulus trace could not be processed. A number of behavioral investigations of infant visual discrimination indicate that there is evidence that infants can, in fact, register most of the information an adult can register but can handle less of the information than adults can. Such results tend to suggest that, at least for visual and auditory input modes, the presentation of sensory input to infants be more slowly paced than it is for adults (e.g., slower speech and slower movement of objects within an infant's visual field).

In addition to the foregoing behavioral investigations of the sensory input duration and perception, electrophysiological methods have also been used to examine various aspects of perceptual functioning. In such studies that have been done with adult subjects, electrodes are placed over the areas of the brain that are considered to be involved in both the brain location where the sensory input is received and the areas of the brain involved in processing the sensory input (i.e., cognitive function). The recorded Event-Related Potential (ERP) is usually divided into categories. The first is exogenous components which are the obligatory responses of the brain to the presentation of a stimulus (i.e., sensory input only). These responses are sensitive to such physical attributes of the stimulus as the intensity or rate of presentation and typically occur in the first 100 to 200 milliseconds after stimulus presentation. The later ERP components, which occur after the first 100–200 milliseconds, are considered to be endogenous components which are influenced by the processing demands of the task rather than the physical characteristics of the stimulus. In adult cognitive ability studies the ERP responses were largest at the parietal pole and were observed in tasks requiring responses to stimulus novelty and uncertainty, task relevance, match-mismatch operations, and categorization.

Although a considerable amount of research has used electrophysiological techniques to investigate cognitive functioning in adults, such research of infant cognitive functioning and related developmental aspects has lagged far behind. In one of the few investigations in this area, Event Related Potentials were recorded from six month-old infants by Nelson and Salapatek (1986) who used colored photographic slides of a male and female face as the stimuli which were presented during three studies of various combinations of familiar and novel exposures with interstimulus intervals of 1200 milliseconds in each study to minimize the possibility of the response in one trial running into the response of the next. The similarity of the early components (exogenous) in the ERPs suggested to the investigators that the infants did not respond differently to the stimuli on the basis of sensory information alone and infants who had no previous experience with either stimulus responded to the stimuli as though they were identical. However, when infants were pre-exposed to one stimulus, they were later able to remember this stimulus and distinguish it from a previously unseen novel stimulus. As the degree of experience with one stimulus increases, the magnitude of the novelty effect increases. Clearly, the infant recognizes the novel situation but the degree to which the increased ERP response reflects the degree of information-processing is not known.

In a comparison of responses observed in infants and those reported for adults, Nelson and Salapatek (1986) noted that the scalp topography for the two populations was similar. In addition, the reported pattern in adults of the magnitude of the ERP diminishing as the probability of the novel stimulus increases relative to the familiar stimulus was duplicated in their series of infant studies. There were, however, differences in the latency and the form of the responses observed in these infants and reported adult responses which might be accounted for by differences in methods of testing and physiological and/or anatomical differences between the infant cortex and the adult cortex. Neurological examinations have clearly indicated there are anatomical differences between the infant and adult cortex and the previously reported behavioral investigations of perceptual functioning in visual and auditory modes support a theoretical model of a longer latency period for information-processing in infants. Moreover, the possibility also exists that different areas of the brain may be differently involved in information-processing of similar stimuli during the maturation process.

An additional aspect of sensory input that may affect the perceptual functioning of the infant is the intensity level of the stimulus. For example, Hershenson (1964) reported that newborns looked more toward patches of light of intermediate brightness than to dimmer or brighter areas. Similarly, the tendency for newborns to turn their eyes toward a sound source increases with increasing sound intensity up to a particular intensity level after which eye turning away predominates for higher intensities (Hammer & Turkewitz, 1975). In a study which combined these two types of sensory inputs, Lawson and Turkewitz (1980) used newborn infants' fixation on a series of graduated numbers of cubes (visual input) under conditions of no sound and white-noise bursts (auditory input) to determine intersensory intensity effects. Under the no sound conditions, the newborns tended to fixate more on the intermediate and higher number of cubes than on the lower number. However, during the noise condition, fixation time tended to be greater on the low number of cubes. To the investigators, these results suggested that the newborns' optimal or preferred amount of stimulation is determined by the total amount of intensity of stimulus input regardless of whether this is contributed by one or more than one modality.

In general, these behavioral and electrophysiological investigations indicate that, for visual and auditory input, the speed of preperceptual processing is slower in very young children than it is in adults. Moreover, the perceptual process also appears to be slower with more attention being given to novel events than to familiar events. In addition, the intensity of the stimulus, or combined stimuli, seems to affect the amount of attention given by the infant to the stimulation. It would seem that the preferential intensity level may have some direct association with the perceptual process but this is an area open for further research endeavors. In short, it would appear that optimal sensory input for perceptual processing by very young children can be achieved through slow paced, moderate intensity and longer duration stimuli which are somewhat different for those with which the child is familiar.

PERCEPTUAL INTEGRATION

In the introductory comparison with computer operation, stress was placed on the unique ability of the human brain to integrate the various sensory inputs. Although the Lawson and Turkewitz (1980) study of the visual fixation time of newborns under conditions of variations in both auditory and visual inputs was designed to measure the effects of intensity level, this study also clearly indicates that there is intersensory functioning in newborns. This close association in intersensory functioning of the auditory and visual systems and the relative ease with which very young infants can be measured in response to these types of sensory stimuli, has produced evidence that these two perceptual systems are unequivocally related by four weeks of age.

In a study of cross-modal transfer of stimulus intensity, Lewkowicz and Turkewitz (1980) used heart rate to measure the responses of 3- to 4-week-old babies and found that their response to sounds of various intensity was affected by the intensity of previously presented light and showed a cross-modal intensity generalization gradient. At this early age such cross-modal equivalence may be based upon primitive, reflexive functions rather than higher perceptual processes but the addition of temporal patterns to the research design would seem to require some perceptual processing on the part of the infant. Regular and irregular rhythm patterns were presented to 4-month-old infants for 60 seconds followed by a 90 second silent film of a puppet opening and closing its mouth in either a familiar rhythm or in a novel rhythm. On the basis of their results, Mendelson and Ferland (1982) hypothesized that two factors influenced looking on the part of the infants, i.e., whether the rhythm of motion was familiar or novel and whether the sound rhythm decreased or increased the interest in the film. Infants in the regular-sound/irregular motion condition had both factors increasing their interest, so they looked longest. The irregular-sound/irregular-motion condition had both factors decreasing the interest of the infants so they looked least. Intermediate looking time was observed in infants who were in the conditions in which one factor increased their interest and one decreased their interest (e.g., irregular-sound/regular motion).

In terms of the way information is processed, infants apparently discriminate the rhythm of sound, discriminate the rhythm of motion, and compare auditory and visual rhythm (Mendelson & Ferland, 1980). Although very young infants appear to be able to remember and make comparisons of regular and irregular rhythms during the short periods of time involved in experimental studies, such studies only point to the potential beginnings of the complex aspects of the development of time concepts. For example, the type of cue and additivity of interfering cues affect children's duration comparisons as indicated by 4- and 5-year-old children who were asked to compare burning times of lights differing in intensity, bulb size, or both. Those who erred tended to attribute longer duration to the brighter or larger bulb with brightness having a stronger interfering effect than size. Levin and Gilat (1983) attributed their results to children's inability to distinguish clearly between time-related and time-unrelated cues and their assumption of direct relationships between dimensions.

Time Concepts

Time concepts develop slowly in relation to the other basic perceptual concepts, perhaps because of their more abstract nature and/or the greater dependence of children upon the development of other concepts before they can make clear conceptual distinctions between time-related quantitative dimensions. According to Piaget (1969), the development of time concepts can be studied meaningfully only in contexts which involve physical movement in space because the young child conceives of an interval of time in terms of speed of movement or the amount of output, such as the space (or distance) traversed or matter moved. For example, when asked to compare the times two cars have been running on parallel tracks, a young child evaluated the relative time durations either by the cars' relative speeds or by the relative distances covered. The child's confusing of time with speed and with distance was explained by Piaget as a conceptual one as young children differentiate time from speed and from distance when dealing with cars running simultaneously on nonparallel tracks.

The concept of time in relation to speed and distance embodies not only the direct relationship (i.e., a perceptually greater value in one correlates with a perceptually greater value in the other) between speed and distance and between duration and distance but also the inverse relationship between speed and duration. For example, as the speed increases the time duration becomes less for a fixed distance. These types of relationships were examined in first- through fifth-grade children who were asked to determine which of two animals ran faster, farther, or for a longer amount of time on the basis of information supplied for the other two dimensions. Acredolo, Adams and Schmid (1984) concluded that their results support the hypothesis that children grasp the direct relationships between speed and distance and between duration and distance before they grasp the inverse relationship between speed and duration. This hierarchy of understanding direct relationships prior to understanding inverse or indirect relationships may represent a general principle of cognitive development. Although a majority of the fourth- and fifth-grade children appeared to understand the relationship between all possible pairs of the three dimensions, the fact that they did not appear to integrate these relationships spontaneously indicates that their comprehension of the relationships between speed, duration, and distance is not yet fully integrated.

Spatial Concepts

In addition to the development of time concepts, Piaget (1962) also considers the concepts of object, space, and causality as central to the child's recognition of the necessary relationships between physical dimensions. The distance dimension of the time concept is one aspect of space concepts and, in keeping with the stress placed by Piaget (1969) upon the role of physical movement distance perception, it is not surprising that studies have been undertaken to investigate the role of passive and active exploration in spatial development. One such study of children aged 20 to 28 months and 36 to 44 months observed and measured the children on the quantity and mode (active vs. passive) of their exploration of an unfamiliar museum room. Later, half of these children were allowed to explore the laboratory playhouse area freely to establish the consistency of their exploration technique and all the children were then taught a specific route through the playhouse and tested on their ability to reverse the route, detour from the route, and reach the goal from other starting points. The results found by Hazen (1982) indicated that active exploration in the playhouse was related to accurate knowledge of its spatial layout. In addition, mode of exploration in the playhouse was correlated with mode of exploration in the unfamiliar museum room and active exploration in the museum was predictive of accurate spatial knowledge of the playhouse. Therefore, individual differences exist in the extent to which children explore actively or passively which may influence their cognitive spatial abilities.

It is possible that there may be developmental limitations on the extent to which activity level affects spatial comprehension. An investigation of the effects of varying levels of motor activity (standing, riding a wagon pulled by the experimenter, and walking) on the ability of kindergarten and third graders to remember the location of buildings in a large model town, indicated that only the kindergartners' accuracy of building placement increased as a function of the amount of motor activity. These results led Herman, Kolker and Shaw (1982) to conclude that kindergartners depended more on motor activity than third graders to learn about the location of objects in an unfamiliar environment.

Other developmental limitations such as sex differences in the hemispheric functioning of the brain may affect spatial cognitive development. Witelson (1976) believes that hemisphere specialization for spatial processing may be critical in human ontogenetic and possibly phylogenetic development of lateralization of function in general. She reports that, in boys, the right hemisphere has the dominant role in processing nonlinguistic spatial information by at least 6 years of age. On the other hand, in girls the right hemisphere is not dominant even at 13 years of age and there is a bilateral representation for spatial information. The greater dominance for spatial processing in the males may account for the superiority of third- and fourth-grade boys in ability to walk out patterns in an expanded spatial field (Keogh, 1971). Moreover, the addition of visual reference in the pattern walking test situation facilitated male performance but not that of females. No sex differences were observed in the hand drawing of patterns which was also a test item in this investigation. The Keogh findings suggest a distinction between gross and fine motor abilities with respect to spatial perception in that walking requires use of large-motor systems whereas the drawing measure requires use of only fine-motor skills. This aspect of spatial perception was tested by Vasta, Regan, and Kerley (1980) who administered pattern copying tasks to 10-year-old boys and girls using arm's length distance from an easel for the large-motor condition and a position closer to the easel where fine-motor hand movements could be used. The additional variable of visual reference cues (gridded or plain background) was also included in this study. Contrary to expectations, there were no sex differences in analysis for the motor condition (i.e., large vs. fine motor) but the study did support the previous findings that males make better use of visual reference cues in that the male performance with the cue stimuli was significantly better than with the unlined materials whereas female performance across cued stimuli was nondifferential.

The interpretation of such variability in results leads to questions associated with the test items (e.g., Is placing a child at arm's length from an easel a large motor condition?) and with the differential experiences of the subjects (e.g., Do noted sex differences reflect differences in socialization experiences or activity preferences?). In a meta-analysis of sex differences in spatial ability, Linn and Petersen (1985) found that sex differences arise on some types of spatial ability but not on others with the largest differences being found only on measures of mental rotation and much smaller differences found on measures of spatial perception. They point out that mechanisms that lead to these differences remain to be established as do the possible influences of these differences on other behaviors and suggest that each individual probably has an assortment of spatial skills rather than a single ability.

To anyone interested in applying our present understandings of perceptual development to the practical situation of child rearing, some knowledge of developmental changes with age is necessary for program development. Although Witelson (1976) reports spatial information processing as being right-hemisphere-oriented in boys by at least 6 years of age, a behavioral study of young and old nursery school children reports consistent sex differences favoring males in ability to infer spatial relationships in a large, familiar environment. In their study, Herman, Shiraki, and Miller (1985) took the children to locations in the nursery school and asked them to point in the direction of known targets they could not see in the school grounds. On the basis of the amount of deviation of the pointed direction from the actual line to the target, older children (mean age of 5 years) were more accurate than younger children on location of nursery school targets. In addition, the sex difference favoring males was much greater for the older than the younger children. Thus, it appears that sex differences in some aspects of spatial conceptual development may have an earlier onset than previously reported.

One aspect of spatial conceptual development, the use of visual cues and visual preferences, have been reported for newborns. Therefore, visual perceptions of space associated with visual sensory input may have their onset in the very young child and such has proven to be the case in a study of reaching by 5- and 7-month-old infants under monocular or binocular vision (Yonas, Pettersen, & Granrud, 1982). The stimuli were photographs of large and small faces with the duration of reaching for the 7-month-olds being greatest in the monocular vision large face condition. Statistical analysis showed that the difference in duration of reaching towards the large and small faces with monocular viewing was significantly larger than the difference in the viewing of the faces with binocular vision for the 7-month-olds whereas the 5-month-olds showed no significant differences in reaching duration time for any of the difference measures. To the investigators, these results indicated that the 7-month-olds perceived the large faces to be within reach and the small faces beyond reach in the monocular condition with the sensitivity to size being indicative of spatial information (i.e., large objects are near and small objects at a distance).

The fact that the 5-month-olds did not show any significant difference in reaching time for the above condition may be ascribed to the fact that depth perception has not been developed in binocular vision or that direct equivalencies between size and space perception have not yet developed. The later explanation would seem to apply as infants of this age are reported to reach reliably for the nearer of two surfaces when sufficient information for relative distance is available. This indicates that the infant has developed perception for depth at an edge which separates the nearer surface from the apparent background surface and raises the question of the infant's sensitivity to accretion and deletion information for depth at an edge.

The effect of accretion and deletion of texture as an effective source of information of the spatial layout of the visual input is illustrated by a white and black spotted dog (dalmation) on a white and black spotted background. When the outline of the dalmation is removed, the shape of the dalmation disappears into the background and the visual input appears as a single surface, white and black spotted area. That is, there is no perception of the outline of the dog (no edge) and hence the whole area appears to be the same distance from the observer (no depth perception). However, as soon as the area which is encompassed within the dog shape (but still not outlined) is moved in one direction, this spotted area is perceived as a dog and appears to be in front of the spotted background area. This process is achieved by the systematic addition of spotted areas appropriate to the motion of a dog walking in one direction and the systematic deletion of the spotted background areas in front of the "dog" spots and the reappearance of the spotted background behind the "dog" spots. This process of accretion and deletion of texture as information for depth at an edge was described by Gibson (1966) and because the visual system functions to extract information for the three-dimensional spatial layout of objects and surfaces in the environment from continuous transformations of the light reaching the eye, the accretion and deletion of texture is an effective source of information for spatial layout.

Granrud and others (1984) tested 5-month and 7-month-old infants on their sensitivity to accretion and deletion of texture using the amount of reaching towards computer-generated kinetic random dot displays. Accretion and deletion of texture (i.e., the appearance and disappearance of moving dots of light) provided the only information for the presence of an edge created by exactly the same rectangular array of dots on one portion of the screen and for the relative distances of the two apparent surfaces. When the entire display was motionless, it appeared as a flat array of dots. As the infants in both age groups showed significant preferences for reaching for the apparently nearer regions in the kinetic display, these results supported previous research that 5- and 7-month-olds reach more frequently for the nearer of two surfaces and are sensitive to accretion and deletion of texture as information for the spatial layout of surfaces.

Object Concepts

The perception for depth at an edge is vital not only to the development of spatial concepts but also forms an integral part of perception and recognition of objects where the structure of an object consists of its surfaces and edges and their relationship to one another. Ruff (1980) bases her lucid review of the development of perception and recognition of objects on Gibson's contention (1966) that an adequate theory of perception must take into account the activity of the observer and the resulting stimulus flow. In order to perceive an object, the observer must perceive the object as unchanging in some respect even though the stimulation caused by the object changes with changes in fixation and with motion of the object. Central to Gibson's theory of perception is the concept of structure. Continuous stimulus change conveys information to the observer about the structure of the objective world around him because the permanent and unchanging aspects within the stimuli reveal the invariant structure of the environment. For example, there is invariance, or nonchange, to specify the arrangements of objects in the entire environment; nonchange to specify the structure of individual objects; and nonchange to specify the structure of the finest texture. Invariance in dot array (texture) in one portion of the kinetic random-dot display in the Granrud et al. study (1984) was used to test for perception of depth at an edge. Therefore, movement and the consequent perception of occlusions help to separate the edges of objects from the background and the edges of one object from those of another.

The amount of information that an infant can acquire from moving objects depends on his ability to follow the objects which move around him. Previously-reported research indicates that even newborns can follow some objects and the infant's ability to follow objects improves greatly over the first three months. However, the age at which infants can extract information from different moving objects undoubtedly depends upon both the complexity of the object's structure and the complexity of the movement. Observers of any age need some overlap of edges to detect structural invariance in an unfamiliar object but the amount of overlap is determined by the speed and/or type of motion. For example, a very fast speed, although it provides a great deal of overlap, may be too fast for proper sensory input processing whereas a very slow speed would result in such a small degree of overlap change that edge distinctions are not made. On the basis of her own work and her review of the literature, Ruff (1980) indicates that younger infants can learn to recognize simpler objects undergoing simpler motions.

The complexity of an object involves another type of change involving the texture on the surfaces of an object which specifies rigidity or elasticity, i.e., the relationship of texture elements on a given surface remains the same when a rigid object moves but changes when an elastic object is deformed. This type of textural change is exemplified by the structural invariants of a cup of milk in that the observations of the cup reveal it as a rigid object with a definite shape whereas observations of the milk reveal that the shape is variable under different movement conditions and its structure is elastic (a liquid).

Observations of objects under moving conditions can be achieved in two ways; i.e., either the object can be moving or the observer can be moving. Initially, the infant's control of relative movement is limited mainly to head and very limited bodily movement so that most early object perception is probably based upon objects being moved within the line of vision of the infant. Later, however, the infant reaches, grasps and manipulates objects and this manipulation can enhance perception of structural properties in two ways. One consequence of manipulation is that the infant can provide himself with facilitative optical changes which will help to establish the invariant structure of the object. For example, manipulative rotation of an object provides changes in edges of the object that help to determine the shape of an object. The other consequence of manipulation is that the infant can obtain tactual and kinesthetic input about the structure of objects. Movement of the hands and fingers over an object results in constantly changing stimulus input and the fingers, like the eyes, can discover nonchange in the character of the edges, the texture of the surfaces, and the relationship of the object's surfaces to one another.

The acquisition of the ability of the infant to reach for and grasp an object results not only in increased sensory input from finger and hand manipulation but enables the child to place the object in his mouth. Both the hands and the mouth are sensitive exploratory tools and Gottfried, Rose, and Bridger (1977) have demonstrated that 1-year-old infants can acquire enough information about shape through either oral or manual exploration to recognize objects visually. In addition, the infant uses circular, waving arm actions which provides auditory sensory input if the object is a rattle and also provides additional kinesthetic input regarding the weight of an object.

As with other aspects of inter-modal perception, the degree to which each of the operant sensory inputs contribute to the development of knowledge of structure of an object depends upon the capabilities of each infant and the opportunities that the infant has for exploration of the object using the various sensory inputs. In keeping with the noted developmental improvement in perception of the basic concepts, there is a decrease in the number of errors for the intersensory judgment of identical forms with increasing age. In a study of intersensory equivalencies, Birch and Lefford (1967) examined children aged 5 through 11 years to determine their ability to make paired matches of information of objects gained through visual, kinesthetic and haptic (combined tactual and kinesthetic) sensory inputs. As the visual stimulus, a block was placed on the table directly in front of the subject. For haptic stimulation, the subject's hand, behind an opaque screen, was placed on the block by the experimenter and the subject actively explored the form with his hand without seeing it. Kinesthetic information was provided by placing the subject's arm behind a screen and, with the arm out of the subject's sight, passively moving it through a path describing the geometric form in the shape of the block. The results, depicted in figure 7.1 indicate there is a marked reduction in errors of judgments of identical forms in the paired comparisons of visual-kinesthetic and haptic-kinesthetic modes with increasing age. The degree of reduction of judgment errors is not as great for the visual-haptic pairing but this is because there are only approximately two judgmental errors in this type of pairing by 8 years of age and older. The higher number of judgmental errors for the kinesthetic mode in pairings with the other two sensory modes may be the result of the test design in that passive kinesthetic input was involved or it may be because the kinesthetic mode is not as sensitive to perceptual requirements for recognition of the types of objects used in the study. Regardless of the reason for the apparent discrepancy in efficiency of object recognition for these sensory inputs, the study does reinforce the fact that all of the inputs can make contributions to object recognition and, in the event of

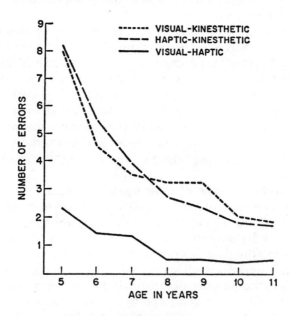

FIGURE 7.1. Mean errors for the intersensory judgment of identical forms at different ages. (From Birch, H. G., & Lefford, A. Visual Differentiation, Intersensory Integration, and Voluntary Motor Control. Monographs of the Society for Research in Child Development. Serial No. 110, Vol. 32, No. 2, 1967. Reprinted by permission of the Society for Research in Child Development, Inc.)

loss of one of these sensory inputs such as the visual, object recognition can still be effectively achieved through the other sensory inputs.

The development of object recognition is considered by Ruff (1980) to be embodied in three principles, all of which are related to the concept of differentiation. The first principle is that object recognition develops from general to specific. There are a number of reasons why the most general aspects of objects should be recognized earlier and more easily than more specific ones. In the first two months, the ability to resolve detail is rather poor with both low acuity and poor accommodation putting limits on the young infant's ability to obtain a sharp focus on boundaries formed by occluding edges or by the meeting of two surfaces. In addition, the consequent restriction on perception of texture elements limits the young infant's perception of occlusions, particularly those involving smaller details within objects. Perceptual learning requires time involving an increasing differentiation which suggests that sheer amount of exposure or experience is an important factor. Moreover, the differentiation of general aspects of objects probably involves fewer invariants than differentiation of specific and unique characteristics and therefore requires less time.

The second principle proposed by Ruff (1980) is that variants are detected, in part, because of the activity the object participates in. Because infants learn to recognize objects in the context of activity, particularly their own, the infant sees and attends to new and different aspects of even familiar objects as his own range of skills widens. For example, the activity of drinking milk from a cup provides the sensory input the infant needs to recognize the invariants relevant to the activity. Although liquids (milk) and containers (cup) are part of the same overall event, they are differentiated both in terms of what happens to them (liquids are ingested, containers are not) and in terms of structural invariants that specify them (containers are rigid, liquids are not). Differentiation therefore parallels the detecting of invariants in objects that belong to the same activity. As the changes in an infant's activity lead him to explore old objects in novel ways he will also be learning new invariants, and when he engages in a new activity the infant is forced to make new discriminations which were not relevant in previous activities. Ruff considers the observer's activity as an essential part of perception even for adults in contrast with Piaget's model (1962) where the motor activity of the infant during the sensory motor period is considered the precursor of cognitive functions.

Ruff's third principle is that object recognition develops from being context-bound to context-free. For infants, recognition is more likely to be tied to the context in which the object is learned whereas older individuals can recognize many objects regardless of the setting or event in which they were first seen. This aspect of development depends upon seeing objects in a variety of circumstances and, when a given object is part of a number of events, the perception of the object becomes richer and more precise. It can also be recognized under widely varying and novel circumstances and, in this sense, comes to exist more as a unique entity with recognition of the object being based on variants which specify many details of the structure (Ruff, 1980). The degree to which this type of object differentiation is achieved would depend upon the quantity of exposure to the object, the opportunity for observation in many different events and undergoing different motions, and the drawing of the attention of the infant. Thus objects very important in the infant's life, such as the mother, probably achieve this unique status long before others.

Causal Concepts

There are several ways in which events and/or actions may be associated and these are the cues that form the bases of the development of causal concept. Once the child has recognized that events have causes, the most important of the cues as to what is the cause of an observed event is the principle of priority; that is, the cause must be an event that preceded the effect. Other cues are based upon the mechanism principle which is based upon the fact that the cause must be linked to the effect. Therefore, the cause is likely to be an event that occurred in spatial and/or temporal contiguity with that effect. This cue is not as strong as that of priority because causes can be discontiguous from their effects but they can never occur prior to those effects in time.

The third kind of cue is derived from repeated observations of an event and is called co-occurrence. In this instance, the cause is likely to be an event that co-occurred with it. However, this relationship is not strictly necessary since an event may have more than one sufficient cause or may require more than one necessary cause to occur. Finally, the amount of experience is important in that children's knowledge of specific kinds of events can provide a rich source of cues as to the cause of observed events (Bullock, Gelman, & Baillargeon, 1982).

On the basis of a series of studies of children's causal judgments, Bullock, Gelman, and Baillargeon (1982) believe that children as young as 3 years already understand that events are caused (their principle of determinism); that causes precede their effects in time (their principle of priority); and that there must be some kind of mechanism linking causes to their effects (their principle of mechanism). Sophian and Huber (1984) examined the responses of 3- and 5-year-olds to conflicts between temporal priority and specific trained knowledge relative to causal judgments. Although both age groups showed some use of temporal priority, the 5-year-olds showed they relied more on temporal order, relative to trained knowledge, in the conflict situation than would be expected from their use of the same cues separately, whereas the 3-year-olds did not. The investigators considered that their findings supported an hypothesized developmental shift in children's causal reasoning with early causal reasoning appearing to be primarily empirical and based on concrete features of the events in question whereas later reasoning may be more logical and involve greater reliance on abstract causal principles that enable children to interpret unfamiliar events.

Motoric Standards and Invariants

Traditional child development behaviorists have been concerned with the development of cognitive and/or reasoning functions associated with the basic concepts of object, space, time, and causality. This approach received its major direction from and was stimulated by the work of Piaget (1962) who described the cognitive processes in terms of schemas with development of each individual progressing through successive levels to achieve maturity. The Piagetian intellectual development model will be discussed more fully later; suffice it here to say that the motor activity of the infant serves as a precursor of cognitive operations in this model. More recently, motion, either of the objects being observed or generated by the observer, is considered to be vital to perception not only during early formative phases (Gibson, 1966) but also during adulthood (Ruff, 1980). In all instances, it is the reaction (i.e., the action) of the observer that is measured regardless of whether it is the object that is moving or whether it is the observer moving the object. The resultant action of the observer is considered to directly measure the degree of perceptual understanding and/or cognitive functioning of the observer. Some motor behaviorists have adapted the Piagetian schema model to describe the process of motor learning. For example, Schmidt's theory (1975) hypothesizes two independent states of motor memory, namely, recognition and recall schemata. The recognition schema is concerned with the evaluation of movement and the recall schema is responsible for response production. As with the Piagetian model, each motor memory state is hypothesized to develop through the formation of rules with initial conditions, sensory consequences, and past actual outcomes leading to expected sensory consequences for recognition of schema while information from initial conditions and past response specifications produce response specifications for the recall schema.

The schema approach, with its emphasis upon each individual progressing through the successive schematic levels to achieve mature cognitive functioning, has been challenged by Gibson's concepts (1966, 1979) of invariant structure and continuous stimulus change. In this model, the child's activity is necessary for the perception of the invariants relevant to the activity and recognition of the invariants of similar situations results in behavior appropriate to the invariants. However, new activities which are not relevant to previous activities required the child to make new invariant discriminations and in this way the model differs from Piaget's model of generalizing assimilation. In addition, continuous change is a vital aspect of the process of recognition in Gibson's model whereas the concept of schemas may, or may not, be units within a developmental framework. Within Gibson's model, all motion that allows for the perception of invariants is important for recognition and/or cognitive functioning.

On the basis of the above discussion of the need for continuous change and the discrimination of new invariants in new activities, it would appear that Gibson's model is not nearly as well structured or as developmentally efficient as Piaget's model of successive schemas. However, central to Gibson's theory of perception is the concept of the structure with emphasis placed upon the permanent or unchanging aspects which reveal the invariant structure of the environment (Gibson, 1966, 1979). Such invariants have been discussed in terms of recognition of an object's structure in the section on object concepts; suffice it here to say that the same invariants which are associated with the structure and motion of objects also apply to humans. In short, all organisms and objects on earth are subject to the same physical laws (such as gravity, force, etc.) so that recognition of the basic invariants (e.g., structural constants) that define these laws is actually a simpler and more efficient model than that of schemas.

Although the basic invariants associated with physical laws have broad, general applications, recognition of the invariants associated with such laws also requires that the child have the opportunity to observe a wide variety of objects entering into the same role of an event to provide the variation which helps the process of differentiation by focusing attention on specific invariants. The maturity of the child with respect to information-processing also is an important factor in the recognition of invariants. For example, the young infant sitting on the floor playing with an object releases it and when the released object consistently drops to the floor, the child shows awareness of what happens to the object by placing it on the floor. Similarly, the young infant sitting in his high chair releases an object outside the area of the chair's tray and, after looking around and locating it on the floor, often makes a game of dropping other items on the floor and watching them as they drop. The child has obviously developed a working knowledge of the effect of gravity on a released object. With increased skill and strength, the young child has the opportunity to observe the effect of gravity on the trajectory of a thrown ball and thus expand his concept of this invariant. Language acquisition enables the child to ask why objects fall down when they are dropped or thrown but the mature understanding of the invariant nature of the law of gravity is not attained until the invariants associated with the logic of mathematics have also been mastered. Therefore, there is a developmental sequence in the basic invariants, or concepts, which is marked by constant change as a result of constant stimulus flow from the experiences of the child and the increasing maturation of bodily functioning especially the brain.

Some of these developmental sequences have received much more research attention than others because the input stimuli are easily measured; the resultant responses are easily measured; and/or the design of the study lends itself to statistical analysis. There are a variety of ways of producing and easily measuring visual and auditory stimuli and responses so that the greatest number of studies has been concerned with these modalities. In general, it is easier to develop ways of assessing and providing information about the external environmental (i.e., visual, auditory, cutaneous, taste, and olfactory systems). The internal sensory systems of kinesthesis and balance are much more difficult to measure in terms of degree of sensory input and output and methods of testing. Yet these, particularly the kinesthetic, play a large role in providing the motion the child imparts to objects as part of the process of determining structural invariants of objects. Moreover, both internal sensory systems are operational during the motion of the child around his environment while he undergoes experiences which will enhance his recognition of the invariants of space, time, and causality.

For the very young infant, the methods of measurement are limited and the movement (i.e., kinesthetic response) of the child often becomes the assessing instrument. Certainly, this aspect of child behavior is a very important feature in the non-laboratory assessment of a child's maturational progress. However, because of measurement difficulties and the tendency for child development behaviorists and motor behaviorists to explore specific aspects of behavior independently, our knowledge of the contributions of the internal sensory systems to the development of invariants is limited. Flavell (1970), who has explored various aspects of the Piagetian model, believes that each individual has standardized evaluative predilections toward differential aspects of his external world and, as a result of his interactions with his environment, develops perceptual and motor constancies. These evaluation tendencies were considered to be concepts with each concept being a system of ordering that serves as the mediating linkage between the input side (stimuli) and the output side (response).

In instances where the stimuli and response involve the same sensory system (e.g., visual input and fixation time response) the concept may be the mediating linkage. However, in events which involve input from one sensory system and output from another, the possibility exists that each of the sensory systems may be functioning in terms of standardized evaluative predilections pertinent to that system. For example, a young infant who has been allowed to play with a round ball of playdough and become familiar with the weight of the dough, is allowed to see that piece of dough reshaped into an "I" form and is again handed the dough. Instead of the usual steady arm and hand position that the infant maintains when the muscle tension is properly adjusted to the weight of the object, the arm and hand move up suddenly upon receipt of the reshaped play-dough. This sudden "flying up" of the arm is interpreted, in the Piagetian model, as indicating that the infant has not yet developed knowledge of the "conservation" of an object with respect to weight; that is, the weight of an object is unaffected by changes in its shape.

Because the young infant at this period in the development of object invariants associates increased size (i.e., o vs. I shape in figure 7.2) with increases in weight, the visual input system's evaluation process signals to the kinesthetic system the degree of change needed but the kinesthetic system must also employ the evaluative process associated with that system to reach an equivalence of degree of adjustment needed for the

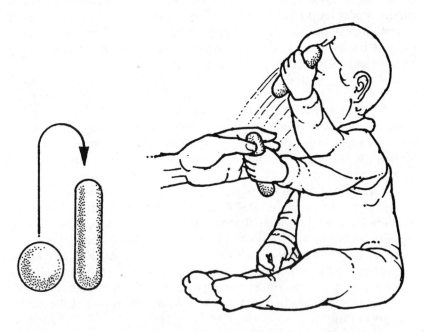

FIGURE 7.2. *When the shape of an object is changed, the young child associates the longer shape with more weight and adjusts the arm muscle tension accordingly. Weight has not changed so the increased muscle tension causes the arm to fly up.*

kinesthetic response to the signalled visual change. Fortunately, by some neural mechanism of which we are not yet aware, the degree of intensity of sensory stimulation seems to be transmitted between the various sensory modalities with a remarkable degree of accuracy and is probably a survival-associated mechanism. However, Flavell's theoretical model (1970) in which each individual has standardized evaluative predilections toward differential aspects of his external world, points to the need to consider individual differences in the evaluative processes for each of the sensory systems which are capable of registering differential aspects. The evaluation process also implies the development of some sort of criteria as the basis for an evaluative judgment. For purposes of this discussion, the criterion developed by each individual to serve as the evaluative base for responses to sensory stimuli is called a "standard." A standard differs from an invariant in that the standard refers to an individual's personal adjustment and/or reaction to his environment whereas invariant refers to those aspects of object, space, time, and causality that are global to all items and events in the environment. In instances where an individual's standard is in high accordance with the relevant invariant (or invariants), the resultant responses are highly accurate. However, we are also aware of many situations where the responses are not accurate.

Just as are all events in the environment, physical performance tasks are governed by the basic physical laws governing objects, space, time, and causality. The only volitional means of movement of the body or any of its segments is muscle action in response to neural stimulation. Fortunately, many of the basic neuromuscular complexes such as reciprocal innervation, in which antagonistic muscles are relaxed while the agonists contract, are genetically predetermined developmentally. However, the degree to which muscles must contract for any specific action is under the volitional control of the individual and, in order to be able to make judgments of the amount of muscle action needed, some sort of standard (or criterion) is required as a basis for such judgments. At the same time the infant is developing knowledge of the invariants associated with the various objects that are manipulated and moved by himself, the actions involved are also providing the infant with internal sensory input (kinesthetic) relative to the degree of force required for the action and of the maximum amount of muscular force the infant can mobilize. Because the maximal available force can be considered to a fixed point at any one time and is personal to the capabilities of each individual, Eckert (1971) proposed that the maximal force is the standard (evaluative criterion) whereby each individual determines the degree of muscular force required for each specific action. This is a simplistic approach to a very complex problem as the force required for any action is dependent upon the basic physical law of Force = Mass × Acceleration and the actions of various muscle groupings also vary. Some of these aspects of muscle action are discussed in the chapter on later childhood; suffice it here to say that we do make judgments as to our capabilities to perform certain actions requiring our personal use of force. For example, how would you respond to this question: Can you move a grand piano?

As with the development of recognition of invariants associated with objects, space, time, and causality, experimental opportunities to interact with objects in the environment play a crucial role in the development of the individual's standard of force. For example, the actions of an 11-month-old girl in playing with various-sized balls is indicative of her conceptual understanding of the muscular force requirements to move these objects in relationship to her previously constructed understanding of her own strength. The girl, Lisa, was a proficient walker and played with a small playground ball by dropping it, watching it bounce, and then picking it up to repeat the process. After a while she tired of this and then noticed a large playground ball (which almost reached her height) in the far corner of the room. She approached the ball at her usual pace but stopped 10 feet short of the ball and looked at it for about one minute. Lisa then turned and went to the security of her mother's arms. Shortly thereafter, Lisa began playing with the medium-sized playground ball which she also picked up, dropped, and watched bounce. This activity soon reached its saturation point and Lisa again spied the large ball in the corner. She then approached the large ball with no hesitation, picked it up, and turned to face the center of the room before dropping it. As the height of the drop was only about three inches, the large ball did not bounce satisfactorily and Lisa abandoned it after the one trial. Lisa had obviously developed some concepts of the basic nature of objects relative to size, weight, and shape and had also developed some standard of her own physical capability to exert muscular force.

Not only the amount of experience but also the type of experience plays a role in the development of the understanding of force application and numerous studies of motor learning report varying degrees of learning based upon varying arrangements of practice trials. A number of the practice variations that usually appear in motor learning studies were part of the design used by Pigott and Shapiro (1984) to investigate the effect of variability in practice and its subsequent influence on transfer performance to a novel variation of the task. Children, aged 6 through 8 years, received varying combinations of practicing tossing four bean bags of varying weights at a fixed target location. Following the series of 24 practice trials, all subjects were given three no-knowledge-of-result trials using different weights to the practice weights. As anticipated all of the practice conditions showed a significant improvement during the practice sessions but the variability group practicing with blocks of three trials at each variation of weight had a slightly lower mean error during the last practice session and significantly superior performance in the novel variation of the task. It would appear, then, that a combination of repetition of an activity requiring the same amount of force together with the provision for experiencing a variety of force demands (weight changes) for the same action provides the most effecient training model for transferring force application to a novel situation (different weight) for the task.

The processes of repetition of actions and participation in a variety of similar and novel actions are crucial to the development of the invariants associated with objects, space, time, and causality. Similarly, they are also crucial to the theoretical model that each individual develops standards applicable to his own performance. Both these theoretical models have similar general orientations and the same actions can contribute to the development of both invariant and standard development. For the example of the bean bag throwing, the invariants associated with space are used in the visual assessment of the distance the bag must be thrown to reach the target whereas the personal force standard of the individual is used to determine the degree of muscular contraction needed to project the bean bag the proper distance. Additional aspects of the action of tossing a bean bag are angle of trajectory which involves space invariants and internal kinesthetic position assessment for the proper point of release of the bag. On the basis of the fact that the same sensory modalities are involved in the development of understandings of the invariants that govern all objects and events in the environment and in the development of personal understandings of the physical capabilities of each individual, it seems logical that similar developmental models apply to both.

One important feature of the invariant model is that the invariant is applicable to many objects and/or events within the environment and thus it provides a criterion for efficient evaluation. Similarly, the standard model should provide for a criterion for the individual to assess the efficiency of his actions. Research undertaken by Hogberg (1952) to determine the effect of stride length variations on the oxygen uptake of a well-trained runner indicated that the most physiologically efficient stride was close to the subject's freely chosen stride length. Subsequent replication of this research by Cavanagh and Williams (1982) using 10 subjects demonstrated that the freely chosen stride length of experienced runners was close to their physiologically optimum stride length. These investigators suggested that this efficiency may be a function of either: (a) the runners altering their stride length due to changes in perceived exertion, or (b) the runners selecting an absolute stride length that subsequently becomes more efficient through repetition (i.e., the physiological training effect). The effect of altered stride length on perceived exertion was examined by Messier, Franke, and Rejeski (1986) using 28 experienced recreational runners. Half of the subjects served as a control group to monitor the result of practice effects of repeated bouts of running and the other half engaged in running trials involving freely-chosen stride length and four variants of this stride length (i.e., two longer and two shorter). The control group's perceived exertion did not change significantly in freely-chosen stride length runs during the six-week testing period. However, significant differences in perceived exertion were registered for the variable stride length group indicating that experienced runners perceive differences in exertion accompanying changes in stride length. Using the standards model, the lack of change in perceived exertion for the control group indicates this measure is consistent enough to serve as a standard. The fact that it can serve as a criterion measure is also indicated by the finding that the changes in physiological demands that accompany changes in stride length are perceived as differences in exertion and the observations that the most physiologically efficient stride is close to the subject's freely-chosen stride length.

It is possible that perceived exertion may reflect not only the personal standard for physiological functioning but may also be associated kinetically with an invariant of motion. The invariant identified by Cutting, Proffitt, and Kozlowski (1978) is the center of moment which is the center for an arc or a system of arcs; for example, a fulcrum is the center of moment of a lever arm, as is an axle for a wheel. Because a moment is the tendency, or measure of the tendency, to produce motion, the center of moment is often called the center of movement in biomechanics. When the principles of structural mechanics are applied to human gait, it is considered to be made up of the rigid motions of four compound pendula (the arms and legs) hinged at the corners of a flat spring (the torso). When all these parts or subsystems are set in motion, the movement is periodic and symmetric about the center of moment of the body as a whole. Although faster and requiring more force exertion, the actions of running are similar to those of gait in terms of structural mechanics.

In their studies of how gait is perceived, Cutting, Proffitt, and Kozlowski (1978) videotaped the gaits of people who had reflecting tape on their joints and used contrasting lighting techniques so that the reflections from the tape remained the only source of information for the viewer. The tapes were taken at right angles to the direction of the walk so that a side view was obtained of the motion of the lights that indicated the location of the subject's shoulder, elbows, wrists, hip, knees, and ankles. The investigators found that subjects could recognize themselves and others from these dynamic point-light displays. In addition, they found that viewers could identify the gender of the walkers using point-light displays which contained no familiarity cues; however, such recognition was possible only from dynamic displays but not from static ones. Analysis of the data, using bodily structure and angular changes, indicated to the investigators that the center of moment was the biomechanical invariant the viewers could use to distinguish between the gait of male and female walkers. The center of moment (movement center) of the body differs from the center of gravity (structural center) of the body and the difference between these two centers is greater for the female than it is for the male during walking so that the center of moment for the female is higher relative to the height of the individual. Although the investigators found that a series of stimulus degradations, such as non-normal variations in walking speed and arm swing, interfered with the perceptual process, the degree of discrimination of the process is indicated by the fact that any pair of lights by themselves (such as on the two ankles) seemed sufficient for gender recognition. However, best recognition performances involved lights on both hip and shoulder.

The ability of an individual to recognize the effect of the center of moment invariant in gait may be related to the individual's standard of perception of his own gait. To illustrate, we often stress to individuals learning a motor skill (e.g., golf) that they try to get the "feel" of the movement of the skill, the object being to develop a kinesthetic standard for the correct movement. When the individual has repeated the movement enough times to get a general movement pattern established, concentration can be placed upon the more specific aspects of the skill and this process can be considered to be a refinement of the kinesthetic standard. A well-skilled individual has little difficulty in consistently repeating a performance (i.e., able to minimize performance error with respect to the standard).

Previous experience, therefore, enables an individual to evaluate current movement in terms of previous movement. In addition, the individual has, from birth, been integrating visual input with kinesthetically-mediated physical responses. Therefore, a strong association has been developed between visual input and the movement responses of the individual. We use this process when we demonstrate the movements of a skill to the learner and the more experience the learner has in the skill (i.e., the better the kinesthetic standard) the more capable the learner is in refining specific aspects of the skill. When we are spectators at a sporting event, such as tennis, in which we have had prior experience, we often find that this integration between the visual and kinesthetic systems enhances our enjoyment of the game. For example, as you watch the player serve the ball during the tennis match, you find your previous experience with tennis allows you to "feel" the action of the serve (i.e., you experience your kinesthetic standard) and, if you are an experienced tennis player, you may even "feel" how the action of the server differs from the action you would use in serving the ball. Similarly, our extensive experience with walking may have so refined our kinesthetic standard that we are able to recognize the very small difference in gait associated with the center of moment invariant and our ability to associate such differences with gender could be based upon the fact that we are fully aware of our own gender.

The center of moment invariant is a spatial and/or patterning invariant and, although some force is obviously required to move the various bodily parts, the recognition of the invariant depends upon the involved movements conforming to normative patterns and speeds (Cutting, Proffitt, & Kozlowski, 1978). The possibility exists, then, that there are at least two invariants associated with movement, namely, center of moment (patterning) and force. A factor analysis of longitudinal data for seven eye-hand coordination tasks available from ages 4½ to 8½ years identified two factors as a patterning or design component and a speed factor (Eckert and Eichorn, 1974). Longitudinal data, because they are derived from the same individuals over a period of time, provide an opportunity to examine age changes in a more precise way than can be achieved with cross-sectional data at the same ages. Thus, the factor pattern, which showed a reduction from three factors to two between 4½ and 5½ years for females and between ages 5½ and 6½ years for males, has potential implications for developmental changes in recognition of invariants. If the assumption is made that a reduction in the number of factors is indicative of a greater understanding (or recognition) of the communalities (invariants) involved in the tasks, then the age difference in factor reduction for the sexes may be a maturational feature of perceptual development consistent with the generally earlier maturing of females. The earlier reduction in the number of factors for the females does not appear to be associated with the level of performance of the sexes as the males tended to be slightly superior to the females on most of the eye-hand coordination tasks and, on this basis, might be expected to develop invariants sooner. However, in only three instances, namely, sorting at 7½ and 8½ years and ball-dropping at age 4½, were there any significant sex differences with the females being superior in the former task and the males in the latter. Although the sorting task was timed (speed and pattern components) and the ball-dropping was based on the number of balls out of 10 dropped into a revolving disk (pattern component), the loadings of these tasks on the two factors was similar for the sexes so that the sex difference in performance level does not appear to affect performance communalities during the age span from 4½ to 8½ years. Therefore, future studies in the area of perceptual recognition of invariants should give some consideration to the possibility that sex differences in neurological maturation may play a role in developmental changes.

Just how the brain processes motion information and is able to register invariants extracted from dynamic events is not known. It is possible that the way the brain organizes movement information may be a factor in the development of the recognition of invariants. The developmental changes in the ability of individuals to organize movements of various lengths was investigated by Gallagher and Thomas (1986) using subjects aged 5, 7, 11, and 19 years. The results indicated that the younger children

(5- and 7-year-olds) were unable to organize unstructured movements. In the experimenter-organized movement situation, the 7-year-olds performed similarly to the 11-year-olds but the 7-year-olds were not able to transfer the strategy to a novel condition as were the older groupings. Only the adult subjects demonstrated the ability to organize the movement information that was presented. To the investigators these results suggested that the difference between adults and children in organization might be due to the children's lack of knowledge base and not due to an inherent inability to produce the strategy.

It seems logical that the process of recognition of movement invariants undergoes developmental changes associated with growth and neural maturation similar to those observed in perceptual development of object, space, time, and causality invariants. Certainly, the center of moment invariant would seem to be integrated with space and time invariants, and perhaps to a lesser degree with other invariants. Ruff's extensive review (1980) of the development of perception and recognition of objects stressed not only the importance of movement in detecting the basic invariants of objects but expressed the opinion that hypotheses about the internal processing involved in recognition would be incomplete without studies which deal with moving objects and active observers. Therefore, the movements, and opportunities for movement, of the child become extremely important for optimal development and integration of the perceptual systems.

MOTOR ACTIVITY AND LANGUAGE

Motor activity has the potential for contributing to language development in that movement plays a key role in the perceptual development of object invariants and objects are defined by nouns. In addition, that other important part of language, the verb, is the part of speech that predicts and is sometimes called the "action" part of the sentence.

The relation of play to language development was examined in 39 infants who were tested by Ungerer and Sigman (1984) at 13½ and 22 months of age. Language was measured by scales which were grouped into five categories. The simple manipulation category included each instance of mouthing, waving, banging, fingering, or throwing of a single toy. Non-functional combinations of objects such as touching or banging two objects, stacking objects, and using one object as a container to hold another was classified as relational play whereas the use of objects in a functionally appropriate manner or in the conventional association of two or more objects was categorized as functional play. Symbolic play included representational-or substitution-object-use during activity and the remaining category of sequences was used to record meaningfully integrated sequences in play. The investigators found that functional play directed toward dolls and other persons and meaningfully-related sequences of functional and symbolic acts at 13½ months were associated with language measured at 13½ months and nine months later at 22 months of age. The consistent relations found between play and language were considered to be derived from the infants' ability to translate experience into symbols that are used as a means for interacting and communicating with others.

In addition to the type of play, the environment in which play occurs would appear to have an impact upon early language development. For example, in a study of 24 children who were videotaped at 15 and 24 months of age in naturalistic interaction with their mothers, Tomasello and Farrar (1986) reported that maternal references to objects that were already the child's focus of attention were positively correlated with the child's vocabulary at 21 months (See figure 7.3). In contrast, object references by the mother that attempted to redirect the child's attention were negatively correlated with vocabulary. An additional experimental study, in which an adult attempted to teach novel words to 17-month-old children, explored the effect of the child's attentional focus. Again, words referring to objects on which the child's attention was already focused were learned better than words presented in an attempt to redirect the child's attentional focus.

Children obviously increase their vocabulary with increasing age but the possibility also exists that there may be developmental changes in the basis upon which children form early word meanings. Although Ungerer

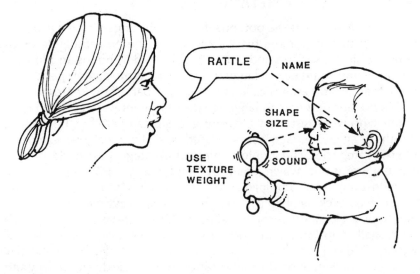

FIGURE 7.3. *Components of object recognition and language association.*

and Sigman (1984) reported that functional play was associated with language at 13½ and 22 months of age, a study of 2- and 3-year-olds to determine whether early word meanings are perceptually- or functionally-based reports somewhat different results. In their series of studies, Tomikawa and Dodd (1980) presented the children with novel objects (toys) in which perceptual and functional features varied independently and the children had choices of how they sorted the novel artificial objects (i.e., either on perceptual or functional features). All of the results supported the conclusion that early conceptualizations and word meanings are perceptually-based when perceptual and functional features are independently available.

There are, however, some types of words for which perceptual features (shape, size, sound, movement, texture, taste) may not be readily apparent and/or applicable and the functional features (i.e., the functional relationships of an object and/or action to the child's behavior) are more appropriate to the understanding of the meaning of a word. For example, the meaning of action words may be more readily comprehended through functional relationships as is illustrated in the following situation in which the age estimate is approximate. A young boy (3 years) and an older girl (5 years) were waiting for their non-English speaking mothers to complete their conversation. The girl said, "Let's play chase." The boy questioned, "What is chase?" The girl responded "It's like this," as she stretched her arms out in front and ran in a circular direction towards the boy. Before she reached the boy, he understood the meaning of "chase" and executed an evasive run to prove the extent of his understanding.

Another aspect of language development may be associated with the sex of the child and the differential functioning of the hemispheres of the brain. Equal numbers of boys and girls in a group of 64 3- and 4-year-olds were asked to identify another's view (spatial perspective) by responding either verbally or by picture selection. In this study, Ives (1980) found that verbalization leads to substantially more correct responses for both boys and girls and the girls were significantly better than the boys across both verbal and pictorial modes. The reportedly better verbal ability for females is in keeping with other findings of sex difference in verbal ability. However, other investigations, such as that of Herman, Shiraki, and Miller (1985) have reported sex differences favoring males in spatial orientation tasks. It would appear that the degree of sex difference in hemispheric functioning of the brain is still questionable as is the interrelationship of the specifically-identified functions of the two hemispheres.

Language is one of the brain's functions that is hemispherically-specific and, for approximately 97 percent of humans, the left hemisphere is the locale for language understanding (Wernicke's area) and for the motor area coordinating speech (Broca's area). Figure 7.4 shows the

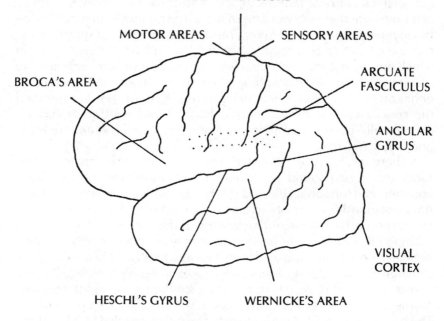

FIGURE 7.4. Left side of the brain indicating language and associated areas.

locations of these areas on the left hemisphere and the location of the arcuate fasciculus which is the nerve bundle joining Wernicke's and Broca's areas. Other areas of importance to language are Heschl's gyrus which is the primary receiver of auditory sensory input and the visual cortex which receives the visual sensory input. The angular gyrus acts as a way station between the auditory and visual regions and is closely associated with Wernicke's area (Geschwind, 1972). For right-handed individuals, other processes governed by the cortex of the left hemisphere are writing and abstract thinking such as mathematical calculations. The right hemisphere cortex is associated with nonverbal concept formation and memory, spatial processing and perception, and with word recognition but poor speech comprehension (Deglin, 1976).

Bilateral spatial representation has been associated with developmental dyslexia in males. The right-handed dyslexic boys studied by Witelson (1977) had normal or better visuo-spatial perception and exhibited bilateral processing of spatial functions. The left hemisphere was also specialized for linguistic function in the dyslexic boys, but their accuracy in tests of function in the left hemisphere was significantly lower than that of normal boys. Witelson speculates that dyslexics may use a spatial, holistic, cognitive strategy in reading and tend to ignore or ineffectually use a phonetic, analytical strategy. Females have a lower incidence of reading difficulty but they also are generally less proficient on spatial tasks. The sex difference in the effects of bilateral spatial representation may be a function of sex differences in neural organization, or it may be a functional reflection of sociocultural influences. Witelson (1977) points out that bilateral representations of spatial functions could overload the left hemisphere and interfere or be incompatible with its specialized role of sequential linguistic processing. This type of overload has the potential of occurring more frequently in males where the social milieu encourages more participation in spatially-oriented activities for males. On the other hand, the bilateral representation for females may be a deficiency condition in that the female may not have had sufficient experience with spatially-oriented activities to develop pronounced right hemisphere spatial-processing.

Similarly, language difficulties, such as the use of spoken language and gesture, is one aspect of autism that seems to be associated with abnormal development of the left cerebral hemisphere with many autistic children excelling at skills associated with the right hemisphere such as visuo-spatial skills (Dawson, 1983). In a study of left versus right hemisphere alpha blocking during verbal and visuo-spatial tasks, Dawson, Warrenburg and Fuller (1982) found that seven of the 10 autistic children tested showed greater right than left hemisphere activation during language processing. In contrast, these children showed normal patterns of hemispheric activation during the two visuo-spatial tasks. Additional evidence of left hemisphere abnormality comes from a neuropsychological study by Dawson (1983) in which right-sided (left hemisphere) sensorimotor and perceptual impairments were more pronounced in a group of autistic children than in a group of mentally retarded children matched for sex, age, handedness, and full scale I.Q. Further study by Dawson and associates (1986) of 17 male autistic children, aged 6 to 18 years, and a matched group of normal children showed that the autistic children's direction of hemispheric asymmetry in response to linguistic stimuli differed significantly from that of normal subjects. The majority of the autistic children showed reversed (i.e., right hemisphere dominant) patterns of hemispheric asymmetry. In their discussion, the investigators proposed the possibility that a shift from right to left hemisphere processing of speech occurs as the autistic child acquires spoken language.

The question of the possible conflict between language and spatial development based upon hemispheric asymmetry is confounded by the findings of Molfese, Freeman and Palermo (1975) that different types of auditory stimuli also have asymmetric hemispheric processing. When these investigators recorded the auditory evoked responses (AER) from the temporal region of both cerebral hemispheres they found that the responses to the speech stimuli was greater in the left hemisphere in nine of the 10 infants tested while the response to the piano chord and noise were greater in the right hemisphere of all 10 infants. As these infants ranged in age from one week to 10 months, the investigators hypothesized that different areas of the brain appeared to be preprogrammed to differentiate between certain types of stimuli very early in life, perhaps at or before birth. However, brain functioning has also been marked by a considerable degree of plasticity which may be reflected in developmental changes. In the study of the ontogeny of the brain lateralization, Molfese et al. (1975) also examined children (age range of 4 to 11 years) and adults (23 to 29 years) and found that the auditory evoked responses were similar for all groups but that the adults did not respond with as great a degree of asymmetry to the speech stimuli as the younger age groups. Moreover, the degree of right hemisphere asymmetry for the nonspeech stimuli was greater for the young infants than for the older age groups. These age differences led the investigators to conclude that the degree of lateralization of both verbal and nonverbal auditory stimuli decreases with increasing age.

It is obvious that the process of language development is very complex and can be affected by both neurological and environmental factors. However, for those individuals with normative neurological functioning and maturation, it would appear that a facilitative environment and involvement by the young infant and child tend to enhance language acquisition. Motoric activities would appear to be one avenue for involvement by the child in developing language understanding.

MOTORIC AND INTELLECTUAL DEVELOPMENT

Although surveys of the literature conclude that there is only a slight or very low relationship between intellectual and motoric performance (Kirkendall, 1986), physical educators and motor behaviorists, during their observations of children, tend to intuitively hypothesize that there is a relationship between mental and motoric development which reflects the unitary nature of the individual. How can one account for these differing conclusions reached by the researcher and the practitioner? And, does further research have the potential for providing new insights which will either reconcile these differences and/or enable the researcher to provide information as to some communalities of mental and motoric development?

The first of these questions may be most readily answered in terms of methods of assessment. The practitioner is more likely to utilize a nonnumerical, qualitative method to derive a hypothesis whereas the researcher is constrained by the "scientific method" to collect numerical data and base subsequent conclusions on the statistical analysis of these data. The analytical constraints placed upon the researcher mean that, although the researcher may personally have the same hypothetical convictions as the practitioner, the researcher must only reach conclusions that are supported by the statistical treatment of the data. Thus, the researcher must be able to justify the validity of the data and, in the instance in question, namely, intelligence, there is a considerable amount of disagreement as to what constitutes intelligence and, accordingly, methods of measurement.

The problems of defining intelligence are pointed out by Sternberg (1985) who identified six theoretical models of intelligence as follows:

1) Geographic model: Intelligence as a map of the mind,—based on factors.
2) Computational model: Intelligence as a computer program,—based on elementary information processing.
3) Anthropological model: Intelligence as a cultural invention,—based on cultural context.
4) Biological model: Intelligence as an evolving system,—based on schemata.
5) Sociological model: Intelligence as the internalization of social processes,—based on mediated learning experience.
6) Political model: Intelligence as mental self-government,—based on internal components of information-processing; external functions of components; facets of experience.

These theoretical models of human intelligence have been cited to indicate not only the complexity of defining and measuring intelligence but they also provide potential avenues for the formulation and testing of new insights concerning the relationship between intellectual and motoric development.

Standardized intelligence tests, such as the Stanford-Binet, and academic performance tests fall almost exclusively within the geographic and computational models as defined above. These types of tests have been the most frequently used in the past to determine the relationship between intellectual and motoric performance (Kirkendall, 1986). The fact that the relationships which have been found have, at best, been slight may be a function not only of the type of tests but may also reflect a lack of cooperative effort between the researcher and practitioner. For example, it is possible that a physical education program which emphasizes the biomechanical aspects of various physical activities may result in a more substantial relationship between physical performance and academic achievement in subjects such as physics and mathematics, especially if the teachers of these subjects have also utilized physical performance situations to illustrate principles.

Three of the other intelligence models identified by Sternberg, namely, the anthropological, the sociological, and especially the political model, are in the early stages of development and/or do not have standardized methods of assessment that are widely recognized so that research based on these models and motoric performance is not possible at present. The political model, which is the one proposed by Sternberg (1985) as appropriate to his definition that "intelligence consists of those mental functions purposively employed for purposes of adaptation to and shaping and selection of real-world environments," would seem to be most in keeping with the various components of physical performance. Certainly this appears to be the interpretation portrayed by the producers of the public television series titled *THE BRAIN* in which the episode on "Vision and Movement" featured the diving skills of Greg Louganis. Unfortunately, the political model is in an embryonic stage and lacks evidence of supporting contextual subtheory and insufficient unification and integration of subtheories thus handicapping research based on this model.

On the other hand, the biological model, which is based upon Piaget's intellectual development hypotheses using schemas, has been well researched and specifications of mechanisms of intellectual development are well documented. Piaget (1962) classifies the first two years of life as the *sensorimotor period* in a child's intellectual development. Although the human can receive stimuli from distant objects via the visual, auditory, and olfactory sense organs, the amount and types of stimuli are greatly increased if the object is brought into contact with bodily sensory processes. The major external sensory processes in the human are concentrated in the head region, which also houses the neural mechanisms for their interpretation, and the anatomical structure of the upper limb is ideal for conveying objects to this great locus of external environmental processors. The newborn infant with its sucking and grasping reflexes has a limited capacity for bringing the external environment to the facial area.

The first month of the sensorimotor period is considered by Piaget (1962) to be the reflex stage in which anything that contacts the mouth is sucked with subsequent rejection of unsatisfactory objects, and objects placed in the hand are grasped but not manipulated. According to Frank (1966), the internal conditions and sensations of the child are becoming increasingly stabilized at this time so that the child can then focus on patternings of external stimuli. During the next three months, the child begins to coordinate the movements of the arm and mouth so the child is able to suck its thumb at will and brings objects placed in the hand to the mouth to suck. Greater attention is given to objects that have become familiar through repeated use than to new objects, and Piaget (1962) considers this to be a stage of simple habits.

The next stage, from 4 to 8 months, is considered to be a repetition of simple habits, but the child has now achieved the neurological development necessary for the early efforts at eye-hand coordination and is able to reach for and bring objects closer to its body. In the process of doing so the child is undoubtedly forming associations which will initiate perceptions of space. In addition, the self-initiation of securing objects affords the child an opportunity for greater exploration of objects in terms of shape, weight, size, and texture. During this stage, there is more association between regularly occurring events and a greater attention to the manipulation of objects which indicates some perception of physical causality. The child also becomes aware that an object will drop when it is released and begins to acquire some knowledge of the permanence of objects. Piaget considers the action of a child who looks back to the position of origin of a movement after the completion of the movement as indicating some spatial and temporal perceptual precursors.

The exploratory field of the child is greatly expanded during the fourth stage from 8 to 12 months which is marked according to Piaget (1962) by the anticipation of familiar events so that the child is able to foresee events connected with his action. Kagan's study (1972) of a number of children supports Piaget's observations of his three children in that Kagan reports the first signs of active mental work (in which the infant tries to generate hypotheses to explain novel events) to occur at about 8 or 9 months. The child's exploratory field is greatly expanded by the acquisition of crawling skill during the early part of this stage and the acquisition of upright locomotion during the later part. The increased external sensory stimuli enhance the perception of object permanence so that a child will now hunt for hidden objects, but spatial awareness is still limited in this regard because the child looks only in the area where the object is first hidden. However, spatial awareness in the manipulative area, where the child has had more exploratory opportunities, is more advanced as the child can now put two objects in relationship to each other—for example, pulling a string tied to an object to secure the object. During the course of manipulative play, the child begins to recall a sequence of ordered events with the action being repeated in temporal sequence, thus indicating increased perceptions of object, spatial relationships, and temporal order. The establishment of object permanence may be a factor in the beginnings of acquisition of speech at this time in that the same auditory stimuli become associated with certain objects.

Trial and error exploration is the approach utilized by the child between 12 and 18 months to solve new problems (Piaget, 1962) and such exploration results in higher perceptual levels of objects, space, physical causality, and time. In addition, the child is now more aware of environmental situations so that the relatively small change that occurred in the behavior of infants of less than nine months when the mother or father left is replaced, in the 18-month-old child, by a marked increase in crying and/or cessation of playing when the mother or father leave (Kagan, 1972). The play and simple games of the child involve use of a number of objects in different spatial and temporal sequences, such as placing a small container in a larger container and then placing a smaller object in the smaller container. The child's play also involves using different types of objects in similar action sequences, such as lifting a ball to arm's length and letting it drop, then lifting a block and letting it drop with further similar variations on the type of object and on the position prior to the dropping of the object. This type of trial and error exploration may have some relationship to the change in schematic organization identified by Piaget (1962) as occurring around 18 months—that is, the change from organized schemas of action, or sensorimotor schemas, to representational schemas. The representational schemas are considered to derive from sensorimotor schemas and are dependent upon a general capacity to represent one thing for another. It is during this period that language development also makes marked gains.

The exploratory experience gained during the stage of trial and error provides an increased level of perceptual understanding of the concepts of object, space, physical causality, and time so that from 18 to 24 months, the child tends to think before resorting to trial and error in the solution of novel situations. For example, the child who has previously been able to remove a chain from a box opened sufficiently so that the hand can be placed in the box will, when presented with a similar situation in which the opening is too small to admit the hands, enlarge the opening of the box to recover the chain. The child's concept of the permanence of objects has advanced to the extent that a ball rolled under a low object which obstructs the view is sought behind the object, and hidden objects are found after several displacements of the object which were invisible to the child. The spatial interrelationships of objects receives more attention from the child as obstructions to the movement of an object, such as a door, will be sought for and removed by the child. The child will also look for the causes of movement in a previously observed immobile object; for example, a stationary ball that is propelled by an observer when the child's attention is directed elsewhere will elicit an inquiring look from the child.

The second period of Piaget's intellectual development model (1962) which is considered as preparation for and organization of concrete operations, corresponds to the period of childhood. As with childhood, which is usually divided into early and late childhood, this period is divided into stages. The first stage, from 2 to 7 years, is called *preoperational representations* and includes the development of representational thought and the world of symbols. It may be hypothesized that the motoric development of the basic physical skills that occurs during this period of early childhood will have a considerable impact upon the development of representational thought and symbols that are related to the basic physical laws governing objects, space, time, and causality. At this time, also, the very simple rules of games are being mastered and the child is, according to Frank (1966), acquiring the sensory experiences which enables the child to gradually learn to stabilize the world around him in terms of the symbol systems, accepted beliefs, and expectations of his group.

The second stage, from 7 to 11 years, is considered by Piaget (Flavell, 1963) to be concerned with concrete operations, and the child develops a stable and orderly conceptual framework particularly as related to the physical aspects of object, space, time, and causality. The corresponding period of late childhood, with its slower growth rate and refinement of basic motor skills, would seem to provide a sensory background during which the development of stable and orderly physical conceptual framework could be maximized.

Formal operations is the designation given by Piaget (Flavell, 1963) to the final period, from 11 to 15 years, of the intellectual development model. This is the period during which the individual learns to deal effectively with reality and with abstract, propositional phrases. The development of the ability to think logically and abstractly occurs during the final stages of the maturation of the cerebral cortex. Physically, the adolescent growth spurt results in marked changes in bodily configurations and physiological functioning, which will affect adult performance levels but have only minor impact upon the patterning of basic motor skills. (See table 7.1.)

The biological model is at present the most viable model for the examination of the relationship between motoric and intellectual development in that the model recognizes the importance of development; has specifications of mechanisms of intellectual development; and has a breadth of theory within the realm of logical-scientific thinking. In contrast with the geographic and computational models where the standardized tests are applicable only to specific age ranges and tend to have different areas of emphasis, the Piagetian model is consistent throughout all age levels in emphasis placed upon the development of object, space, time, and causality concepts. When the schema approach of the Piagetian model is modified by the Gibson concepts (1966, 1979) of invariant structure and continuous stimulus change, the correspondence between the biological model of intellectual development and motoric development becomes even greater. Although research in this area has been minimal, recent developments in research instrumentation and methodology now make it possible to examine the relationships between motoric activity and physical changes in the brain (and hence potential intellectual function).

TABLE 7.1. Summary of intellectual and motoric development

Intellectual Development*	Motor Performance Aspects	Primary Concepts*	Motor Performance Aspects
I. Sensory Motor Intelligence (0–2 years)		1. Object	Size, weight, shape, texture ⎫ Use of
1. Use of reflexes (0–1 month)		2. Space	Distance, force, range of ⎭ strength
2. Simple habits (1–4 months)			movement
3. Repetition of motor habits (4–8 months)	Prehension	3. Causality	Feedback, coordination, balance
4. Anticipate familiar events (8–12 months)	Walking skills	4. Time	Speed, acceleration, endurance
5. Trial and error exploration (12–18 months)	Beginning language		
6. Think before trial and error (18–24 months)			
II. Preparation for and Organization of Concrete Operations (2–11 years)			
1. Preoperational representations (2–7 years) Representational thought, world of symbols	Basic skill development (run, jump, throw, catch) Very simple rules		
2. Concrete operations (7–11 years) Stable and orderly conceptual framework	Refinement of basic skills More organization and rules		
III. Formal Operations (11–15 years)			
1. Deals effectively with reality and with abstract, propositional phrases	Good skill level		
2. Thinks logically and abstractly	Well-organized activities after puberty: Adult skill, championship performance		

*Based on J.H. Flavell, *The developmental psychology of Jean Piaget.* Princeton, N.J.: Van Nostrand Co., Inc., 1963.

One approach to investigating this relationship is by examination of the brain to determine the effect, if any, that activity level will have on the anatomical structure. The work of Marian Diamond, which is reported in "The Two Brains" segment of THE BRAIN series and elsewhere (Rosenzweig, Bennett, & Diamond, 1972), clearly indicates that an enriched environment results in anatomical changes such as increased weight of the occipital cortex of rats, greater thickness of cortex, increased number of glial cells and cross-section of neuron cell bodies as well as larger synaptic junctions. The enriched environment for the rats included a larger cage, more rats per cage and various types of objects such as ramps, walking bars and hoops, or objects that stimulated a natural environment. The enriched environment brain structure was compared only to brain structure under environmental conditions where the standard-sized cage containing only feeding apparatus was occupied by one rat (impoverished condition) and the normal number of two rats per cage. Therefore, it is not possible to determine precisely which of the changed environmental variables, i.e., larger area in which to move around, more objects to explore, or interaction with larger number of rats, contributed most to the noted structural change in the occipital cortex. However, it may be assumed that the opportunity for increased motoric behavior was the prime factor as this is the primary mode of exploration and expression for the rat.

Similar types of studies are, of course, not possible with humans but it should be recalled that a great deal of our present knowledge about the human brain was derived by postmortem examination of individuals with known conditions prior to death. Using this research model, Witelson (1985) made postmortem measurements of the corpus callosum (the bundle of nerves connecting the two hemispheres of the brain) in individuals who were tested for handedness prior to death. The subjects in the study included 27 consistent right-handers and 15 who showed mixed-hand preference but no left-handers. The corpus callosum of the mixed-hand group was found to be about 11 percent larger than in the right-hand group with the sex of the subject not being a significant factor even though the brain of males is larger than that of females. Witelson, who has also done research on the patterns of hemispheric specialization, concluded that the larger corpus callosum of the mixed-handers may be associated with the greater bihemispheric cognitive functions in mixed-handers. In other words, individuals who have the same types of cognitive functions in both hemispheres of the brain may have also developed more connections between the two hemispheres and these are individuals who are motorically adept at using either hand.

The effect of environmental activity on neurological functioning has also been examined using electroencephalograms (EEGs). As part of a longitudinal study of 53 pre-term infants, Beckwith and Parmelee (1986) used sleep state organization and EEG patterns at term date as an index of maturity and integrity of neurophysiological organization. These children were then tested at 4, 9, and 24 months on the Gesell Developmental Scale; at 5 years by the Stanford-Binet Intelligence Scale; and at 8 years by the Wechsler Intelligence Scale for Children. The rearing environments of the infants were also assessed when the infants were 1, 8, and 24 months. In general, the results showed that children who, at term date, showed less 407-Trace Alternant EEG pattern (particularly in quiet sleep) had lower IQs beginning at 4 months and continuing to age 8. The exception to this trend occurred for children being reared in a consistently attentive, responsive environment. These children, even though they showed decreased amounts of 407-Trace Alternant earlier, had higher IQ scores (equal to those of infants with more 407-Trace Alternant) by 24 months of age and continuing to age 8. Therefore, the rearing environment of infants is extremely important and can have a buffering effect in ameliorating early risk factors expressed in brain activity in young infants. Whether an enriched environment can markedly improve brain activity beyond normal limits is conjectural on the basis of our present knowledge.

The development of non-invasive measuring devices promises to greatly enhance our ability to research the relationships between all aspects of bodily functioning. For example, knowledge of developmental changes in the brain with growth is now being reinforced by using positron emission tomography (PET) which uses compounds labelled with radioactive substances to provide an x-ray-like image of specific activities. The nerve cells of the brain utilize glucose as the fuel source for neural activity and PET scans based on radioactive glucose utilization provide a pictorial image of neuronal functioning. Based on data for nine infants ranging in age from 5 days to 1.5 years and whose status at the time of the PET procedure was judged to be nearly normal, Chugani and Phelps (1986) noted that, at 5 weeks or younger, glucose utilization was highest in the sensorimotor cortex, thalamus, mid-brainstem, and cerebellar vermis. By 3 months, glucose metabolic activity had increased in the parietal, temporal, and occipital cortices and the basal ganglia, with subsequent increases in frontal and various association regions occurring by 8 months. The investigators concluded that the functional changes measured by PET were in agreement with behavioral, neurophysiological, and anatomical alterations known to occur during infant development.

Not only does PET provide an image of the location in which the glucose is utilized by the neural tissue, it also provides a method for assessing the amount of glucose that is utilized. This is done by programming the computer, which analyzes the amount of radioactive glucose, to depict the varying amounts of glucose in different colors. Thus it is possible to determine not only the areas of primary function but also areas of associated neuronal activity. In their report of PET as an analytical imaging technique for testing anatomical distribution and rates of glucose utilization in human brain functions, Phelps and Mazziotta (1985) depict PET images when normal subjects respond to various stimuli such as visual, auditory, motor, and cognitive. As may be expected, the visual stimulus showed the highest concentrations of glucose in the visual cortex and lesser concentrations in associated areas. Similarly, the greatest utilization for the auditory stimuli was in the area of Heschl's gyri with associated lesser utilization areas. A sequential finger movement of the right hand was the motor task and, as expected, the greatest concentration of glucose was in the left motor strip and supplementary motor cortex. However, in this instance, areas of lesser glucose utilization were spread over a much wider area than for the visual and auditory stimuli. These PET images raise such questions as: What is the nature and role of the less activated neural areas? and, Does the extent and/or degree of these areas of activation reflect the nature and/or the complexity of the task?

Phelps and Mazziotta (1985) report that studies of the human auditory system indicate a correlation between the distribution of glucose usage and the content of the stimulus and, in some cases, the strategy used by the individual. For example, subjects who were asked to recall specific aspects of auditory stimuli had activations of the mesial temporal lobe that were not seen in situations where auditory perceptions without memory tasks were required of the subjects. With non-verbal stimuli, such as musical chords where subjects who listened to the sequence of musical notes were asked to determine whether notes of one sequence differed from those of another, the pattern of glucose utilization correlated with the strategy of the subject. Those individuals who used specific imagery and analytical strategies (i.e., visual musical scales for comparing note sequences) had predominately left hemisphere asymmetries and increases in glucose utilization in the posterior temporal region. On the other hand, subjects who used non-visual imagery as a comparison technique had activations in the inferior parietal and temporal-occipital regions of the right hemisphere.

It is obvious that the use of PET instrumentation opens immense possibilities of resolving some of the questions of interrelationship among the various sensory inputs at both the developmental and individual differences levels. The Piagetian intellectual development model with its well-documented indicators of cognitive competencies can now be examined in terms of locus of neural activity and degree of biochemical reactions to determine if there are "developmental patterns" such as are exhibited in the various types of motor performance. Moreover, our well-documented motor development patterns can also be subjected to

PET analysis and comparisons made with cognitive competency patterns to determine the degree of relationship between these series of developmental patterns. The use of PET instrumentation for assessing these two aspects of human development would be the first time that the same device has been utilized for both intellectual and motoric performance to provide the same standard of interpretation. Moreover, it is one that can be applied over the entire life-span as opposed to the previously-used age-specific measuring devices for cognitive functioning.

Although it may be some time before we can expect such research to be undertaken, some inferences can be made regarding the relationship between physical activity and anatomical and physiological neural parameters on the basis of available data. The work of Phelps and Mazziotta (1985) on PET imaging of various auditory stimuli indicates that neural connective strategies used by individuals vary thus suggesting that physical educators must organize their programs so that individual differences in learning styles are accommodated and the physical educator must also be prepared to recognize that a variation in response on the part of the student may be a feature of such differences in neural connective strategy.

Witelson (1985) presents two possible interpretations for the noted anatomical differences in the corpus callosum based on the handedness of the individual and both of these interpretations have decided ramifications for physical educators from a developmental aspect. One hypothesis that could account for the noted differences is that the greater bimanual experience of mixed-handers and/or the representation of language and of sensorimotor functions of the dominant hand in opposite hemisphere, as exists in most left-handers, may result in the growth of more axons and a larger callosum. The other hypothesis is based upon findings in developmental neurobiology that during the early stages of neurogenesis there is an overproduction of neurons and fibers followed by the death of neurons and elimination of axon collaterals which do not make functional connections so that there are fewer neurons and axons in the final stages of neurogenesis. On the basis of this hypothesis, Witelson theorizes that "if more fibers do exist in the larger callosa of mixed-handers, the neuroanatomical difference between hand groups may be related at least in part to axonal elimination, which occurs prior to most environmental influences." However, she also points out that "it remains to be determined whether the larger callosum of mixed-handers contains a greater number of fibers, thicker axons, more myelin, or just fewer fibers per unit area."

The corpus callosum does not become heavily myelinated until approximately 5 years of age so that the hypothesized neurogenic changes are occurring during the time period in which the child is learning the basic motor skills and movement patterns. The relationship between neural development and motoric function appears to be reciprocal during the developmental years with neuromotor functioning enhancing myelinization and myelinization enhancing functioning. Therefore, regardless of which of these hypotheses is applicable, it is vital that each child have the opportunity to develop his or her own motoric abilities to the optimal level of his or her own capabilities. In addition, until it is proven otherwise, we should assume the hypothesis that increased experience may result in neural modifications is a viable one and strive for the optimization of each individual's motoric abilities at all age levels.

Physical educators can contribute markedly to this developmental process by ensuring that children are encouraged to participate in activities appropriate to their neuromotor development. Young children should not be expected to perform basic skills using adult motor performance patterns. Rather it is the responsibility of the educator to recognize age-appropriate skill performance patterns and provide the opportunity for the child to gradually develop more mature patterns.

The extent of the glucose utilization in the previously defined anatomical areas associated with specific sensory inputs has served to reinforce such knowledge and also provide the scientific verification of the use of PET for analysis of brain functioning. Sensory input must be analyzed by the brain and concepts developed on the basis of input from various sensory systems as one aspect of intelligence. The strong possibility exists that the associated glucose utilization areas of the brain revealed by PET may be involved in such concept development.

A great deal of attention is given to the five external sensory input systems (i.e., visual, auditory, cutaneous, olfactory, and taste) but physical educators seem to be among the few groups which also stress the internal sensory input systems, namely, the proprioceptive (kinesthetic) and vestibular (balance). Hence, physical educators have a unique opportunity to contribute to the enhancement of concept development by providing additional sensory input for the brain and encouraging their students to use such input where possible. For example, judgment of an object to be moved is based not only upon size, shape, and texture which is determined by external input systems (visual and cutaneous) but also by weight (internal proprioceptive system). Therefore, the individual who has had the opportunity to develop concepts of objects that incorporate all of the sensory input modalities has the potential for making better judgments and, hence, experiencing fewer injuries and "accidents" and may even utilize such knowledge to make a more economical purchase of a cabbage which is priced by the head rather than the pound.

Although visual input is one of the pirmary means of supplying information in physical education classes, auditory explanations by the instructor are usually incorporated with the visual demonstration. As the work of Phelps and Mazziotta (1985) on PET imaging of various auditory stimuli indicates that neural connective strategies used by individuals vary, physical educators must organize their programs so that individual differences in learning styles are accommodated. In addition, the physical educator must be prepared to recognize that a variation in response on the part of the student may be a feature of such differences in neural connective strategy. In short, the instrumental program should allow for individual creativity and place minimal emphasis upon "rules-oriented" activities during the period of early childhood.

The types of programs which seem to provide the greatest opportunity for exploratory, creative, and experimental behavior for children during the early developmental years are movement education and/or exploratory programs. These programs also allow for individual differences without placing undue emphasis upon such individual differences. Tradition, lack of equipment, and previous ambivalence of research evidence supporting the desirability of such programs has delayed their widespread use. However, equipment is being developed to meet the needs for more flexible instructional programs designed to encourage creativity and individual performance capabilities of children. The research evidence of PET imaging which shows a high degree of associated neural function with motor tasks points to the need for physical educators to become adept at maximizing the creative and exploratory aspects of motor development of children.

It is, then, the responsibility of the individual physical educator to determine whether to remain within the traditional program mode or to venture into the realm of creative, individualized programming. Hopefully, it will be the latter decision as the future of the child depends upon the ability of the practitioner to apply the new knowledges we are gaining about that unifying structure of the body—"the brain."

SUMMARY

1. The process of perception is governed by sensory input(s); the length of time the resultant stimuli persist in the brain; the speed and degree of integration between sensory systems; and the interpretation of the integrated information Table (7.2).

2. The latency period (i.e., the length of time a stimulus persists in the nerves) is longer in very young infants than in adulthood. Therefore, time between stimuli must be greater to enable the infant to process the information; for example, use of slower speech and slower movement of objects within the infant's visual field.

3. It takes longer for very young infants to process information. However, once a stimulus becomes familiar, a novel stimulus attracts more attention.

TABLE 7.2. Perceptual schedule

Age	Event or Activity	Author
Neonate	Greater attention to intermediate intensity stimuli than extremes	Hershenson, 1964 (light) Hammer & Turkewitz, 1975 (sound)
	Summation of intensities (vision and sound); intensity response same as for 1 mode	Lawson & Turkewitz, 1980
1 week – 10 months	Speech stimuli response in left hemisphere; nonspeech acoustic responses in right hemisphere	Molfese et al., 1975
3–4 weeks	Cross-modal intensity gradient transfer (visual and auditory)	Lewkowicz & Turkewitz, 1980
8–9 weeks	Longer auditory latency period than in adults	Cowan et al., 1982
4 months	Distinguish familiar from novel rhythm (auditory and visual)	Mendelson & Ferland, 1982
5 months	Visual preperception of longer duration than in adults	Lasky & Spiro, 1980
	Reach for nearer of two surfaces when kinetic information shows which is closest (i.e., depth perception)	Granrud et al., 1984
6 months	Remember repeated stimuli and distinguish from novel stimuli	Nelson & Salapatek, 1961
	Size of object associated with spatial distance (i.e., large objects within reach, small objects are not)	Yonas et al., 1982
13 months & 22 months	Functional play and meaningfully related sequences of functional play, symbolic acts related to language	Ungerer & Sigman, 1984
1 year	Can acquire enough information from either oral (mouthing) or manual exploration to recognize object visually	Gottfried et al., 1977
10–28 months & 36–44 mos.	Active exploration related to accurate knowledge of unfamiliar area	Hazen, 1982
3 years	Child understands 1) events are caused; 2) causes precede effects; and 3) causes are linked to effects	Bullock et al., 1982

4. Intermediate-intensity stimuli are attended to for longer periods of time by young infants than low- or high-intensity stimuli.

5. When sensory input is from more than one modality, the intensities of the stimuli are summated and the young infant responds to the summated intensity in the same way as intensity from one modality alone. Therefore, persons in charge of the child should monitor the stimulus level of the learning situation.

6. Cross-modal transfer of visual and auditory stimulus intensities occurs in very young infants and the equivalence of intensity of transfer persists into childhood (i.e., high intensity in one mode directly related to high intensity in another mode).

7. Infants can distinguish familiar from novel rhythm patterns at 4 months of age and greatest attention occurs when a novel situation occurs in only one modality (i.e., visual or auditory rhythm).

8. Although rhythm has a time component, time-related concepts such as duration, speed and distance develop slowly. Children grasp direct relationships between duration and distance and between speed and distance before they grasp the inverse relationship between duration and speed. That is, direct relationships are understood before indirect or inverse relationships.

9. By 7 months, the infant associates size with spatial distance; that is, a large size is considered to be within reaching distance whereas a small size is not.

10. Children who actively explore an unfamiliar area (e.g., a playroom) develop a more accurate knowledge of the spatial layout of the area. As children become older than kindergarten age, they may rely more on other types of sensory input to gain knowledge of spatial layout.

11. There may be sex diffferences in spatial aspects such as spatial directional orientation. Spatial abilities are mediated by the right hemisphere of the brain and the noted differences may be due to sex differences in hemispheric development or as a result of sex differences in spatial experiences. Males appear to make better use of visual reference cues in visuospatial tasks.

12. When kinetic information (i.e., one object moving in front of another) is available to show which of two objects is closest, the 5-month-old infant will reliably reach for the closest object, thus indicating depth perception.

13. Change (i.e., movement) conveys information to the observer about the structure of the objective world around him because the permanent and unchanging aspects within the stimuli reveal the invariant structure of the environment.

14. Nonchange aspects (i.e., invariance) specify the arrangement of objects in the entire environment (e.g., close objects overlap more distant objects); the structure of individual objects (e.g., curved or straight-

line objects); and the structure of the finest texture (e.g., rigid or elastic surface).

15. Rate of speed and complexity of an object are factors affecting the recognition of the structural properties of objects. Simpler objects undergoing simpler motions are easier to recognize than complex objects moving quickly. These factors should be kept in mind in selecting toys and in providing a favorable learning environment for children.

16. Once the infant can reach for and grasp an object, manual (finger and hand) and oral (mouthing) exploration augments visual and auditory input to provide optimal sensory modality input. The extent of intermodality integration is shown in 1-year-olds by their visual recognition of objects previously explored using either mouthing or hand-finger manipulation.

17. With increasing age, intersensory integration results in fewer errors in intermodal object recognition indicating increasing ability to recognize structural invariants. The developmental change is governed by capabilities of each individual, maturation rate, and environmental conditions.

18. Principles of object recognition (Ruff, 1980): 1) recognition develops from general to specific; 2) variations are detected, in part, because of the activity the object participates in; and 3) object recognition develops from being content-bound to content-free.

19. Factors associated with causality concepts are: 1) priority (i.e., cause precedes the effect); 2) mechanism (i.e., the cause must be linked to the event); 3) co-occurrence (i.e., repeated observation of events that occur together); and 4) amount of experience of the child.

20. A "standard" refers to an individual's personal criterion for assessing external and internal sensory stimuli whereas "invariant" refers to those aspects of object, space, time, and causality that are global to items and events in the environment.

21. A combination of repetition of activity (same force) together with varying force (weight changes) in the same action provides the most efficient training for transfer of force application.

22. For the experienced runner, perceived exertion may be the standard for physiological functioning with the freely-chosen stride length being the most physiologically efficient length.

23. The center of moment, which is the center for an arc or a system of arcs, has been identified by Cutting et al. (1978) as a biomechanical invariant of motion.

24. Factor analysis of longitudinal eye-hand coordination data from 4¼ to 8¼ years shows two factors: namely, patterning (an aspect of center of moment invariant) and speed (an aspect of force invariant).

25. The ability to organize similar unstructured movements increases with age from 5 through 19 years.

26. Functional play and meaningfully related sequences of functional play and symbolic acts have been associated with language at 13½ and 22 months.

27. Attentional focus of the child on the object being named is important in language acquisitions.

28. The differential functioning of the hemispheres of the brain (i.e., verbal in left and spatial in right) have been associated with sex differences in verbal ability (females better) and spatial ability (males better).

29. Studies examining the relationship between degree of activity level and anatomical differences in the brain tend to show enhanced neurological development with increased amounts of activity.

30. Longitudinal studies showed a relationship between EEG patterns and IQ but children reared in consistently attentive, responsive environments had higher IQ scores than expected for EEG pattern.

31. Non-invasive techniques, such as PET, show primary and secondary sensory activation areas of the brain and may provide clues as to the integration of perceptual, motoric, and intellectual development.

SUGGESTED ACTIVITIES

1. During early infancy (0 to 5 mos.), a mobile suspended above the crib provides the motion to objects that is necessary for the accretion and deletion of information at an edge involved in object, shape, and depth perception. Mobiles should be changed periodically and each change should be moderate to maintain interest.

2. Games using an object stimulate ocular control as well as spatial, causal, and time perceptions. Some examples include Simple Dodge Ball, Tether Ball, and Hot Potato.

3. Games that involve imitation stress not only visual input but also require appropriate kinesthetic adjustments during the imitated movement. Thus, such activities encourage optimal development of visual-kinesthetic equivalencies. Imitative types of games include Simon Says, Follow the Leader, and Do This-Do That.

4. All types of activities in which the child must move, and especially those which involve rapid changes of direction and/or levels, enchance balance development. Examples of such activities are Musical Chairs and Freeze (where the moving child must "freeze" in position in response to a signal).

5. Spatial, especially distance concepts, can be enhanced by having children run to and from objects. Having children run to, identify, pick up, and carry objects of different geometric shapes from one location to another, adds additional concepts of object (especially shape) as well as language to such activities.

6. Having children follow and/or write directions for obstacle courses, exercise stations, or mazes combines movement associated concepts and language. This is especially applicable to "action" words but also contributes to object perceptions.

7. Object concepts can be enhanced by having children participate in activities using different sizes and textures of the same object. For example, using balls of different shapes and sizes (i.e., footballs and playground balls) in the same game not only increases perceptions of size, texture, and shape but also enhances kinesthetic awareness of amount of force required to project different types of balls over the appropriate distances.

8. Time concepts can be enhanced by rhythmic activities such as marching to the beat of various types of percussion instruments beaten at various rhythms. Movement patterns such as hopping, galloping, and skipping can be added to such types of activities.

9. In an unobstructed space, children can be asked to close their eyes and move either toward or away from a voice or other auditory signal to enhance intersensory equivalency between auditory input and kinesthetic responses. Children can also be asked to move about without touching each other while making their own sounds—the scoring in this instance being the least number of contacts made by the child with other children. The level of difficulty can be increased by reducing the size of the area for movement.

10. Language can be enhanced by developing relays in which children, who have been assigned letters from the alphabet, run to a designated area in the proper sequence to form specific words.

11. Letters can be placed in hopscotch or grid patterns and children asked to spell words by hopping or jumping to the letters in proper sequence.

12. Spoken language can be enhanced by asking children to describe the movements of another child and/or describe the rules for a game they are playing or have devised.

13. Children can be asked to write and/or diagram the rules for a game they have played and/or devised.

8

Motor Behavior in Early Childhood

The period of early childhood is usually considered to encompass the age range of 2 to 6 years. Although some investigators have placed the beginning of childhood at 18 months as this is the average age of independent walking, the variations among individuals are great and at no time is there a clear-cut break in human growth characteristics. Therefore, the figure of 2 years is just as acceptable a division between infancy and early childhood and is more frequently used as it lends itself to age comparisons more readily. Furthermore, at about 2 years of age, the relative rate of growth of the child tends to level off in comparison with the rapid growth prior to this time (figure 8.1).

PHYSICAL GROWTH

Although gains in height and weight progress at fairly uniform rates during the period of early childhood, the rate of gain in height is nearly twice that in weight. The lower limbs grow rapidly in proportion to the trunk length but neither shoulder nor pelvic breadth increase rapidly, so that the total configurational change during childhood is toward a more rectilinear and relatively flat bodied child (See figure 5.1 in chapter 5). The male tends to be somewhat taller and heavier at all ages, but the proportional rate of growth remains similar for both sexes during this period. Girls maintain their relatively longer leg length in comparison to stem length until the end of early childhood. During this period also there is no difference between the sexes with respect to the ratio of shoulder breadth to pelvic breadth, although the measurements for males are slightly larger than for females.

The proportional increases in bone, muscle, and fat that occur at this

183

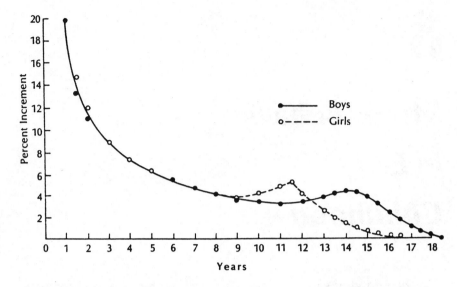

FIGURE 8.1. *Relative growth rate. (From Leona M. Bayer and Nancy Bayley,* Growth diagnosis. *Chicago: The University of Chicago Press, 1959. By permission of the publisher.)*

time do not parallel the distribution of these tissues during either infancy or adulthood. The rate of height gain and the rapid ossification of the bones indicate that bone tissue plays a significant role in weight increase. The proportion of muscle tissue remains fairly constant at 25 percent until the beginning of the fifth year when 75 percent of the gain in weight is attributed to muscle tissue. First bone and then muscle tissue make their gains at the expense of a reduced rate of gain in fatty tissue. Subcutaneous tissue measurements, before 6 years of age, show a similar pattern for both sexes (Boynton, 1936). The more rapid increase in muscle tissue during the fifth year makes available a larger potential of effective muscular energy for movement in the expanding number of physical activities of the child.

GENERAL DEVELOPMENT

With the start of walking, the world of the child expands rapidly. Quite literally he goes anywhere and everywhere paths are open to him. Since he has increasing amounts of energy available as he grows older and much of this energy is directed into gross motor activity, he needs a safe and, if possible, spacious place to play. In the years from 2 to 6 all of the usual locomotor patterns are perfected and a variety of eye-hand coordinations are learned. The latter are more dependent upon opportunity than the former and are almost certainly more influenced by instruction and encouragement. The child will walk and run, for example, and push furniture about and climb onto it in the ordinary course of development. He does not learn to catch or bounce balls nor to strike or bat them as readily without help.

The child usually begins to speak as well as to walk in the second year and, by the age of 2, has a mean vocaulary of 29.1 different words. Comprehension of the meaning of what others are saying increases rapidly, as does vocabulary (Terman & Merrill, 1937). At 3 years the child has acquired, on the average, a vocabulary of 62.8; at 4 years, 92.6; and at 5½ years, 99.5 words (McCarthy, 1930). The gain in new words is not linear but is greatest between 2 to 3 years of age. This coincides with the beginning of walking. A limited correlation of .39 had been found between the onset of talking and that of walking (Baylet, 1935). To Landreth (1958), these observations suggest that children are ready to make gains in both speech and walking at the same time but do so at the expense of each other, so that the motor skill of upright progression would appear to take precedence over, or develop at the expense of, speech during the period from 15 to 18 months. She also believes that further support is given to the theory of generalized conflict between motor skills and language by the observed sex differences in favor of language in girls and of motor skills in boys.

The manipulative activity of the young child is as constant and all encompassing as time and circumstances will permit. Children want to touch, feel, pick up, carry, and play with every object on which they can get their hands. Through continuous explorations of both space and things, they learn the nature of objects, of space, and to some extent themselves.

The critical nature of early childhood as a period of acquiring motor skills has been stressed by a number of investigators (Hurlock, 1953; Rarick, 1954; Frank, 1966). Overprotection may hamper a child's motor development by instilling fear in the child of possible bodily harm or by preventing practice during the maturation of particular abilities. Later on, the child may be unable to participate satisfactorily with peers because of this deficiency or retardation. Such an effect may snowball in that the child's inability to play on equal terms with others further limits his opportunities for practice and so he falls still further behind.

The need for ample opportunity and acceptable means for children to exercise their emerging motor skills is illustrated through an experiment by Johnson (1935). The social behavior of nursery school children was compared with the behavior of the same children after one-half of the equipment had been removed from the playground. A significant increase occurred in the amount of asocial play and physical assault among the children in the more barren surroundings. To Landreth (1958), such results suggested that the children solved the problem of equipment shortage for exercising their newly acquired and developing motor skills by using each other. She strongly recommends that the motor developmental aspect of the child not be neglected at this age level but be encouraged and enhanced as much as possible.

The significant role of motor skills in social development, even at these very early ages, should be noted. The child gains approval from his parents as he learns to do things for himself. His early contacts with other children are frequently through parallel and manipulative play in which objects may circulate among the group. By the fourth year he wants to be with others and to share more vigorous activities. Special skills become important. There would appear to be a reciprocal action between the motor behavior of a child and his emotional responses in that activity promotes a child's well-being and this, in turn, coupled with success in the performance of the activity, leads to expansive action on the part of the child (Landreth, 1958). This reciprocal action between motor behavior and pleasurable feeling is illustrated in reports of numerous investigations that the young child tends to repeat his most recently acquired or developing motor skills. Furthermore, the most frequent cause of smiling in children from 18 to 48 months is their own activity (Ames, 1949). This reaction is not confined to young children, certainly, since many adults experience exhilaration and expansiveness after successfully performing a challenging motor activity.

The examination of the development of specific motor patterns in early childhood reveals increased facility and complexity with increased age.

WALKING

The relatively slower rate of growth during the period of early childhood, coupled with the changes in bodily proportions, results in conditions that are increasingly conducive to the development of skill in the recently acquired activity of upright, bipedal locomotion. The child's eagerness to increase his facility in this activity and his contacts with his resultant constantly expanding environment are marked by determination and persistence despite many a tumble and bump.

The pattern of walking undergoes a transition from the first, hesitant, full sole steps with feet widely spread apart to the adult style of walking with a smooth, easy transition of weight in a heel-toe progression from one foot to the other. The rate of walking tends to stabilize at approximately 170 steps per minute between the ages of 18 months and 2 years while, in comparison, the range of steps for four briskly walking adults has been found to be 140 to 145 steps. Of course, adults have a much greater length of stride so that over the same period of time the 2-year-old child, even with a higher step rate, covers only a little more than half the distance traversed by an adult. Since the rate of stride does not increase as rapidly as the amount of distance covered within any period of time, the length of stride must increase from the age of 18 months to 2 years to account for the noted increase in traversed distance (Shirley, 1931).

Along with the increase in the length of stride and the development of a relatively consistent step rate, there is a changing pattern in the use of the foot. During the early stages of walking, toeing out is typical but is gradually replaced by a straighter placement of the foot so that foot alignment in the line of progression is fairly common by the 18th month. Although the length and width of the step become quite uniform between the 20th and 22nd months, the stride of the child is still jerky because of the continued use of the full-sole step. However, by the age of 2 years, and in some instances sooner, the transfer of weight from the heel to the toe of the foot upon contacting the ground results in a much smoother walk.

By the time the child is 3 years old, walking has become so automatic that little attention needs to be given to it even when the walking surface is slightly uneven. The 3-year-old has developed a good deal of uniformity of length, height, and width of step, with heel-toe weight transfer being well established and a certain amount of individuality beginning to appear in the manner in which the child carries his head and trunk. Around the age of 4 years, the child has almost achieved an adult style of walking in his easy, swinging, rhythmical stride and in the smoother transfer of weight in traversing both a straight line or in turning a sharp corner so that the act of walking is now a graceful movement. The use of the foot as both a source of propulsive power and as a rocker to receive and support the body weight has almost approached the adult level of coordination. Although there is great variation among children in the age of accomplishment of mature methods of upright locomotion, in general it is not until approximately 3 years after the first step is taken, or at around 50 months, that the art of walking may be considered to be perfected in the child (Rarick, 1954.)

Some of the differences in foot patterning for the beginning walker and for the adult are illustrated in figure 8.2. The foot size and step length are not in direct proportion and the line of walk of the beginner may be more erratic than illustrated. The shading at the heel and toe of the adult pattern indicates the areas of greater contact force as may be seen when an individual walks on firm sand. The full-sole step of the early walker does not show this type of rocker action.

The problems associated with the acquisition of walking skills revolve largely around the building up of sufficient strength to support the

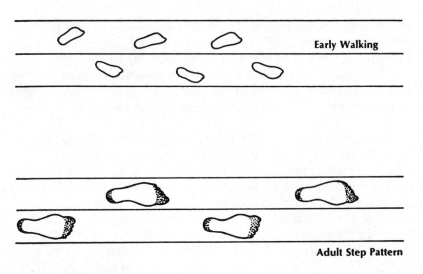

FIGURE 8.2. *Step patterns by a child during early walking and by an adult. Shaded area indicates contact force areas.*

weight of the body temporarily on one leg and the development of the finely adjusted balance mechanisms required for upright locomotion. The wide base of support and the outstretched arms coupled with the uneven, jerky steps of the beginning walker, often more appropriately called the toddler, is indicative of the struggle with the force of gravity. Even at 2 years of age when some facility in walking and running has been achieved, the child is still only able to maintain balance on one foot for a very few seconds. Increasing facility in the maintenance of balance is reflected in the ability of the child to walk in a straight line in a given direction. The toddler tends to weave about in progressing from one point to the next with the ability to walk in a straight line in a given direction not being established until the average age of 31.3 months, according to one study (Bayley, 1935). In another instance, only one-half of the children tested at the age of 37 months were able to walk a one-inch wide line for a distance of 10 feet without stepping off (Wellman, 1937). Greater balance difficulties are presented by the task of walking a circular path, for one-half of a group of children tested were not able to master a circle of 21½ feet without any step-offs until the age of 45 months (Wellman, 1937).

Growth in stature and increasing age both influence gait patterns and a quantitative analysis of gait development in children, with an age range of 13 to 69 months, indicates developmental patterns of alteration in velocity, stride length, and cadence closely paralleled previously made observations (Hennessy et al., 1984). The efficiency of gait was also assessed and, contrary to the adult pattern of optimal efficiency of energy expenditure, a child may choose either to increase gait velocity while maintaining the same cadence; maintain the same velocity and decrease cadence; or choose some combination of the two in violation of the energy-governing regulatory mechanism utilized by adults. Walking speed or gait velocity consistently varied with stride length and the stride length in turn was linked to leg length and total body height. The strength of the relationship between gait velocity and measures of stride length and body height after 18 months suggested to Hennessy et al. (1984) that these bodily proportions as well as neuromuscular maturation were a basic deteriminant of locomotor development in the young child. Some evidence of minimization of energy expenditure was seen in the trend for older children with decreased cadence and increased velocity to spend slightly more time in single leg stance and less time with weight shift in double leg support as occurs in adults.

In the adult gait pattern a relatively fixed relationship exists between stride length and cadence, with both increasing with walking speed and with any deviation from freely-chosen walking speed resulting in increased energy expenditure. Winter (1983) examined the motor patterns in normal human gait under conditions of slow, natural, and fast walking and found that:

1. Over the stride period, joint angle patterns were very consistent and did not change with cadence from slow to fast walking.
2. The ankle moment of force patterns were least variable and most consistent for all walking speeds.
3. Support moment patterns are also consistent for all speeds.
4. The moments of movement at the hip and knee are highly variable at all cadences but the amount of variability decreases with increasing cadence.
5. Mechanical power patterns at all joints are consistent in timing and are closely correlated with speed of walking.
6. Although the amplitude of the EMG pattern for the five observed muscles increases with increasing speed, the profiles of these muscles shows a consistent timing over the stride period.

Winter (1984) concluded that the findings support the concept that walking speed is largely controlled by gain and the timing of motor patterns, which is extremely tightly synchronized with anatomical position, is under major afferent control.

Variations on Walking Patterns

Other locomotor activities also require, as does walking, a sufficient degree of strength and the development of the necessary sensory-motor balance mechanisms in addition to the new neuromotor coordinations necessary for successful performance in the new activity. A new activity radically different from the skills already achieved by the child would necessitate tremendous adjustments in these areas. Therefore, it is not surprising that variations of the original basic walking or creeping patterns are gradually established. However, the desire for experimenting with new modes of achieving locomotion is very great during infancy and early childhood, as evidenced by the wide variety of form in the basic modes of prone and upright locomotion. The constant quest for control of the body by children is reflected in the variations of walking achieved very shortly after the establishment of upright locomotion. Walking sideways has been noted to occur at the average age of 16.5 months, walking backwards at 16.9 months, while the more complicated feat of walking on tip-toes is not normally attempted until after 30 months of age (Bayley, 1935). Furthermore, anyone who has ever watched young children at play has seen them pivoting around and around until they become so dizzy they can hardly stand, especially upon a soft, grassy surface where a tumble is such fun that it is usually the climax of such activity.

RUNNING

Since the basic limb movements in running are similar to those in walking, little adjustment is required with respect to neuromuscular patterning, but this mechanism must be capable of adjusting to the increased tempo of the run with its quicker interaction of **agonists** and antagonists in a coordinated fashion. Strength must also be greater to propel the body off the ground for a short period of time and better balance is required to receive the weight of the body on one foot after its momentary free flight through the air between the steps of the run.

The early type of run which many children adopt at approximately 18 months of age is not a true run but rather a modified walk as there is no period at which the body is not supported by one foot. As heel-toe progression has not become established at this time and the walk itself is stiff legged, the modified run is performed on the entire sole of the foot with the lower limbs being relatively stiff so that the movement is jarring and has an uneven length of stride. The child achieves a smoother stride and run between the ages of 2 and 3 but is still lacking control in the ability to stop or turn quickly. Continuing improvement in the power and form of the run results in the gradual accomplishment of control over starting, stopping, and turning by the ages of 4 to 5 years. Between the ages of 5 and 6, skill in running has advanced to the level where the adult manner of running is reasonably well established and the child is now able to use running skills effectively in play activities (see figure 8.3.)

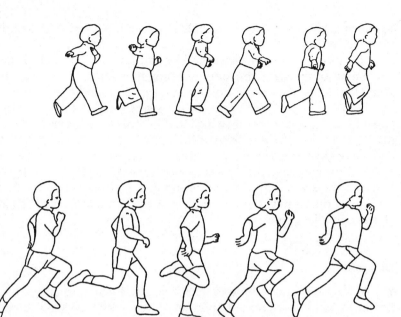

FIGURE 8.3. *Upper: Running form of a 15-month-old child. Lower: A 5-year-old boy demonstrating more advanced arm and leg movements. (Reprinted from Ralph L. Wickstrom,* Fundamental Motor Patterns. *Third Edition. Philadelphia: Lea & Febiger, 1983. By permission of the publisher.)*

An analysis of running patterns of 2-, 4-, and 6-year-old children by Fortney (1983) indicated that running speed improved with age. Although height and weight gains influenced improvement in running performance, biomechanical variables, such as displacement, velocity, and magnitude of forces, also contributed to the development of the running pattern. Differences between the 2-year-old group and the two other groups accounted for the majority of the significant age differences in the selected kinematic and kinetic variables. At contact, the support ankle was slightly less than 90 degrees for the 2-year-olds and 98 degrees for the other ages. Also, at contact, the swing knee angle of the younger group placed the heel lower than the swing knee while for the other age groups the joint angle of the swing knee placed the heel higher than the swing knee. The developmental trends at take-off showed that, with age, the support knee was more extended and, in both the swing knee and ankle, there were developmental trends in the direction of greater knee flexion and greater plantar flexion with age. The measures of height, leg length, and closely related step length showed significant differences between all age groups but in running speed and running speed indices significant differences occurred only between the 2-year-old group and the other groups.

Sex differences were also noted by Fortney (1983) with the range of movement of the swing hip and peak angular velocity of flexion of the swing leg being greater for boys than for girls. In addition, there was a significantly greater joint angle for the swing knee at takeoff in males. Possible explanations for the swing hip differences are suggested as structural (pelvic girdle differences) or functional (strength and/or flexibility differences in hip and lower spine area). Although sex differences did not occur in running speed, it was suggested that the significant difference between the swing hip of the boys and girls is a forerunner of the step frequency differences which exist between the sexes in older children and also in elite runners.

CLIMBING

At about the same time that an infant is learning to creep, he also begins to pull himself up onto his feet so that, with the establishment of creeping, it is not surprising that the infant will attempt to progress up stairs. This behavior begins shortly before the time the child has learned to walk (Gesell & Ilg, 1946) and a study of the cinema records of 12 infants by Ames (1937) indicates that the movement patterns used in ascending stairs at this time are almost identical to those used by the same infants in creeping on a level floor.

Soon after independent walking is established, the young child will attempt to ascend stairs in an upright position if supported by an older person and shortly thereafter will attempt ascent alone if there is a hand rail available to offer some support. The foot pattern used by young children just beginning to climb stairs differs from the alternating foot method used by adults in that the young novice will advance the same foot each time with the trailing foot brought up and placed on the riser beside the lead foot before the next step is taken. Thus the initial stair climbing pattern involves marking time on each step and is normally continued by most infants for several months until strength, balance, and coordination have developed to the extent that the adult alternate foot pattern can be negotiated successfully.

As with walking, a considerable variability exists among children as to the time when they are able to climb stairs. With help, young children will usually ascend stairs in an upright position between 18 and 20 months of age. The problem of descent, however, is not mastered at the same rate as is ascent so that it is not unusual for a child to creep or walk up a short flight of stairs if such is available, and then cry indignantly because he does not know how to get down. In general, descent, when it is first mastered, consists of crawling down the stairs backwards and, even when the child has achieved the skill to ascend stairs independently in the upright position, it is not unusual for him to make his descent by crawling down backwards.

A number of investigators have made independent observations of the development of stair climbing skill in youngsters and report similar types of activities used in the progressive development of the skill. After observing 98 children ranging in age from 26 to 74 months, Wellman (1937) noted that 50 percent of the children were successful at negotiating the various performance levels involved in stair climbing at certain ages. These she referred to as the "motor age" at which one might normally expect such a performance level. Her achievement levels and ages at which they were found to appear in 50 percent of her subjects are listed in table 8.1. The youngsters were tested on their ability to negotiate both a short flight (three steps) and a long flight (11 steps) of stairs.

The sequential stages listed by Wellman give evidence of successively more mature methods of negotiating stairs and are substantiated by the observations of Bayley (1935). However, the latter investigator noted that the children whom she observed tended to reach the various levels of achievement at a slightly earlier age. This finding is not out of line with the earlier reported differences in the ages in which the various progressive stages in walking were observed to occur in children in Minnesota (Shirley, 1931) and in California (Bayley, 1935). In this comparative instance, the California infants tended to achieve the skills necessary for both prone and upright locomotion at a slightly earlier age than those in Minnesota. These findings, in conjunction with the earlier achievements of stair climbing skills by the Californias children, would seem to indicate

TABLE 8.1. Stair climbing achievements of preschool children*

Stages in Ascending and Descending Steps	Motor Age in Months			
	Ascending		Descending	
	Short Flight	Long Flight	Short Flight	Long Flight
Mark time, without support	27	29	28	34
Alternate feet, with support	29	31	48	48
Alternate feet, without support	31	41	49	55

* From Beth L. Wellman, Motor achievements of preschool children. *Child. Educ.*, 1937, 13, 311–316. Reprinted by permission of the Association for Childhood Education International, 3615 Wisconsin Avenue N.W., Washington, D.C.

that there may be some regional differences in the onset of motor skills. Were comparative height and weight data available, it would also be interesting to analyze these data in terms of regional differences.

Considerable variability is reported to exist among studied children with respect to the age at which the various sequential stages are mastered by the children. Also there are considerable differences in the amount of time a child may utilize a certain technique as the primary means of negotiating stairs until the adult pattern is achieved (Wellman, 1937; Bayley, 1935). Moreover, there are inherent levels of difficulty in the length of the stairs to be negotiated and also in the height of the stair risers. Stairs with lower risers, so that they are more in proportion to the child's size, are mastered at an earlier age than stairs of adult size. Using an experimental staircase, Gesell and Thompson (1934) found that stair climbing behavior of the creeping type began in children between the ages of 40 to 50 weeks and, by 56 weeks of age, 53 percent of the infants were able to creep up a staircase constructed of four shorter risers. On the basis of these observations and the fact that studies tend to report averages based on group data, the standards of stair climbing performance established by various investigators should not be regarded as a rigid developmental schedule for the normal child but rather as a guide to the sequence and general time of appearance of such patterns in the motor development of children.

In general, studies of the development of ability in stair climbing indicate the following:

1. Ascending skill at a given level is achieved prior to descending abilities at the same level of achievement.
2. The child is able to accomplish an activity of a given level with help before he is able to perform the same activity alone.
3. At each level of achievement, the child will be able to negotiate a shorter flight of stairs before he is able to do so with a longer flight.
4. Stairs with lower risers can be mastered, at each level of achievement, prior to those of adult height.

In ladder climbing, as in stair climbing, the developmental sequence involves leading with the same foot and marking time on each rung before the more mature technique of alternating feet is attempted. The skill of ascending a ladder is achieved before the youngster attempts to descend a ladder of equal length and rung placement. The distance between the rungs of the ladder seems to have a marked effect upon climbing performance and this is to be expected, since the normal distance separating the rungs of a ladder is greater than that of stair risers. Furthermore, a ladder may be placed at varying angles and the greater the inclination the greater the height and the greater the strength requirement in both the arms and legs to support and propel the body. An apparent association that seems to be made by all children is that of the height of the climb with the difficulty of ascent. Children who employed advanced climbing techniques when operating at low heights have been noted to revert to more cautious movements on all fours when the heights they are to climb are materially increased (Guttridge, 1939).

When general climbing ability is studied using such equipment as stairs, packing boxes, inclined planks, jungle gyms, and similar apparatus, a steady increase in climbing proficiency is noted between the ages of 3 to 6 years. Guttridge (1939) used such equipment to survey the climbing performance of approximately 2,000 youngsters ranging in age from 2 to 7 years and found that by the time these children were 6 years old, over 90 percent of them could be classified as reasonably proficient climbers. There were wide differences among the children in climbing ability at every age, with the boys being slightly superior to the girls at 2, 3, and 6 years while the sexes tended to be equal ability at 4 and 5 years of age.

JUMPING AND HOPPING

The development of jumping and hopping involves fairly complicated modifications of the walking and running movement patterns. Since the jump necessitates elevation of the body off the ground for a longer period than is required for the run, greater strength is required to exert sufficient force and more complicated balancing adjustments are required both to maintain an acceptable body position while the body is in the air and to accommodate the body to the immediate deceleration of landing. Jumping occurs when the body is lifted completely off the ground by the action of one or both legs and the landing is made on one or both feet. Hopping, then, is a more complicated version of the jump for the body is lifted off the ground by the action of one foot and the landing is made on the same foot so that a higher degree of strength is required and a finer adjustment of balance is necessary to achieve a successful landing on the relatively small one-foot base. The leap is a specialized version of the run with the take-off being made from one foot and the landing on the alternate foot. However, the distance covered is so much greater in the leap than in any step of the run that the strength and balance requirements are closer to those of the jump.

Jumping

The first stage in jumping is considered to be the exaggerated step down from a higher level to a lower one so that the onset of jumping and descending stairs has the same origin and, of course, the same occurrence in time. When a momentary period occurs during which the child is not supported in his progress from a higher to a lower level, a downward leap or a one-foot jump is executed (figure 8.4). Here the child must have achieved enough strength and balance to accommodate the gravity-generated force of his descent to immediate deceleration on a narrow one-foot base.

At about the same time that the child is experimenting with one-foot jumps from heights with help, he has been independently jumping up and down on the floor with both feet used simultaneously. Although a two-foot landing is more stable, the two-foot take-off presents coordination problems that are new to the child since all his previous locomotion

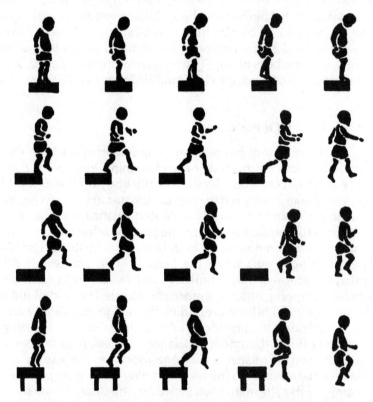

FIGURE 8.4. *Illustrations of the inability of the very young child (Willie) to jump from two feet simultaneously.* **Rows 1 and 2:** *stepping off an elevation at 17 months of age.* **Row 3:** *momentary suspension during a jump made at 18 months.* **Row 4:** *signs of incipient two-footed jumping at 21 months. Observe beginning shoulder girdle and arm retraction. (From F. A. Hellebrandt, G. L. Rarick, R. Glassow, and M. L. Carns, Physiological analysis of basic motor skills. I. Growth and develoment of jumping. Amer. J. Phys. Med., 1961, 40, 14–25. By permission of the publisher, Williams and Wilkins.)*

techniques have been based upon single, not simultaneous, limb propulsion. It is not surprising, therefore, that the one-foot take-off and landing is replaced by the one-foot take-off and two-foot landing. However, the young child must first develop enough strength to produce the necessary body elevation and speed of limb movement that is required for the take-off and two-foot landing. Clearly, also, a higher level of neuromuscular coordination is required for this latter type of jump. On the basis of its ontogenetic development, the most difficult type of jump for distance would appear to be the standing broad jump with its two-foot take-off and landing (figure 8.5.)

The developmental sequence for the standing broad jump was examined by Clark and Phillips (1985) on the basis of four hypothesized levels of leg action; namely, 1) stepping out or one-foot take-off; 2) propulsion with both feet and knee extension preceding heels up; 3) knee extension and heels up simultaneously; and 4) knee extension follows heels up. In addition, arm action was examined on the basis of the hypothesized developmental sequence of: 1) no arm action or "winging"; 2) shoulder flexion only (some shoulder abduction may also occur); 3) incomplete biphasic arm action; and 4) complete biphasic arm action. In their sample of 3- to 7-year-old children, Clark and Phillips did not find any of the children operating at level 1 for the leg action but suggested this might be a factor of the age of their subjects. Similarly, the lack of congruence between the hypothesized curves for levels 3 and 4 for leg

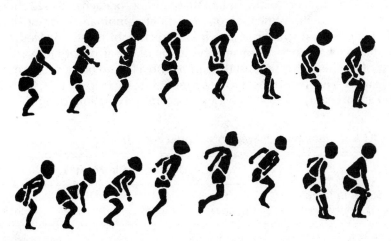

FIGURE 8.5. Row 1: *the earliest jump from a two-footed take-off observed in David at 32 months of age.* **Row 2:** *standing broad jump at the age of 3 years. Note the same shoulder girdle and arm retraction seen in figure 8.4. (From F. A. Hellebrandt, G. L. Rarick, R. Glassow, and M. L. Carns, Physiological analysis of basic motor skills. I. Growth and development of jumping. Amer. J. Phys. Med., 1961, 40, 14–25. By permission of the publisher, Williams and Wilkins.)*

action and the sample curves may have been a function of the selected sample. For arm action, however, the observed curves for arm sequence during the jumping performance of the children demonstrated not only the proper ordering of all hypothesized developmental levels but also the appropriate sign of the function.

There would appear to be almost a parallel development in both stair climbing and jumping off heights, which may have its basis in the similar origin of the two activities or may be just a reflection of the expansion in the variety of activities with which the child is experimenting at this time. The "motor age" at which 50 percent of the youngsters observed by Wellman (1937) were able to successfully perform the various achievement levels of jumping from various heights is reproduced in table 8.2. It may be noted that the earliest efforts were executed with the modified step-down movement and that the children were able to perform the activity at a given height and level of achievement with help before they were able to execute the skill alone. The more mature method of jumping with two feet together did not appear until some time after successful one-foot take-off had been achieved at the same height.

The technique of asking the child to jump and touch a long red balloon held horizontally by an adult was used to elicit a jump-and-reach for children at ages 23 to 35 months (Poe, 1976). Analysis of the filmed jumps indicated that 16 of the 22 children were able to meet the requirements of a jump by pushing off with one or both feet and landing on both. Analysis of the filmed record of the best of three jumps for each of the 22 children resulted in the identification of six distinct combinations of movement characteristics or patterns. The least effective of these involved a very shallow crouch; extension and abduction of the arms with forward flexion of the head throughout the jump; and a flexed body configuration. The most effective jumps involved a moderate to deep crouch; both arms flexed forceably upward with lower extremity extension; deep backward

TABLE 8.2. Jumping achievements of preschool children*

Stages in Jumping (From Heights)	Motor Age in Months			
	8 Inches	12 Inches	18 Inches	28 Inches
With help			27	36
Alone, one foot ahead		27	31	43
Alone, feet together	33	34	37	46

* From Beth L. Wellman, Motor achievements of preschool children. *Child. Educ.*, 1937, 13, 311–316. Reprinted by permission of the association for Childhood Education International, 3615 Wisconsin Avenue, N.W., Washington, D.C.

flexion of the head; and near complete extension in flight (Poe, 1976). The trends in the jumping patterns were:

1. From a very shallow crouch to a moderate or deep crouch during action of the legs
2. From extension and abduction of the arms or one arm reaching prior to take-off and throughout the jump to the use of the arms as augmentors, that is, flexed prior to take-off then extended with extension of legs to augment the jumping action
3. From a forward flexion of the head throughout the jump to deep dorsiflexion of the head during the entire sequence
4. From a flexed body configuration in flight to complete extension after take-off

Sixteen of the 22 children in Poe's study (1976) were able to meet the requirements of a jump by pushing off with one or both feet and landing on both. The youngest of these was less than 2 years of age. Six of the children exhibited almost adult-like jump and reach patterns leading Poe to conclude that most 2-year-old children can perform a jump-and-reach task when an overhead target is provided. She also points out that the group differences were so great that description of a "typical" 2-year-old jump-and-reach pattern would be virtually meaningless.

Observations by other investigators indicate that many different types of jumps are being explored by the child at about the same time. Normal progress in the various types of jumps is illustrated in figure 8.6. It may be noted that jumping over a barrier, in this instance a rope, appears

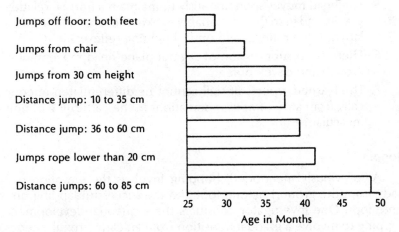

FIGURE 8.6. *Progress in various jumping skills. (Adapted from date by Nancy Bayley, The development of motor abilities in the first three years. Monogr. Soc. Res. Child Develpm., 1935, 1(1), 1–26.)*

to occur somewhat after jumps from height and jumps from distance have been mastered to a certain degree. Another investigator, Guttridge (1939), has observed that these types of jumps appear to be a complicated problem for youngsters and found it was not uncommon for 4-year-old children to have difficulty with jumping over barriers. This same study revealed that, in general, 42 percent of preschool children are able to jump well at 3 years of age while 72 percent may be considered to be skillful jumpers at 4½ years, with 80 percent of them having reasonably good mastery of jumping skills one-half year later.

The development of jumping has been summarized by Hellebrandt et al. (1961), with special emphasis on the standing broad jump, on the basis of the cinematographical records of 47 boys ranging in age from 14 months to 11 years. These investigators conclude that:

1. Jumping is a phylogenetic acquisition which unfolds progressively *pari passu* with growth and development of mechanisms capable of mobilizing the mechanical forces required.
2. Stepping off elevations precedes ability to jump by simultaneously extending both lower extremities.
3. Protection of the integrity of the weight-bearing limbs is ensured from the onset of jumping by automatic alignment of the lower extremities to receive the impact of landing most advantageously.
4. The upper extremities serve first as brakes by moving in a direction opposite to the line of motion, then as coronal plane stabilizers, and finally as augmenters of the momentum generated by the extensor thrust of the the legs.
5. The head moves spontaneously to maintain a normal relation to gravity and in so doing probably evokes the tonic neck reflex and labyrinthine reflexes and optical righting reflexes.
6. There is no suppression of sagittal plane head movement with growth and development.
7. The learned aspects of skill cannot be differentiated unequivocally from autonomous modulations in the patterning of neuromuscular response.*

Hopping

As previously mentioned, hopping involves the elevation of the body from the ground by one foot and the successful landing on the same foot. One investigator considers the sequential development of hopping to involve a gradual transition from an early irregular series of

---

* Excerpt from F. A. Hellebrandt, G. L. Rarick, R. Glassow, and M. L. Carns, Physiological analysis of basic motor skills; I. Growth and development of jumping. *Amer. J. Phys. Med.*, 1961, 40, 14–25. By permission of the publishers.

jumps to a more coordinated, regular pattern and manner of movement (Guttridge, 1939). Another believes hopping on two feet, which occurs earlier than hopping on one foot, to be part of the sequential development of this skill (McCaskill & Wellman, 1938). It is obvious that the development of balance, as well as the necessary strength to elevate the mass of the body with one foot is required before any skill may be achieved in hopping. Table 8.3 clearly indicates that hopping on both feet is mastered some time before the child is able to hop an equal distance using only one foot.

Static balance on one foot is according to Bayley (1935), not achieved until the infant is approximately 29 months old; and it is not until almost 21 months later, at approximately 50 months, that the average performer is able to hop up to two meters on the right foot. The intricacies of hopping, however, are not fully mastered at this time, for Breckenridge and Vincent (1949) point out that it is not until 6 years of age that most children can be considered to hop with skill and, even at this age, the range of skill varies from those extremely inept or refusing to make the effort to those children who are excellent performers. Once some skill has been mastered in hopping, the child tends to experiment with a large number of variations, such as hopping sidewise, backwards, and changing facing, and incorporates these into such games as hopscotch.

A prelongitudinal screening technique was used by Halverson and Williams (1935) to test proposed developmental steps in hopping for distance. The hopping performance of children, ranging in age from 2 through 5 years, was photographed and analyzed in terms of leg and arm actions. The leg action developmental steps included all observed leg movements and were accepted as comprehensive. The steps within this developmental sequence for leg action are labelled: 1)momentary flight; 2) fall and catch: swing leg inactive; 3) projected take-off: swing leg assists; and 4) projection delay: swing leg leads. The proposed develop-

TABLE 8.3. Hopping achievements of preschool children*

| | Motor Age in Months | |
Hopping, Steps	Both Feet	One Foot
1 to 3	38	43
4 to 6	40	46
7 to 9	41	55
10 or more	42	60

* From Beth L. Wellman, Motor achievements of preschool children. *Child. Educ.*, 1937, 13, 311–316. Reprinted by permission of the association for Childhood Education International, 3615 Wisconsin Avenue, N.W., Washington, D.C.

mental sequence for arm action was revised on the basis of the data with the revised developmental sequence for arm action being: 1) bilateral inactive; 2) bilateral reactive; 3) bilateral assist; 4) semi-opposition; and 5) opposing assist. The validity of these developmental steps was supported by the finding that children used less advanced movement patterns when hopping on their non-chosen leg as compared with their chosen leg. Fuller descriptions of the actions within each of the steps in the developmental sequences for leg and arm action are included in the published research study (Halverson & Williams, 1985). These investigators found that the children in their study were classified predominantly at low and intermediate developmental levels indicating that development of hopping may take longer than previously suggested. However, their results also confirmed previously reported sex differences in hopping with girls, by age 5, being placed at advanced developmental steps more frequently than boys.

The general sequence in the development of hopping includes:

1. The nonsupport leg is lifted in front of or to the side of the body and is held high while the arms are held near shoulder height. The propelling leg flexes quickly and little force is produced so that the hop is short.

2. The thigh of the nonsupport leg is more vertical and the bend of the knee brings the lower leg behind the body which leans forward during the extension of the propelling leg. Arms swing upward bilaterally to act either as a balancing reaction or slight propulsive force.

3. The thigh of the nonsupport leg is held vertically and there may be some movement of the lower leg which is held at a knee angle of 90 degrees or less. There is a greater forward body lean and greater flexion and extension of the propelling leg with the arms aiding in force production by moving up and down bilaterally.

4. The position is much the same as before but action of the propelling leg is much smoother and the nonsupport leg swings freely to augment force production. The arms swing alternately to the action of the nonsupport leg or are carried close to the body.

GALLOPING AND SKIPPING

The skills of skipping and galloping are built into the walking and running patterns by the additional introduction of modified jumping movements. Galloping combines the basic patterns of the walk and the leap; the skip consists of a hop interspaced in the walk pattern with the familiar "step-hop" of so many folk dances being a rhythmic variation of the skip pattern. The relatively late appearance of these skills in the motor behavior of the young child may be expected in view of the fact that they require the development of the balancing mechanisms at, or above, the level of hopping and that the movement sequences involved in their successful performance are new to the child even though their separate components have already been mastered.

Galloping is learned by most children by pounding to the strong beat of the music with the same foot or by periodically introducing a leaping step into their run. Gradually, the children will master the technique and degree of balance required to consistently throw their body weight onto the forward foot and then they begin to experiment with sidewise and backward variations in addition to the first learned forward progression. Guttridge's observations (1939) reveal the relatively late acquisition of this skill although it tends to appear slightly sooner than skipping. This investigator noted that 43 percent of the children at 4 years of age could be classified as having learned to gallop with the percentage increasing to 78 by 5 years, although skillful galloping is not achieved by most children until they are approximately 6½ years of age.

A type of shuffle, which is performed by the child at approximately 38 months, may be considered to be a forerunner of the first skipping movements. More frequently, the early skipping movements are considered to be those which involve a skip on one foot while the other performs only a walking pattern. Such activity has been noted as occurring around 43 months with the full blown alternate foot pattern of skipping not being achieved until the child is approximately 60 months old (Wellman, 1937). Children, however, are not content with the mere acquisition of the basic alternate foot pattern of skipping but also explore variations involving changes of direction and tempo. The relatively complex nature of skipping is indicated by the fact that only 14 percent of 4-year-olds and 22 percent of 5-year-olds were considered by Guttridge (1939) as skipping well. By the time the observed children were 6 years old, 90 percent of them were classified as being able to skip well but, even at this time, the variation in performance among the children was still very great.

KICKING

By the time the child is two years old, his balancing mechanisms have developed to the extent that he is able to maintain an upright position when balanced on one foot and still impart some degree of force to an object, such as a ball, with the other foot. During the early attempts, the range of action of the propulsive leg is very limited and the first kicks are executed with no backswing and very little follow through so that the object to be kicked must be directly in front of the foot or contact will not be made. Gradually as a higher degree of balance and strength are developed, the range of movement increases, first with a backswing originating from the knee, then the hip joint, and finally with a full leg backswing which includes a concomitant forward body lean by the time the child is 6 years old (Deach, 1951; see figures 8.7 and 8.8).

As the range of the backswing increases and amount of force generated increases, the follow through must naturally also be augmented to absorb the generated forces and maintain balance. Therefore, from the early beginnings of a stationary upper torso with arms at the side, the arms become increasingly used for maintenance of balance, with marked arm-foot opposition being evident at the age of 6 years (Halverson &

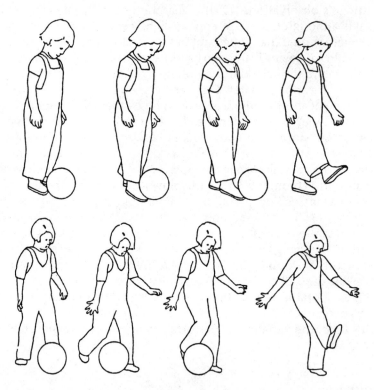

FIGURE 8.7. *Upper: Stage I in Deach's sequence. The girl keeps her kicking leg nearly straight and scarcely involves the rest of her body in the movement. Lower: Stage II. Additional leverage for the kick is gained by lifting the lower leg backward and upward in preparation for the kick. There is a small amount of opposition from the arms and slight backward trunk lean. (Drawn from film loaned by Deach.) (Reprinted from Ralph L. Wickstrom,* Fundamental Motor Patterns. *Third Edition. Philadelphia: Lea & Febiger, 1983. By permission of the publisher.)*

Roberton, 1966). Furthermore, the body increasingly tilts backwards during the follow-through to compensate for the increasingly greater termination angle of the propulsive leg.

THROWING

In a sense, the beginnings of the throwing pattern may be considered to originate in the first releases of an object held by an infant. However, the skill of throwing effectively, namely, the ability to project an object accurately and with sufficient force through space, requires coordination of many distinct mechanisms which require many years of

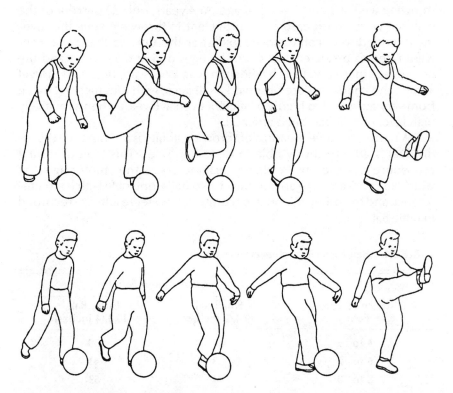

FIGURE 8.8. *Upper: Stage III in Deach's kicking sequence showing increased preliminary extension at the hip, greater arc in the leg swing, and additional body adjustments. The lower leg is slightly overcocked. Lower: Stage IV. Effective cocking at the hip and the knee, forceful kicking action requiring backward trunk lean, and extensive arm adjustments during follow-through. (Drawn from film loaned by Deach.) (Reprinted from Ralph L. Wickstrom,* Fundamental Motor Patterns. *Third Edition. Philadelphia: Lea & Febiger, 1983. By permission of the publisher.)*

experimentation and practice on the part of the child before a mature pattern is developed. At approximately 6 months of age, many children are able to perform a crude and unrefined throw involving limited and isolated use of the throwing arm when the child is in a sitting position. In general, children are able to give a reasonably well-defined direction to a thrown ball shortly before the first year. Further observation reveals that both distance and direction improve during the second year but that the throwing pattern tends to remain quite immature, consisting mainly of stiff, jerky movements of the arms with little or no effective use being made of foot or trunk movements (Gesell & Thompson, 1934).

Using a number of trained observers to rate the children included in her study, Guttridge (1939) noted that none of the children was rated as throwing well at 2 and 3 years of age. At 4 years, only 20 percent of the children were considered to be proficient in throwing while improvement tended to become more rapid after this time so that 74 percent were rated as proficient between the ages of 5 and 5½ years and the percentage increased to 84 by the sixth year. Wide variations in skill level among the children were observed at all ages, with judgments ranging from very awkward to highly proficient even at 6 years when a relatively high level of skill had been attained.

A more objective measure of throwing ability is the distance the individual is able to throw objects of certain sizes. This type of testing procedure was used by Wellman (1937) to assess the "motor ages" at which 98 children were able to throw two balls, one of 9½-inch circumference and the other 16¼-inch circumference. Her results are recorded in table 8.4.

TABLE 8.4. Ball-throwing achievements of preschool children*

	Motor Age in Months	
Distance of Throw Feet	Small Ball (9 1/2 inches)	Large Ball (16 1/4 inches)
4 to 5	30	30
6 to 7	33	43
8 to 9	44	53
10 to 11	52	63
12 to 13	57	above 72
14 to 15	65	
16 to 17	above 72	

* From Beth L. Wellman, Motor achievements of preschool children. *Child. Educ.*, 1937, 13, 311–316. Reprinted by permission of the association for Childhood Education International, 3615 Wisconsin Avenue, N.W., Washington, D.C.

An exhaustive study was made by Wild (1938) of development of throwing behavior in which the combinations of movement patterns of the arms and body were analyzed by means of cinematographic records taken of children during the performance of a throw. Although the study was of the cross-sectional type, the children at each age level were carefully selected on the basis of the achievement of normal physical, motor, mental, and personality development at the time of the study. This selection involved a total of 32 children comprising a boy and a girl at each 6-month-age level within the age range of 2 to 7 years. Each subject was asked to perform three overhand throws which were filmed and subsequently carefully analyzed (figures 8.9 and 8.10).

Analysis of the data revealed four distinct types of throws which appeared to be closely associated with particular age groups. The least mature type of throw predominates at the ages of 2 and 3 and involves movements of the arm and body which are confined mainly to the anterioposterior plane. In starting the first phase of this throwing pattern, the

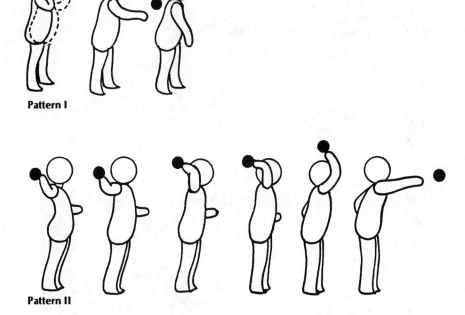

Pattern I

Pattern II

FIGURE 8.9. *Overhand throw. Pattern I: 2–3 years. Little force to anterioposterior action. Pattern II: 3½–5 years. More force to anterioposterior action. (Redrawn from Wild, M. The Behavior Pattern of Throwing and Some Observations Concerning Its Course of Development in Children. Doctoral Dissertation. University of Wisconsin, Madison, 1937.)*

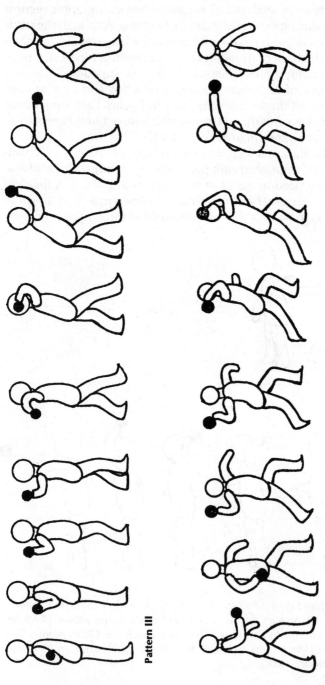

Pattern III

FIGURE 8.10. *Overhand throw. Pattern III: 5–6 years. Horizontal arm action and step forward on ipsilateral foot. Pattern IV: 6½ years and older. Horizontal arm action; trunk rotation; and step forward on contralateral foot. (Redrawn from Wild, M. The Behavior Pattern of Throwing and Some Observations Concerning Its Course of Development in Children. Doctoral Dissertation. University of Wisconsin, Madison, 1937.)*

arm is drawn up either frontally or obliquely with a corresponding extension of the trunk until the object to be thrown is at a point high above the shoulders. With the delivery, the trunk straightens with a forward carry of the shoulders as the arm comes through fairly stiffly in a downward motion. During the entire throw, both feet remain firmly in place and the body facing toward the direction of the throw is also maintained.

The second pattern of throw was typical of the 3½- to 5-year age range and was distinguished from the first type of throw by the execution of both the arm and the body movements in a horizontal plane rather than the previously used anterioposterior plane. Although the feet continue to remain together and in place during the entire throw, rotation of the body is first to the right in preparing to throw and then to the left as the ball is delivered with the right hand. The arm action is slightly flatter than the previous arm pattern but greater in force attained from the forward and downward follow-through.

The most conspicuous change in pattern during the fifth and sixth years involves the introduction of a step forward with the right foot as the ball is delivered with the right hand. This marks the third stage. In the preparatory phase of the throw, the weight is retained on the left, or rear, foot while the body is rotated to the right and the arm is brought obliquely upward and over the shoulder so that it is in a flexed and retracted position. During delivery, the child steps forward on the right foot while the body rotates to the left and the arm swings forward in either an oblique or lateral movement about the shoulder joint. Upon completion of the throw, the body facing is partially to the left in contrast to the earlier forward facing in the preceding throwing patterns.

The mature throwing pattern is the fourth in the sequence identified by Wild and was used by all the boys in this study of 6½ years and older. Again the main change from the preceding pattern is in the use of the base of support to provide opposition of movement so that greater power can be obtained from the throw. In this instance, the weight is transferred to the right foot during the preparatory phase and the left foot moves forward and receives the weight during the delivery phase of the throw. Such action enables a marked trunk rotation to occur and this, coupled with the horizontal adduction of the arm during the forward swing, enables the child to achieve the maximal use of body leverage for attaining speed at the most distal segment, in this instance, the hand. Although the boys achieved the adult pattern of overhand throw, the girls in Wild's study did not progress beyond the third stage in either arm or foot action or both. It is not uncommon for even adult women never to achieve the mature overhand throw pattern although it is usually found in skilled females.

In general, Wild (1938) concluded that there were two main developmental trends in the sequential movement patterns of throwing: namely, (1) the gradual shift of movements from a predominantly anteri-oposterior plane to a horizontal plane; and (2) the transition from the use of an unchanging base of support to a shifting base on the same side as the throwing arm followed by the transference of weight in a much more stable and functional arm-foot opposition relationship. Wild further noted that each of the successive throwing patterns exhibited a more effective means of mechanical projection on the basis of marked increase in the ability to develop acceleration in the ball.

The stability of the throwing pattern over repeated trials was investi-gated by Roberton (1977) through an examination of the filmed records of 10 successive overhand throws by 73 first-grade children. Analysis was in terms of arm action categories and pelvic-spinal categories with the observed frequencies of occurrence being recorded. For the children in this study, 52 percent were completely consistent across all trials in their arm category and the average modal category contained 8.97 trials. The frequency distribution for modal categories of pelvic-spinal action was similar to that of arm action with the children also averaging 8.9 trials within their modal category. The results of this component analysis of the overhand throw indicated to the investigator that development within component parts may proceed at different rates within the same individ-ual or at different rates in different individuals. Moreover, the degree of stability of performance of the component parts may vary within any one individual and is different for each individual.

Gender differences for 5-year-olds in the overarm throw for distance were examined by Nelson et al. (1986) in terms of various biological and environmental variables. The results indicated that boys threw further than girls and were rated as having more mature trunk rotation and foot action. The correlation between distance throw and trunk rotation was .67 and between throw and foot action was .64. Of the seven biological variables, boys were significantly better only in greater joint diameters (sum of elbow and knee) and had smaller sum of four skinfolds (triceps, subscapular, iliac, and calf) than girls. In the other measures they did not differ significantly but when the slightly longer boys' arm length and the boys' greater shoulder/hip ratios were added to the discriminate regres-sion equation, which also included the joint diameter and skinfold mea-sures, these biological variables became significant discriminators. The unadjusted comparison of throwing performance indicated girls' per-formance was only 57 percent of that of boys but adjustments for a linear composite of the biological variables increased girls' throwing perfor-mance to 69 percent of the boys' distance. Of the environmental variable, only the fact that boys played more with other children significantly dis-criminated between gender. On the basis of their results, these investigators concluded that some of the gender differences in throwing performance appear to reflect biological characteristics even as early as 5 years of age.

CATCHING

The child has become very proficient in reaching for and grasping stationary objects by the time he is 2 years old but moving objects require adjustments for, and some understanding of, time-space relationships before any proficiency is achieved in catching them. Attempts at stopping a rolling ball or other moving objects can be considered to be initial attempts at catching. Perhaps the most successful of these early attempts at catching occurs when a ball is rolled toward the child as it is seated on the floor with legs spread apart. The ball may then be stopped by the hands or corralled by the legs fairly readily. With sufficient practice the child will gradually be able to synchronize the movements of the arms with the speed of the ball and the hands can then reach around the ball and stop it.

A ball tossed into the air is influenced by the effects of gravity so that catching an aerial ball presents a more complicated task than the relatively simpler adjustments to variations in speed and direction in the horizontal plane such as is characteristic of a rolling ball. The first attempts at catching an aerial ball usually consist of simply holding the arms stiffly out-stretched in front of the body. Little or no effort is made to move the body to adjust to the flight of the ball and, even when the toss lands directly on the arms, their stiffness or delayed shoveling action usually results in failure to retain possession of the ball. Gradually the child begins to develop a sense of timing and the arms are relaxed slightly so that tosses directly into the arms are scooped up against the body with the arms and hands working as a unit. Very gradually, also, the child begins to be able to judge and adjust to increasingly greater deviations in the position of the aerial ball and will move his body to try to get into the most favorable catching position (figures 8.11 and 8.12).

With increasing age, the catching pattern changes to one in which the elbows are still kept in front of the body but the hands are positioned in opposition to one another in a similar manner to the position of the jaws in a vise. Gradually this pattern gives way to the mature form where the elbows are to the sides of the body and the hands are cupped with either the thumbs or little fingers together, depending upon the position of the ball, to receive the ball. The arms at the sides position allows for a greater degree of "give" in arm movement in absorbing the force of the ball. As with throwing, some girls never acquire the mature two-handed

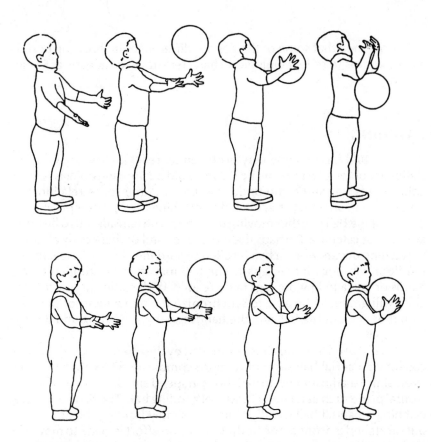

FIGURE 8.11. *Upper: Unsuccessful attempt to catch a large ball which shows apprehension by turning the head to the side and by leaning backward slightly. The arm action, which is quite common, frequently causes the hands to strike the ball and knock it upward. Lower: A 33-month-old boy extends his arms before the ball is tossed. He waits for the ball without moving, responds after the ball has touched his hands, and then he gently traps it against his chest. It is essentially a robot-like performance. (Reprinted from Ralph L. Wickstrom,* Fundamental Motor Patterns. *Third Edition. Philadelphia: Lea & Febiger, 1983. By permission of the publisher.)*

catching pattern and tend to use the vise positioning of the hands to catch the ball, although the predominating trend involves arms at the side of the body. Depending upon the size of the object, variations such as one-handed catching are attempted as soon as some confidence is achieved in judgment of speed and direction.

The relatively slow acquisition of catching skills is illustrated by the findings of a study by Wellman (1937) with the same size small and large

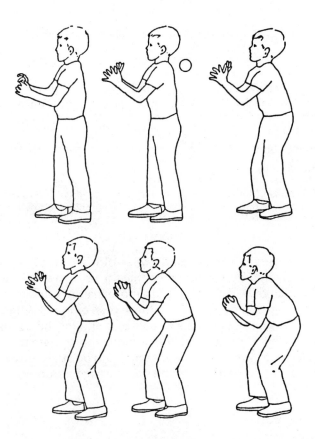

FIGURE 8.12. *The form used by a 5-year-old boy to make an effective hand catch of a ball thrown softly from a short distance. (Reprinted from Ralph L. Wickstrom,* Fundamental Motor Patterns. *Third Edition. Philadelphia: Lea & Febiger, 1983. By permission of the publisher.)*

balls that were used for throwing (table 8.5). As may be expected, skill is attained at a certain level of performance with the large ball before the same level is achieved with the small ball. In general, proficiency in catching is achieved by only 29 percent of 4-year-olds, 56 percent of 5-year-olds, while at 6 years the proportion has increased to only 63 percent (Guttridge, 1939).

In an examination of ball catching proficiency among 4-, 6-, and 8-year-old girls, Du Randt (1985) reports that age, ball size, and ball flight trajectory; the interaction of age and ball flight trajectory; and the interaction of ball size and ball flight trajectory all significantly influenced ball-catching ability among all three age groups. On the basis of her data, Du Randt estimated that the average percentages of balls that might be

TABLE 8.5. Ball catching achievements of preschool children*

Method of Catching the Ball (Success in 2 or 3 trials)	Motor Age in Months	
	Larger Ball (16 1/4 inches)	Small Ball (9 1/2 inches)
Arms straight	34	37
Elbows in front of body	44	50
Elbows at side of body	68	—

* From Beth L. Wellman, Motor achievements of preschool children. *Child. Educ.*, 1937, 13, 311–316. Reprinted by permission of the association for Childhood Education International, 3615 Wisconsin Avenue, N.W., Washington, D.C.

expected to be caught by 4-, 6-, and 8-year-olds are more or less 20, 40, and 80, respectively. She also observed that the use of a small ball (tennis ball size) stimulated the occurrence of a more mature catching response in the older age groupings but not in the 4-year-olds. In addition, a low flight trajectory is more favorable to ball-catching for the youngest age group whereas the medium trajectory is more appropriate for the older age groupings. The older age groupings may also be expected to advance to higher trajectories sooner than the younger age grouping.

BALL-BOUNCING

Ball-bouncing has its origins in the casual or deliberate dropping of the ball to cause it to bounce. From this simple, single bounce a very gradual improvement occurs in the number of times a child is able to tap the ball until control is lost or the taps no longer impart enough force to the ball for it to bounce to any reasonable height. The mature, multiple, controlled bounce requires that the proportionate size of the hand and ball are such that some control over direction is forthcoming in the placement of the hand in the relation to the center of mass of the ball. Furthermore, the hand should meet the ball on the upward portion of the bounce for a maximum contact period rather than "chase" the ball when on its downward path as is typical of the unskilled performer (figure 8.13).

Although the two-hand bounce would seem to offer advantages in that a bigger hand surface is available for contact, and hence control, of the ball and more force could also be applied to the ball, it is in fact inferior to the one-hand bounce in that the use of two hands restricts the positioning of the ball in relationship to the body to a position directly in front of the body. Furthermore, the time of contact and the amount of

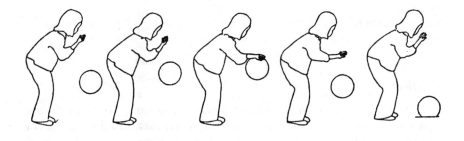

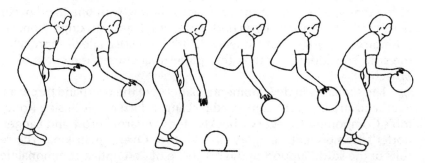

FIGURE 8.13. *Upper: Hitting motion that is characteristic of unskilled dribbling. Lower: Skilled form in stationary dribbling. The pushing action is clearly demonstrated. (Reprinted from Ralph L. Wickstrom,* Fundamental Motor Patterns. *Third Edition. Philadelphia: Lea & Febiger, 1983. By permission of the publisher.)*

force exerted by each hand must be extremely concise and well-synchronized for the achievement of any degree of control over the direction of the ball. Therefore, it is not surprising that the one-hand multiple bounce is mastered by children prior to a two-hand bounce.

However, the size of the ball in relation to the size of the hand is an important consideration in the development of ball-bouncing. In addition, children do not have the strength to bounce a large ball with one hand as soon as they are able to bounce a small ball. A small ball of 9½-inch circumference can be bounced a distance of one to three feet at approximately 27 months using one hand and the distance is increased to four to five feet by the age of 40 months. Bouncing a larger ball with a circumference of 16¼ inches is mastered first with both hands where a distance of four to five feet is achieved by 46 months. However, bouncing the larger ball with one hand presents problems of control as well as sufficient strength for the young child and it is not until approximately 71 months of age, or 44 months after bouncing a small ball for a distance of one to three feet, that the child is able to bounce a large ball a similar distance using one hand (Wellman, 1937).

STRIKING

Striking develops from a throw action in the anteriuposterior plane and is generally associated with anger or resentment on the part of the infant. It is not unusual to see angry children throw "nothing" at each other or even at an adult. Gradually such action is restricted to situations in which contact can be achieved with an object, but the type of contact has the texture of a push rather than an actual hit. The overhand arm action tends to be used at the time actual hitting with one hand occurs but is gradually replaced by an underarm, or sidearm, striking action. The position of the object does, however, influence the angle of approach of the arm. The addition of the other patterns augments the range of approach.

The similarity in developmental patterns in the overhand throw and overhand striking were compared by Langendorfer (1987) using Roberton's Component Category Checklist for Overarm Throw and Langendorfer's Component Category Checklist for Overarm Striking. The results of the study supported the existence of descriptive commonalities across the changing levels of several motor sequences within the two tasks. The relevant component sequences with their levels are: a) trunk action (no rotation; spinal or block rotation; and differentiated rotation); b) humerous action (oblique humerous; aligned but independent; and lagging humerous); and c) forearm action in throwing and racquet action in striking (no forearm or racquet lag; forearm or racquet lag; and delayed forearm or racquet lag). For these component sequences, there was evidence that most subjects moved synchronously in the primitive levels of the two skills. However, the commonalities across levels within the motor sequences of the different skills also demonstrated pronounced temporal asynchronies, especially at the intermediate and advanced levels of each sequence. The results also showed a lack of support for horizontal structure in stepping action (no step; ipsilateral step; contralateral step; and long contralateral step) across throwing and striking. On the basis of his results, Langendorfer suggested that developmental status may be characterized as relatively generalized at primitive levels and in intermediate levels but more specialized at advanced levels.

A study by Halverson and Roberton (1966) shows that—at the age of 3 years—a directional goal such as "Can you hit the ball to your dad?" elicits a sidearm striking pattern with a light plastic paddle when a tennis ball is suspended at waist-high level. Furthermore, at this same age, children can successfully contact a softly tossed aerial ball with a one-hand sidearm swing but experience difficulty in contact using a two-handed sidearm swing for, although the pattern is well-defined, the swing is initiated too early. In general, well-defined sidearm striking patterns are used by children beginning at approximately 3 years of age as long as successful contact is achieved. However, substitution of a less mature form of pattern or of another pattern is almost immediately made when failure results under stress, the problem is beyond the ability of the youngster, or the equipment is too long or heavy. Children of this age also appear to experience less difficulty in contacting a ball tossed with an underhand pattern than one with an overarm pattern even when the velocity of the toss is as constant as possible. This type of experience is limited for children of this age since the cooperation of an adult is required. It assumes importance in the peer group when the child becomes of school age.

SWIMMING

One of the earliest ages at which training in swimming has been attempted was undertaken by McGraw (1935) in her experiments with Johnny and Jimmy, the former being the twin receiving training while the latter received no training. Instruction in swimming for Johnny was begun when he was 231 days, or approximately 8 months old, with the aid of a strap support to prevent his complete submersion so that he was able to hold his head out of the water. However, lowering the supporting strap so that greater use could be made of the arms revealed that Johnny preferred to swim with his face under the water. Therefore, at the age of 290 days, or around 9½ months, Johnny was submerged without artificial support and by the time he was 17 months old was able to swim from 12 to 15 feet, which was the distance permitted by one breath.

Observations of primitive children who are allowed to play in the water from early infancy indicate that there are few, if any, who are not able to swim well at 5 years (Mead, 1930). Some recent work with preschool children indicates that it is not unusual for 3-year-olds to develop reasonably good swimming skills and it is possible that there may be real advantages with regard to physique for the introduction of swimming at this time. Rarick (1954) points out that the remaining baby fat would tend to add to the bouyancy of these younger children and the short legs would reduce drag. Furthermore, the early introduction of swimming would preclude, or offer less opportunity for, the development of negative attitudes to water which become more dominant as the child becomes older. However, when observed in situations without formal instruction, children under five years of age seem to prefer to splash and play in the water with little concern for learning to swim, whereas after this age interest in learning to swim increases greatly as does the rate of progress in learning to swim.

OTHER ACTIVITIES

Once the child has learned to walk, most of his physical activities during the next four years are concerned with play, to the extent that investigators in the field of child development consider play to be the most important business of childhood. Toys are, at one and the same time, the instruments of play and the tools by which children develop their gross and fine motor abilities. Kawin (1934) has classified toys on the basis of five types of play situations in which they can be used and suggests that an adequate selection of each type of toy is vital to the development of the child in each of the five areas. Selections should, therefore, include:

1. Toys for developing bodily strength and growth in a variety of physical skills;
2. Creative constructive toys, such as blocks, clay, hammers, nails, and saws;
3. Toys for dramatization and imitation, such as miniature houses, automobiles, stores, forts, and farms;
4. Toys emphasizing the artistic, such as toy musical and rhythmic instruments, and art and handicraft materials;
5. Toys for promoting intellectual development which might include animal or bird games, anagrams, map puzzles, and travel games.

Early toy preferences, based upon parental recall of their child's toy preferences, was examined by Thomas (1984) for a group of 4-year-old readers and nonreaders. According to the parents' reports, there were significant differences in the toy preferences of the two groups with the readers reported as playing, enjoying, and valuing reading readiness toys, such as books and alphabet cards, significantly more than nonreaders. On other hand, nonreaders preferred gross motor, construction, and fantasy toys significantly more than 4-year-old readers. As the groups had been matched for sex, family background, and the General Cognitive Index Score on the McCarthy Scales of Children's Abilities, Thomas concluded that the results indicated that early readers cannot be differentiated by IQ or family demographic information alone and that consistent toy preferences precede the acquisition of early reading skills.

Children tend to respond to different play materials in a different manner at various age levels. Between the ages of 2 and 6 years the most frequently used indoor play materials are, according to Van Alystne

(1932), blocks, clay, and doll-corner materials. Furthermore, children tend to use the same materials in different ways with advancing years, indicating a continuity of preference for favorite toys which points to a recommendation of a smaller number of well-selected, durable toys in preference to a large number of limited-use, easily broken toys. From the previous discussion of throwing, catching, bouncing, kicking, and striking, it is quite obvious that balls are also a favorite toy of children of this age and have many uses as well as being reasonably durable.

Wheel toys are very popular and extensively used by children when available. These include the push and pull type of toy, the kiddie car, wagon, tricycle, roller skates, and bicycle. Recently a large number of the push and pull type of toys have become battery operated, which, although they may create an incentive for the child to chase the toy, do remove a great deal of the opportunity for using the back and leg muscles for propulsive power as well as reducing the exploratory learnings of the child into the manner in which such propulsive force has to be applied. Fortunately the larger wheel toys still allow such developmental opportunities until late childhood when the mechanized go-cart again is a temptation.

An extensive investigation of the developmental sequences which occur during the process of learning to operate a wagon has been made by Jones (1939). He noted that children of 21 to 26 months will manipulate the parts of the wagon and push it back and forth repeatedly in an unskilled manner. The next two months may see the child getting into the wagon in the typical propulsive position with one knee on the wagon bed and the other on the ground but no effort is made to propel the wagon. Subsequent to this period and until the 36th month, practicing of the propelling skill is undertaken in the typical propulsion position. There is a gradual unification of the skills involved into an increasingly skillful pattern so that by the time the child is 4 years old the specific skills of propelling and manipulating a wagon are well established. The child then is able to operate in terms of ideas he wishes to effect rather than simply concentrating on the motor act involved in the operation of the wagon.

Similar behavioral changes have been observed in children learning to ride tricycles. If children have been exposed to wheel toys from an early age, it is not surprising to find them showing a marked facility in their operation, and under these circumstances, 2-year-old youngsters may exhibit considerable skill in handling tricycles, being able to steer, back, and manage sharp turns with speed and accuracy. In general, most children can ride a tricycle proficiently at 3 years of age and it is not infrequent for youngsters of this age to have some ability in the management of two-wheeled scooters; reasonable skill in the operation of foot-operated automobiles is achieved by the age of 4 years. Bicycle riding is usually an achievement of later childhood when the child is more capable of handling the vehicle in traffic. Children of 5 and 6 can ride small bicycles, however, if they have the opportunity to do so.

Although Johnny was trained by McGraw (1935) to roller-skate at 2 years, it is more usual for children of 5 and 6 years to attain some proficiency in roller-skating if they are given adequate opportunity to practice. Similarly, in cold climates, ice-skating is an activity in which some degree of mastery is possible at this age level and bob sleds, toboggans, and skis replace wagons and tricycles in the snowy, winter months.

BALANCE

As with the acquisition of walking, running, and jumping and the numerous locomotor variations of these skills, the problem of balance is vitally important in the acquiring of skill in roller-skating, ice-skating, skiing, and operating two-wheeled vehicles. The development of balance itself has been the subject of numerous studies. The complexity of balance and the wide range of ability from one age level to another has resulted in very low intercorrelations between various measures of balance and no single measure of balance has been generally accepted as indicative of balance performance over a wide age range.

Static balance, as measured by balancing on either foot as long as possible, was used by Morris et al. (1982) to assess performance of 3- to 6-year-old children and improvements in balancing ability were noted at each successive age level for both sexes. Balancing ability was slightly better for girls at ages 3 and 4; similar for the sexes at 5 years; but significantly better for the girls than boys at 6 years of age although the girls were also more variable in balancing ability at this age. A stabilometer was used by Erbaugh (1984) to measure static balance in 3- and 4-year-old children and she also related balancing performance to anthropometric measures of body size, body composition, and somatotype. Regression analysis indicated that five physical growth measures (height/age; biacromial diameter; abdominal circumference; fat area/arm area; and ectomorphy) accounted for 28 percent of the variation in performance on the stabilometer test.

Dynamic balance, which is the ability to maintain balance while moving, is usually measured by performance on a walking board or balance beam. An elevated beam, on which performance was scored on the basis of distance traversed on the beam divided by the time, was used as a dynamic balance measure in the Erbaugh (1984) study. Regression analysis was also used to determine the association between dynamic balancing ability and the physical growth measures with the result that 55 percent of the performance variance on the elevated balance beam test was accounted for by seven physical growth measures (estimated leg length/

tibial length; foot length; abdominal circumference; chest circumference; foot breadth; leg muscle area; and ectomorphy). Erbaugh noted that, for performance in dynamic and static balance, physical growth independently explained a significant percentage of performance variation which could not be explained by age and sex. In addition, it was found that the relationships between age, sex, and stability performances were similar to those reported in previous research; i.e., dynamic stability performance improved with age and there is little evidence of sex differences.

Erbaugh (1984) reports that the relationship between the elevated beam measure of dynamic balance and the stabilometer measure of static balance was only .13 and concludes the relationship between physical growth and performance on the two tests was different because two types of balance were tested. Little or no relationship is generally reported between measures of static and dynamic balance. Similarly, relationships among various static balance tests and among various dynamic balance tests are frequently low due, in part, to administrative differences. For example, although the walking board has been used over a wide age range as a measure of dynamic balance, differences in the size of the board, manner of scoring, and general procedures have been such that comparisons of results obtained by different investigators is often not feasible. In general, developmental sequences of dynamic balance and age placement of the various levels obtained by Bayley using a walking board 2.5 meters long, 6 cm wide, and 10 cm high are typical of those obtained by other investigators (table 8.6).

The balance subtest items of the Bruininks-Oseretsky Test of Motor Proficiency were used by Ulrich and Ulrich (1985) to measure balancing

TABLE 8.6. Dynamic balance on a walking board*

	Age in Months
Tries to stand on walking board	22.5
Walking with one foot on board	27.6
Standing on board with both feet	31.0
Attempts to step	32.8
Alternates feet part way	38.0
Alternates feet full length	56.0
Length in 6 to 9 seconds	59.5
Length in 3 to 5 seconds	66.0
Length in less than 3 seconds	80.0

* From Nancy Bayley, A scale of motor development. Institute of Child Welfare, University of California, Berkeley. Used by permission.

ability of 3-, 4-, and 5-year-old children. In addition, these children were assessed on their developmental level in six fundamental gross motor skills (overhand throw, kick, strike, horizontal jump, hop, and skip). When these data were analyzed, a linear relationship was found among all three ages for developmental level scores for the fundamental skills of throwing, kicking, striking, and hopping. Boys were significantly more advanced than girls in throwing, kicking, and striking whereas girls were significantly more proficient in skipping than boys. Balancing ability was found to be significantly related to developmental levels in hopping on the preferred and nonpreferred foot, jumping, and striking. However, balance accounted for only a small proportion of the variance in the developmental levels of those fundamental skills to which it was significantly related.

INTEGRATIVE ASPECTS

During the period of late childhood, objective measures of basic motor skills reveal little difference between the sexes except in the throw for distance. There has been considerable speculation that the performance differences that do exist between boys and girls at this level may be a product of socio-cultural milieu; the relatively high degree of variability in performance level within any one sex may be considered to support this point of view. However, examinations of individual variability indicate that this aspect of performance may be conditioned by a number of factors. An investigation of relative intraindividual variability, which is the ratio of the intraindividual variability over the mean, indicates that developmental variability in reaction time may be mediated by maturational components as there are only minor changes in relative intraindividual variability with age (Eckert & Eichorn, 1977). On the other hand, a learning component is exemplified by skill acquisition in tasks such as the **pursuit rotor** where relative intraindividual variability decreases with age and increases with task complexity at any specific age level (Eckert, 1974).

The nature and degree of variability is a vital aspect of development, learning, and performance. Bruner (1973) has defined the development of skilled action as the construction of serially ordered acts whose performance is modified towards less variability, more anticipation, and greater economy of effort. On the other hand, Fiske and Rice (1955) have emphasized that "not only must the individual respond differently to different situations but he must also vary his response to the same situation in order to adapt, i.e., to improve his adjustment to the situation." Statistical analysis of objective data using relative intraindividual variability would seem to accommodate the hypotheses of Bruner (skilled performance is less variable) and of Fiske and Rice (need to vary to improve) with respect to specific tasks. However, this statistical model has not been tested in analysis of performance where the individual must respond differently to different situations nor has it been tested with respect to pattern development in skill acquisition.

In her examination of the stability of the overhand throw, Roberton (1977) tested the hypothesis that children would be more consistent in early stages of throwing due to the availability of limited movement patterns and have more movement patterns available with increasing age. However, as the child reached advanced stages there would be an increasing tendency for the child to use the most successful option under stable conditions. Thus, the consistent movers would be found to be using primitive or advanced stages of arm action in the throwing pattern. This hypothesis was supported by the data for the earlier and intermediate patterns, but the small number of subjects with advanced pattern prohibited statistical confirmation. Longitudinal collection of similar data (Roberton, 1978) gives promise of resolving further aspects associated with pattern development.

Flavell (1970) believes that an individual interacts with his environment by breaking it down and organizing it into meaningful patterns congruent with his own needs and psychological make-up. The orderliness of pattern development for basic motor skills would seem to support the theoretical conclusion of Bruner (1973) that a great deal of the orderliness of early skilled behavior comes from internal biological sources and is shaped, but not constructed, by the environment. Gardener (1965) defines skill as "the putting together of simple natural movements, of which we have only about two hundred, in unusual and complex combinations to achieve a given objective." If this definition is accepted, then the meaningful patterns could be the two hundred simple natural movements. However, during the early phases of skill development, many of the simple natural movements are still being developed or modified and Gardener's definition does not account for the mechanism whereby these simple natural movements are put together in unusual or complex combinations to achieve a given objective.

Attempts to identify common aspects of movement have been of concern to researchers and practioners as such identification could greatly simplify recognition and remediation of movement problems. Fleishman's identification (1964) of 11 factors from more than 200 psychomotor tasks administered to thousands of subjects in a series of interlocking studies would seem to indicate that a considerable amount of communality, as reflected in the 11 factors, exists in psychomotor tasks. An additional investigation by Fleishman (1964) of 30 physical performance tests resulted in the identification of nine factors. After analyzing the filmed records of 18 fundamental movement tasks for children, aged 2 to 6 years, C. B. Sinclair (1971) identified the following seven characteristics: dynamic balance; opposition and symmetry; total body assembly; rhythmic locomotion; eye-hand efficiency; agility; and postural adjustment. Factor analysis was used by Rarick and Dobbins (1975) to extract six basic components from 47 motor performance and physical growth measures obtained on children ranging in age from 6 to 9.9 years. The six factors that accounted for a major portion of the variance in both sexes were tentatively identified as: 1) strength-power-body size; 2) gross limb-eye coordination; 3) fine visual motor coordination; 4) fat or dead weight; 5) balance; 6) and leg power and coordination.

These studies indicate that communalities or basic components of performance can be identified on the basis of either performance scores or analysis of movement characteristics. If the communalities inherent in a factor can be translated into concepts, then it becomes feasible to identify such factorial concepts in terms of the basic physical components (or invariants) of object, space, time, and causality concepts as presented in chapter 7. Bruner (1973) has defined skilled action as the construction of serially-ordered skilled-action and in this regard is in accord with the definition of Gardener. According to Bruner (1973), skill acquisition, following the initial preadapted stages, suggests a capacity for appropriate construction of skilled behavior, and the role of learning is to shape and correct these constructions to meet the idiosyncratic nature of particular tasks encountered. Eckert's proposed theoretical model (1965), i.e., the development of a standard of maximal available strength as a mediator of tasks involving volitional muscle action, can readily be expanded to accommodate Bruner's model of construction of skilled behavior when it is considered as a construct standards model. In addition, the standards theoretical model can incorporate the basic physical components of object, space, time, and causality concepts in terms of each individual's personal standard of motoric capabilities.

The construct standards model is appropriate not only for the developmental changes occurring during early childhood but is applicable to motor performance at all age levels. For example, if the reader is asked to move an iron bar, there is an assessment of the individual's strength in terms of the individual's concept of the weight of the object. The reader has obviously developed a concept (or standard) of maximal available strength and utilizes this individually specific standard to assess ability to move the known or estimated weight of the iron bar. Although the term "standard" is used, the construct standards model does not assume a fixed standard but only the standard that is used at the time of assessent. The standard is subject to fluctuation and to readjustment. For example, an individual who has been bedridden for a period of time must readjust the strength standard as bed rest is debilitating. Moreover, the trained athlete tends to have less fluctuation in standard assessment than does the untrained athlete, and this accounts for the reduction in variability and greater economy of effort associated with more precise assessment in the activity for which the athlete has trained.

The construct standards model is supported not only by examples of precision in adjustments to idiosyncratic demands of a task but also by improper adjustment due to irregularities which do not conform to established standards. For example, an individual who is asked to lift a block of wood tends to assess the amount of force required to lift the wooden block on the basis of previously constructed standards of size, shape, and composition (i.e., wood and not iron). The more experience the individual has had in developing these standards the more accurate the individual tends to be. However, there are irregularities in the weight of wood with balsa wood being much lighter than hardwoods and, in instances where the individual does not have much experience with wood texture and graining or where these are obscured, that individual will invariably exert too much force in lifting the wood. In this instance, the standards upon which force assesssments were made were either erroneous or incomplete information was provided.

Experiments by Held (1965) indicate that movement experiences are vital to the development of a spatial orientation and that the plasticity of the sensory-motor systems allows for learning adaptations. Observations of newborn infants for a total of eight hours each during the two days following birth indicated that the 14 males exhibited significantly greater scores in low-intensity motor and facial activity and were awake more than the 15 females in the study (Phillips et al., 1978). Heart rate monitoring of the activities of prepubescent children, aged 6 to 7 years, indicated that boys are more physically active than girls (Gilliam et al., 1981). The work of Rosenzweig et al. (1972) with rats in enriched and impoverished environments wherein the environmentally enriched rats displayed more favorable brain changes would indicate that an enriched neural system is associated with an enriched environment. Keogh (1971), after observing that third- and fourth-grade boys were superior to girls in ability to make patterns by walking in an expanded spatial field, attributed the observed sex difference to greater experience of males in such situations. If spatial orientation can be assumed to be a construct, then the results of these investigations may be interpreted as indicating that enriched environmental experience enhances the development of a spatial construct and the breadth of environmental experiences would increase the precision of construct standard assessments for idiosyncratic situations. Using this model, it may be possible to explain the sex difference in throwing on the basis of enriched spatial experiences for boys. These experiences develop an enriched spatial construct thereby encouraging young boys to experiment more readily with modifications to available throwing patterns to develop the increasing lever involvement, and hence more force, that are necessary for maximal distance in an overhand throw.

The stability of movement patterns reported by Roberton (1977) in primitive throwers may not be only a reflection of the limited movement patterns available but also of the more primitive level of spatial construct development. On the other hand, the relatively greater variability of the intermediate stage throwers could be indicative of an expanded spatial construct and the experimental adjustments of the child to meet that expanded construct. The greater stability noted for advanced throwers under stable conditions can be considered to reflect the development of a fairly stable spatial construct standard as well as the selection of the most successful option for that situation. It would appear, then, that some consideration should be given to the conceptual understandings of the child in addition to the analysis of overt actions and patternings of motor development.

If the construct standards model proves viable in terms of future investigations of intellectual and motor development, then the identification of the constructs central to motor performance could enhance potential ability to assist those children who either have been deprived in their environmental experiences or lack facility in developing constructs appropriate to good motor performance. It is extremely important that the child develop adequate levels of motor performance during infancy and early childhood as this is the period encompassing the greatest changes in pattern development for the basic motor skills. The facility of an individual in the basic motor skills has a tremendous impact upon the individual's willingness to participate in motor activities. Moreover, it has been well documented that physiological functioning is influenced by the degree of physical activity participation. Therefore, the degree to which the individual masters the basic motor skills has the potential of influencing the individual's life style and affecting the health of that individual as it relates to physiological functioning.

GENERAL MOTOR DEVELOPMENT

The tendency for certain phases in the developmental sequence to be achieved by children at approximately the same time has led a number of investigators to develop motor scales of performance indicating normative behavior in a wide variety of activities. The California Infant Scale of Motor Development, published in 1936 and based upon a somewhat select group of approximately 50 children, is indicative of this type of scale, which attempts to assess a general motor development rather than separate the various skills as has been done in the foregoing discussion (table 8.7).

Although no distinction is generally made in the motor performance of boys and girls in most activities during infancy and early childhood because the differences are not very great, there are some events in which one sex tends to exceed the performance of the other in either maturity of pattern development or in objective measure. In the case of reports involving pattern development or subjective rating of skill level, there will, in the very nature of such procedures, be a substantial variability in the criteria of judgment so that this type of study will more frequently report sex differences. In one such investigation of skill levels of children ages 2 to 7 years, girls are reported as tending to excel in hopping, skipping, and galloping while boys are superior in jumping and throwing (Guttridge, 1939). A cinematographic study of children, aged 2 through 6 years, of the performance of throwing, catching, kicking, striking, and ball-bouncing indicated that the boys were about one year in advance of the girls in pattern development and showed greater ability to move with an integrated body pattern in all activities except the multiple ball bounce (Deach, 1951).

The analysis of filmed records of 18 fundamental movement tasks for 2 through 6-year-old children by C. B. Sinclair (1971) indicated girls had higher movement scores in jumping, rhythmic locomotion, and balance at about age 4 or later whereas boys scored higher in catching and in

TABLE 8.7. California Infant Scale of Motor Development*

Months	
16.5	Walks sideways
16.9	Walks backwards—several steps
20.3	Walks upstairs with help
24.3	Walks upstairs alone—marks time
28.0	Jumps off floor—both feet
29.2	Stands on one foot alone
30.1	Walks on tiptoe
32.1	Jumps from chair—16 cm high
35.5	Walks upstairs—alternating forward foot
37.3	Distance jump—10 to 35 cm
49.3	Hop on one foot—2 or 3 hops

* Excerpts from Nancy Bayley, *The California Infant Scale of Motor Development*. Berkeley: University of California Press, 1936. By permission of the publisher.

those tasks requiring strength and speed. The greatest sex difference occurred in throwing where boys scored higher than girls at age 3 years and at succeeding ages with the observed sex differences being attributed in part to the social environment.

Preschool children were examined by Broadhead and Church (1985) in gross movement tasks (throwing, catching, jumping, hopping, skipping, standing still, and balancing) and in fine movement tasks (matching, building, cutting, copying shapes, copying letters, touching fingers, and clapping hands). Significant linear trends for age occurred for all fine and gross motor tasks. In addition significant sex differences favoring girls occurred for hopping, skipping, copying letters, touching fingers, and clapping hands. Significant racial differences were also observed with black children being better in jumping, hopping, and skipping and white children better in catching, standing still, balancing, and in five of the fine motor tasks.

With a view to developing quantitative norms, Morris and three of her associates (1978) at the University of Arizona administered seven motor performance test items to 269 boys and girls aged 3 to 6 years. The test items were: catching, scramble, speed run, standing long jump, tennis ball throw for distance, softball throw for distance, and balance. The investigators found that boys were superior to girls at all age levels for all the motor performance items except balance in which the girls were superior. In general, the boys' performance scores appeared to be equal to those of girls who were in an age group one year older than the boys. The conclusion of the investigators was that, in selected motor skills, boys' performance capabilities develop a full year in advance of girls' motor performance capabilities.

The University of Arizona investigators (Morris et al., 1978) also recorded 23 **anthropometric** measurements for each child. Analyses of these data indicated that the physical growth of boys and girls was closely paralleled in height, weight, and leg length at each age. Of all the anthropometric measures taken, only the leg length classified children according to their appropriate age groups. This finding is in keeping with previously established differential growth rates, with leg length increasing more rapidly than trunk length or head size from birth to late childhood.

The general developmental characteristics associated with motor development in early childhood are summarized in tables 8.8 and 8.9. The early manipulative and locomotor development of infancy is expanded to include all of the large muscle, basic motor skills within the human repertoire table (8.8). To assist in the development of these basic motor skills, general needs have been identified and suggestions are made for physical activity experiences appropriate to meeting those needs table (8.9). As a result of prior experiences, or concurrent experiences over which the teacher has no control, some children will require more attention to some aspects of general development than will others. The discerning observer, who has a good grasp of the developmental sequences and patterns discussed in this chapter, should be able to develop situations and experiences which will be of greatest value for the motoric development of the individual child.

TABLE 8.8 Summary of Motor Skill Development

Skill	2–3 years	3–4 years	4–5 years	5–6 years
Walking	Rocker action of foot. Step pattern smoother. Walk backwards easily. Walk with 1 foot on balance board. Walk on tiptoe.	Well coordinated walk. Walk along line without stepping off. Alternate feet part way on balance board.	Stabilized gait pattern. Walk length of balance board. Walk along circle without stepping off.	Stand on tiptoe for 10 sec. Balance on 1 foot 4–6 sec. Increase speed of walk on balance board.
Running	Jerky action: changing from full sole to rocker action.	Run smoother and can do on toes.	More control and power. Increased length of stride and non-support period.	Control turn and stop. Use run effectively in games.
Hopping Galloping Skipping	Balance on 1 foot. Jump off floor with both feet.	Consecutive jumps off floor with 2 feet. Early gallop by varying beat of run.	Hop on 1 foot. Master gallop beat. Skip on 1 foot.	Hop with better form for 10 or more hops on 1 foot. Hop on either foot. Good galloping skill. Alternate foot skip.
Climbing	Walk upstairs alone: mark time.	Walk upstairs alone: alternate feet. Descend stairs with help, alternate feet.	Descend stairs alone: alternate feet. Ascend ladders: mark time.	Ascend short ladder: alternate feet. Descend ladders: mark time.
Jumping	Jump from 12″ height one foot ahead. Rudimentary jump and reach.	Jump from 12″ height feet together. Jump rope lower than 20 cm. Distance jump: 10–35 cm. Arms used as stabilizer. Better jump and reach form.	Increased distance jump, height in jump and reach and over obstacle. Better form with arms used to augment action.	Continued increase in height jumped and distance jumped. Continued improvement in form.

Kicking	Contacts ball during "walk."	Contacts ball directly in front. Little leg backswing or follow through.	Adjusts to ball. More backswing and follow-through.	Full backswing; forward body lean. Better foot contact.
Throwing	Some force in anterior-posterior hand release.	Anterior-posterior throwing action of arm and trunk. Feet stationary.	Horizontal arm. Some trunk rotation. Ipsilateral step forward.	Horizontal arm action and trunk rotation. Ipsilateral step but also some alternate step during throw.
Catching	Extended parallel arm with no or little action to trap ball (large).	Scooping action with parallel arms with large ball.	Smaller ball catch with vice grip and elbows in front of body.	Large ball catch with vice grip and elbows in front of body.
Ball bouncing	Bounce small ball with one hand 1–3 ft. Tapping action of hand.	Bounce larger ball with both hands.	Bounce smaller ball further distance. Use chasing action of hand.	Bounce larger ball with one hand 1–3 ft.

TABLE 8.9 Summary of general developmental characteristics during early childhood

Characteristics
1. Rapid acquisition of large muscle, basic motor skills
2. All skills developing concurrently but at different rates
3. Amount of variability between individuals increases with increasing age
4. Rapid increase in strength for both sexes—65 percent between 3 & 6 years
5. Limb length increasing proportionately more than other body parts
6. Increased limb length results in greater leverage for speed
7. Increased coordination and use of leverage allows for maximal application of strength
8. Increased balance development allows for increased range of movement in executing a skill
9. Cephalocaudal development of control and coordination, e.g., overhand throw, striking
10. Development of basic concepts of object, space, force, causality, and time for conscious control and coordination of movement
11. Manipulative skills need refinement, e.g., catching balls
12. Very active; great deal of energy in short spurts
13. Increased wakeful period provides more time for skill development
14. Short attention span
15. Imaginative, imitative, curious
16. Individualistic or egocentric; noisy
17. Like rhythm, moving to and/or singing
18. Some sex differences in performance, particularly in the distance throw
19. Begin to judge others on the basis of motoric performance

Need	Experiences
Vigorous exercise requiring use of large muscles	Running and chasing games; hanging and climbing; large apparatus; stunts (self-testing)
Simple games with short explanation, simple class organization and change activities quickly	Hide and seek; stunts; simple singing games (Mulberry Bush)
Opportunity to try things and to "pretend"	Movement exploration using basic skills and small apparatus; creative dance; story plays (animals)
Learn to share, engage in parallel play with others	Small group work; self-testing activities; exploration of movement
Opportunities to use medium-size objects such as balls	Ball handling games, bean bags, hoops, wands, etc. Start with larger objects at 2-3 years and work to smaller objects at 5-6 years

9

Motor Behavior in Later Childhood

The relatively slow and constant growth trend of later childhood, extending approximately from 6 to 10 or 12 years of age, is terminated by the pubescent growth spurt. Although these years are ones of slow developmental change, it is a time of rapid learning (Goodenough, 1945) and what may be thought of as growth consolidation, characterized more by the perfection and stabilization of previously acquired skills and abilities than by the emergence of new ones.

It is also the period in which the child moves from the sheltered home environment to the involved social climate of the school. Major adjustments are required to cope with the three outward thrusts that are the developmental tasks of this period, namely (1) the thrust from the home into the peer group; (2) the thrust into the realm of work and games, each of which requires added development of neuromuscular skills; and (3) the thrust into the world of adult concepts, which requires the gradual acquisition of the skills and art of logic, symbolism, and communication (Havighurst, 1950).

INDICES OF GROWTH AND MATURATION

The most commonly used indices for assessing the developmental age or physiological maturity of a growing child are skeletal age, dental age, secondary sex character age, and morphological age. Skeletal age is one of the more generally used indicators of physiological maturity as its effective range extends from birth through 18 years of age. Roentgenograms (or x-rays) of the wrist and hand are used most frequently for assessing the amount of ossification and amount of epiphyseal fusion as these anatomical structures contain a great concentration of bones that mature at different rates. The amount of ossification and amount of epiphyseal fusion are related to skeletal maturity and standardized procedures have been developed for such assessment. Figure 9.1 clearly illustrates that girls are more skeletally mature than boys from birth and they maintain this status to achieve maturity approximately two years earlier than boys.

On the average, **skeletal** age and **chronological** age coincide, but any one individual may be normal, advanced, or retarded in skeletal age with respect to chronological age. There may also be fluctuations in the rate of skeletal maturing such as those illustrated in figure 9.2.

The relation of chronological or skeletal age to performance depends to a great extent upon the range of age included, the sex, and general maturity level of the subjects. Correlation coefficients ranging from .42 to .56 were obtained between seven performance measures and skeletal age of primary school children (Seils, 1951). However, Rarick and Oyster (1964), studying elementary school children, obtained different results in calculating the relationships between chronological age, height, weight, and skeletal age and performance items including the run, standing broad jump, distance throw, and weight strength measures.

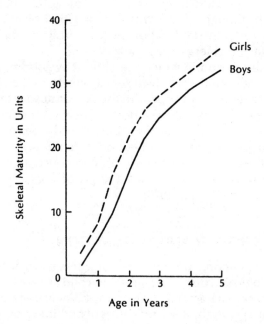

FIGURE 9.1. *Skeletal maturity of the hand. (From R. M. Acheson, A method of assessing skeletal maturity from radiographs. A report from the Oxford Child Health Survey. J. Anat., 1954, 88, 498–508. By permission of the author and publisher, Cambridge University Press.)*

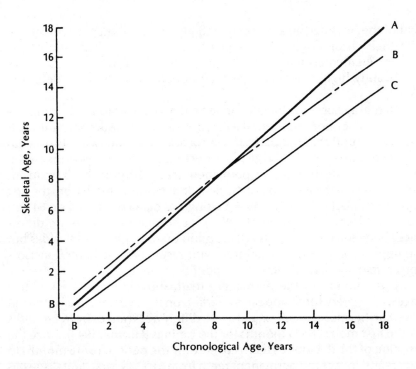

FIGURE 9.2. *Skeletal age plotted against chronological age for three hypothetical persons. A, average of standardizing group throughout all growth period; B, initially skeletally mature above average, but passing later to below average; C, consistently below average maturity (a late maturer). (From J. M. Tanner,* Growth at adolescence. *Oxford, Eng.: Blackwell Scientific Publications, 1955. By permission of the publisher.)*

By holding the maturity measures constant and computing partial correlations for each of the various measures, it was found that neither skeletal age nor any of the other three maturity measures accounted for a major part of the variance in any of the strength or physical performance measures. After further partialling, it was found that chronological age, which gave the highest third order correlation values, accounted for, at most, 15 percent of the variance in strength measures. Rarick and Oyster concluded that skeletal maturity was a factor of little consequence in accounting for individual differences in strength and motor performance, while chronological age was the most important maturity indicator in explaining the variance in strength.

Skeletal maturity is, however, an important factor in superior athletic performance of boys in later childhood. Krogman (1959) reports that of the 55 boys who participated in the 1957 Little League World Series, 29 percent had a skeletal age less than their chronological age while 71 percent of the boys had an advanced, or higher skeletal age, in comparison with their chronological age. Similarly, outstanding school athletes, at both the elementary and the junior high school level, were found to have significantly higher skeletal ages than nonathletes (Clarke & Petersen, 1961).

Dental age uses a principle similar to that of skeletal age and employs the eruption or noneruption of each tooth as the measure of maturity. It has been found that the pattern of appearance of the two sets of teeth vary for the sexes. Although girls are more mature than boys as measured by skeletal ossification and by permanent teeth eruption, boys are in advance of girls in the eruption of the first, or deciduous, teeth from the first tooth to the last (Meredith, 1946). Using the data completed on 64 Fels Study children, Robinow et al. (1942) found that there were no differences between deciduous teeth eruption on the right and left sides but the upper-lower eruption differed with respect to the central incisors (lower first) and lateral incisors (upper first).

The eruption of the permanent teeth showed marked sex differences, with every tooth appearing earlier, on the average, in girls than in boys. Furthermore, the timing of these differences ranges from 2 months for the first molars to 11 months for the canines (Hurme, 1949). Since the eruption of the deciduous teeth covers only the period from 6 months to 2 years and that of the permanent teeth from 6 to 13 years, dental age has not been used extensively for gauging maturity.

Secondary sex character age is based upon ratings for the stages of maturation of genital, pubic hair, and breast development and, as such, is applicable only to the periods of preadolescence and adolescence. Although the determination of secondary sex character age requires reasonably complicated procedures, this method of assessment of development has been frequently used and will be discussed more fully in dealing with the period of adolescence.

Morphological age employs height, weight, and various other anthropometric measures or combinations of these in relation to norms based upon chronological age. The charts of growth in height (figure 9.3) and for weight (figure 9.4) are examples of this technique for assessing growth. These types of measurements are the most easily obtained and the most obvious indicators of individual variations in development. Both of these factors have contributed to the extensive development and use of height-weight tables for the prediction of normal growth.

A relationship between body size and level of motor performance has long been recognized by individuals interested in physical abilities. One of the first systems of classifying children into homogeneous groups for games and athletic activities involved the use of chronological age, school grade, height, and weight (Reilly, 1917). Two commonly used methods of classifying children and youth were developed independently

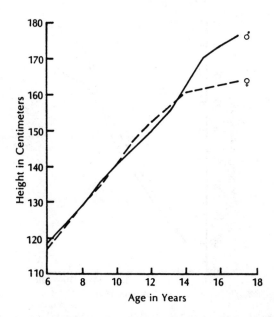

FIGURE 9.3. *Age changes in height for white males and females. (Adapted from 50th percentile data at ages 6 to 11 in R. M. Malina; P. V. V. Hamill; and S. Lemeshow,* Body dimensions and proportions: White and Negro children 6-11 years. *Washington, D.C.: U.S. Government Printing Office, Series 11 (143), 1974; also adapted from 50th percentile data at ages 12-17 in P. V. V. Hamill; F. E. Johnston; and S. E. Lemeshow,* Body weight, stature, and sitting height: White and Negro youths 12-17 years. *Washington, D.C.: U.S. Government Printing Office, Series 11 (126), 1973.*

by McCloy (1945) and by Neilson and Cozens (1934) with both using the factors of age, weight, and height. Each subjected records of thousands of children to statistical analysis and obtained multiple correlations ranging from .40 to .67 between various events and age, height, and weight. The classification formulae developed by these investigators were very similar, as follows:

McCloy: Classification Index I = 20 (Age) + 6 (Height) + Weight
Neilson and Cozens: Revised Formula = 20 (Age) + 5.5 (Height)
+ 1.1 (Weight)

Subsequently, these investigators modified their formulae for special age or sex groupings. McCloy (1945) concluded, for example, that height of elementary school boys added little to the prediction formula. He suggested that increases in body weight would normally reflect increases in the amount of muscle tissue if its proportion of approximately 40 percent of the body weight is retained. Furthermore, this increase in muscle

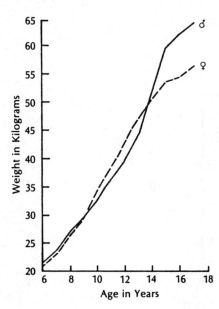

FIGURE 9.4. *Age changes in weight for white males and females. (Adapted from 50th percentile data at ages 6 to 11 in R. M. Malina; P. V. V. Hamill; and S. Lemeshow,* Body dimensions and proportions: White and Negro children 6–11 years. *Washington, D.C.: U.S. Government Printing Office. Series 11 (143), 1974; also adapted from 50th percentile data at ages 12–17 in P. V. V. Hamill; F. E. Johnston; and S. E. Lemeshow,* Body weight, stature, and sitting height: White and Negro youths 12–17 years. *Washington, D.C.: U.S. Government Printing Office, Series 11 (126), 1973.)*

tissue coupled with increased lever length resulting from growth in height should result in greater power and thus in higher motor achievement. Growth in height in the elementary school years is apparently reflected adequately by increase in weight so that the latter alone, with age, is predictive of performance.

In all of these earlier studies designed primarily to develop classification for physical activities, a wide range of performance measures were used and various age ranges were included. More recent studies, where computer analysis has been possible, have given more precise results. The importance of weight as an indicator of strength has been reaffirmed by Clarke and Carter (1959) who found—after experimenting with chronological age, weight, and anthropometric measures—that weight and age gave the highest multiple correlation with strength as measured by the Roger's Strength Test.

Nonlinearity has been reported in the relationship between age, height, and weight and the athletic events of standing broad jump, softball throw, and six-second run on the basis of tests of 882 boys and 900 girls ranging in age from 9 to 17 years (Cearley, 1957). Actual correlations are very high, however, as would be expected for such a wide age range. When age is held constant, the relationships of a number of physical performance measures to height and to weight are generally low at all ages 10 to 17 for both boys and girls. The relationships of height and weight with various performance items do vary markedly, however (Espenschade, 1963).

No significant relationship has been found between performance and body build (Breitinger, 1935; Barry & Cureton, 1961) and body size is not as significant in distinguishing athletes from nonathletes at the elementary school level as it is at the junior high school level (Clarke & Petersen, 1961).

It may be well at this time to point out certain limitations that exist in the various measures of maturation. Available norms in all areas are based on cross-sectional studies of relatively homogeneous populations. All physical growth patterns, including those of the timing and sequence of ossification of the skeleton (Reynolds, 1943) and the eruption of teeth (Tisserand-Perrier, 1953) are to some degree hereditary in character. Thus norms for dental age especially, which are based on a relatively small sample, may be biased.

Studies of various racial groups confirm the fact that human development follows a common pattern. Racial differences do exist, however, in actual size, proportions, and possibly timing. For example, data by Malina et al. (1974) and Hamill et al. (1973) indicate that black males are taller than white males at all ages from 6 through 17 years except at ages 9, 10, 15, and 17. However, black males are heavier only at ages 8 and 17 years. Similarly, black girls are taller than white girls except at ages 8, 12, 14, and 17 but white girls are heavier at ages 7, 8, 9, 14, and 15 years. The apparent disparity in height and weight increments is probably a function of racial differences in proportional growth which were mentioned in the previous chapter and will again be referred to in the section on changes in body proportions. Norms, therefore, are appropriate only for populations comparable for those on which they were developed. One other limitation should be noted. Cross-sectionally developed norms all show straight-line growth, whereas longitudinal studies demonstrate clearly that individual growth shows cycles of rapid and slow progress.

CHANGES IN SIZE AND BODY PROPORTIONS

Growth during the period of early childhood is relatively slow and constant in comparison with the previously rapid growth of earlier periods and the rapid growth of the following adolescent period (see figures 8.1, 9.3 and 9.4). This is an important factor in improved motor functioning and coordination. Body size and proportions change gradually and a nearly constant relationship is maintained in bone and tissue development. Therefore, the energies of the child can be directed towards perfecting the basic movement patterns that have been established during the period of early childhood and adapting and modifying them to meet an increasing variety of situations.

The limbs continue to grow proportionately more than the trunk and this is particularly true for boys so that the relatively longer leg length of the girls during infancy and early childhood tends to disappear in later childhood. Thereafter, the boys exhibit comparatively greater leg length. This growth pattern is illustrated by the ratio of sitting height to stature shown in figure 9.5. Here the decline in the ratio indicates that the legs are growing longer relative to the sitting height up until the age of 11 years for the girls and 14 for the boys. The subsequent slight rise in the ratio for both sexes after these times marks the increase in trunk length which occurs toward the end of the adolescent growth spurt.

The comparative data supplied by Malina et al. (1974) and Hamill et al. (1973) for a much larger national survey of 6- to 17-year-olds supports the earlier data of Bayer and Bayley for the sitting height/stature ratio. In addition, the data from the national survey indicates a very definite racial difference between blacks and whites in the ratio of sitting height to standing height. At all age levels from 6 through 17 years, the blacks have longer legs than do whites, but the patterning of the sex differences par-

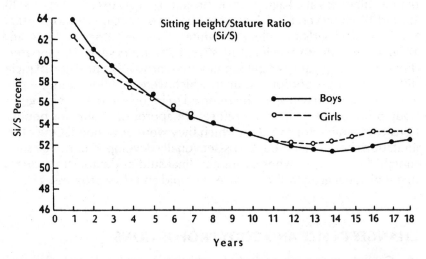

FIGURE 9.5. The ratio of sitting height to stature at ages 1 to 18 inclusive. As the legs grow relatively longer, the ratio falls, rising again after puberty. (From Leona M. Bayer and Nancy Bayley. Growth diagnosis. Chicago: The University of Chicago Press, 1959. By permission of the publisher.)

allels that of the whites. Therefore, if the sitting height/stature curves for blacks were added to figure 9.5, the curves would be exactly similar in shape to those illustrated but paralleling them at a slightly lower level. Although females for both races have proportionately shorter legs than males after 11 years of age, the racial difference in proportional leg growth is marked enough that black females have proportionately longer legs than white males at all age levels (Malina et al. 1974; Hamill et al., 1973).

Another sex difference that becomes more noticeable after the age of 6 years is that of the hip-shoulder ratio. During infancy and early childhood, boys have larger overall measurements of the pelvis while girls tend to be either relatively or absolutely larger in measurements of the inner structure of the pelvis (Reynolds, 1945, 1947). The proportional change in the hip-shoulder ratio after the age of 6 (figure 9.6) is caused by a sex difference in the growth pattern of the shoulder and the hip. While the relative amount of gain in shoulder width is approximately the same for both sexes from 6 to 10 years, the girls make consistently higher gains in hip width during this time. Subsequent changes are attributable to the adolescent growth spurt, where girls continue to have greater gains in hip width while the boys increase markedly in shoulder width.

Other sex differences that have been noted during the growth years include larger thighs for the girls from the ages of 3 to 18 years and larger

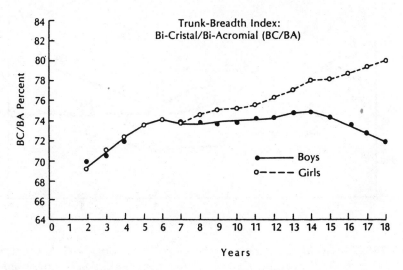

FIGURE 9.6. *The ratio of bi-cristal diameter to bi-acromial diameter at ages 1 to 18 inclusive. As boys' shoulders grow relatively wider, their ratio falls. As girls' hips grow relatively broader, the BC/BA curve for girls rises. (From Leona M. Bayer and Nancy Bayley. Growth diagnosis. Chicago: The University of Chicago Press, 1959. By permission of the publisher.)*

thoracic circumference and girth of the forearm in boys (Boynton, 1936). The larger length of forearm for boys that becomes noticeable during early childhood is maintained through adulthood. However, the sex differences that have been cited are slight in late childhood, and there is little difference with respect to physique between boys and girls until preadolescent changes are manifested.

BODY BUILD

Closely allied to measures of morphological age is the body build of the child as it is based upon the interrelationships of height, weight, and various anthropometric measurements. Bayley and Davis (1935) found that the index of weight/length^2 was the most valid measure of lateral-linear tendencies in body build during the first three years of life but that the indices obtained at these early ages were not predictive of what an individual's body build would be later in life. Figure 9.7 clearly indicates

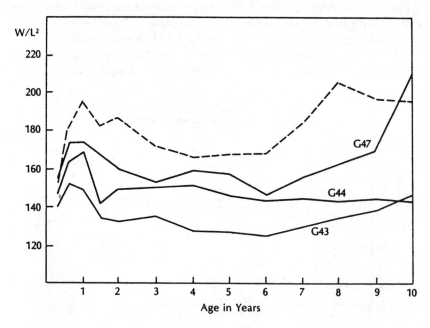

FIGURE 9.7. *Individual changes in weight/length^2 index with age. Girls G43, G44, and G47 are taller than average but of different body build. G43 is underweight for age and height; legs proportionately long. G44 approximates normal proportions. G47 is overweight for height; pelvis wide for body length. Dotted line represents index changes for short stocky girl. (From Helen Thompson, Physical growth. In L. Carmichael (Ed.), Manual of child psychology. New York: John Wiley & Sons, Inc., 1954. By permission of the publisher.)*

these changes in the growth pattern based upon the weight/length^2 ratios of three girls who were taller than average. Here, as Bayley and Davis also found, chubbiness reached its peak between 9 and 12 months of age. Furthermore, although the curves do not cross from 28 weeks to 9 years, G43 was more chubby at 28 weeks than G44 at 5 years, and G44 was decidedly more chubby at 28 weeks than G47 at 5 years. With regard to general body build, G43 was underweight for her height and age and had proportionately longer legs; G44 was of approximately normal proportions; while G47 was overweight for her height and age and had a comparatively large pelvis for her body length (Thompson, 1954).

Although weight increase is a correlate of growth, it is not necessarily indicative of growth since weight changes may be merely the result of changes in water content or of fatty deposits, both of which may be transitory modifications (Simmons & Todd, 1938). Weight has been found to be more variable and more indicative of nutritional status than any other physical measurement. In spite of the fact that the optimum weight of an individual depends upon the age, body build, and stature of an individual as well as on his nutrition, age norms for weight alone have been used as indicators of a child's development and nutritional status, particularly during the period of infancy.

Because of changing body proportions with growth (Hejinian & Hatt, 1929), no scheme of body typing developed to date has proven satisfactory for use over the entire span of growth. It has been found that indices such as stem length/recumbent length ratio are valid only at certain periods of growth and tend to lose their significance at other ages. An investigation of the whole period of physical growth was made by McCloy (1936) in which he employed a factor analysis technique to isolate the most useful items in appraising body type. He concluded that the two most useful indices were the weight$^{1/3}$/height and chest girth/height ratios, but even these were satisfactory only after the period of infancy. When McCloy's weight $^{1/3}$/height ratio is applied to data by Malina et al. (1974) and Hamill et al. (1973), the resultant patterning (figure 9.8) indicates that the changes in the ratio closely parallel the changes in height (figure 9.3) and weight (figure 9.4) during the years 6 through 17.

A grid technique devised by Wetzel (1941, 1943) provides seven different growth channels for individuals of varying body builds. Placement in a channel results from plotting height and weight on the coordinates. Wetzel (1941) points out that certain combinations of height and weight tend to produce characteristic contours which are typical of different body types. Children of average physique fall into the middle channel of the grid; the channels to the left are for those who were obese and of progressively more stocky frame; and channels to the right for thin children of more linear frame. Wetzel believes that the body build for all children placed in the same channel on the basis of height and weight is

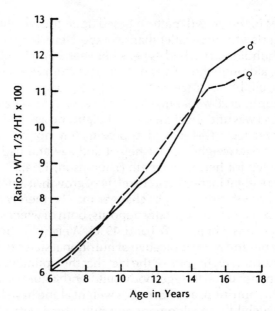

FIGURE 9.8. *Age Changes in weight* $^{1/3}$/*height ratio for white males and females. (Adapted from 50th percentile data at ages 6–11 in R. M. Malina; P. V. V. Hamill; and S. Lemeshow, Body dimensions and proportions: White and Negro children 6–11 years. Washington, D.C.: U.S. Government Printing Office. Series 11 (143), 1974; also adapted from 50th percentile data at ages 12–17 in P. V. V. Hamill; F. E. Johnston; and S. E. Lemeshow, Body weight, stature, and sitting height: White and Negro youths 12–17 years. Washington, D.C.: U.S. Government Printing Office. Series 11 (126), 1973.)*

essentially the same irrespective of their level of development. Furthermore, once a child's channel can be established at about 6 or 7 years, healthy children should be expected to maintain growth close to the limits imposed by the channel and thus to show consistent body build.

Since growth failure in the Wetzel technique is assessed from height and weight alone, it is subject to marked limitations (Thompson, 1954). A more satisfactory technique developed by Pryor and Stolz (1933) used age, sex, height, and bi-iliac width for the prediction of optimum weight of children 6 to 16 years of age. No specific body typing results from the latter method, however.

A more comprehensive approach to body typing was undertaken by Sheldon and co-workers (1940), based upon adult male somatic characteristics, and using three main components and four second-order variables. These investigators relate the three components to the embryonic tissues, namely: the endoderm, the mesoderm, and the ectoderm. The first component, endomorphy, is regarded as characteristic of the viscerally-dominated body as evidenced by soft, rounded body regions. Mesomorphy is characteristic of the bone, muscle, and connective tissue-dominated body such as is shown by a heavy, hard, and rectangularly outlined body. Ectomorphy, the third component, is considered to be characteristic of the body type dominated by the central nervous system as shown by a linear, fragile body with relatively large surface area. Within these three main components, the second order variables are texture, or coarseness or fineness of the structure; dysplasia, or disharmony between the various parts of the body; hirsutism, or amount of body hair; and gynandromorphy, or degree of bisexuality. All these traits, both components and second-order variables are rated on a seven point scale by anthroscopic and anthropometric methods.

Sheldon himself **somatotyped** the boys and girls of the Oakland Growth Study. His final typing represented a composite for each individual developed from the serial photographs taken throughout the study for he considered this would better represent the genotype. A grouping of boys and of girls who were consistently superior or the reverse in motor abilities was made from these same subjects (Espenschade, 1940). Somatotypes of these latter individuals are summarized in table 9.1. The superior performers among boys are high in mesomorphy and low in endomorphy in comparison with the poor performers. Differences are less marked for girls as both groups are below average in mesomorphy. The poor performers are decidedly more endomorphic, however.

Still another approach to rating has been that of Bayley and Bayer (1946) who devised a five-area classification by which young adults may be evaluated according to the sex-appropriateness of their builds. The profile rating for **androgynic** patterns of body form developed by these investigators involves 14 items of measurement from photographic records which serve to categorize the individual into the five areas of hypermasculinity, masculinity, intermediate or bisexual, femininity, and hyperfemininity. The most obvious feature of differentiation in this androgynic rating system is the shoulder width/hip width ratio. The hypermasculinity grouping has very broad shoulders in comparison to hip width, whereas the hyperfeminine grouping has very narrow shoulders in comparison with hip width. The male and female intermediate, or bisexual, groupings are characterized by similar breadths in the shoulder and the hip areas.

TABLE 9.1. Mean Sheldon somatotype ratings of adolescent boys and girls high and low in physical performances

	High			Low		
Boys	3.0	5.2	3.1	4.6	4.5	2.9
Girls	4.9	3.7	2.7	5.6	3.0	2.8

This classification system has received very limited use in comparison with Sheldon's somatotyping and variants thereof.

The Heath-Carter somatotype rating system (1967) utilizes skinfold measurements of the **triceps, subscapular, suprailiac,** and calf to determine the relative fatness or leanness associated with the first component, or endomorphy. The relative musculoskeletal development of the second, or mesomorphic, component is assessed by measures of the height, the **humerus** and femur **biepicondylar** diameters, and the flexed upper arm and calf girths less the relevant skinfold thickness, that is, calf triceps from the arm girth and the calf skinfold from the calf girth. The weight and ratio of height/$\sqrt[3]{\text{weight}}$ are used to assess the relative linearity of the ectomorphic, or third, component. The Heath-Carter system appears to be more sensitive as a physique rating system to changes in body shape and composition resulting from growth and training changes than the Sheldonian systems. Moreover, it also appears to have more practical application for the somatotype rating of children (Hebbelinck et al., 1972). Using the Heath-Carter system, 18 percent of early maturing boys had endomorphic dominance whereas less than 3 percent of late maturers had endomorphic dominance. Mesomorphic components were similar for the two groups.

The Sheldon somatotyping technique has been utilized extensively to assess the body builds of champion athletes (Cureton, 1951) (see figure 9.9), and more recently, similar analyses have been made using the Heath-Carter rating form (de Garay et al., 1974). However, the adaptability of these methods to the assessment of body build as it relates to the performance of children may be more equivocal. Slaughter et al. (1977) examined the association between somatotype, as measured by Sheldon's trunk index method and Heath-Carter's anthropometric method; body composition, estimated as fat and lean body mass from ^{40}K measures and two skinfold thicknesses; and physical performance measures consisting of three tests of running and two types of jumps. On the basis of the data collected on the three variables for 68 boys ranging in age from 7 to 12 years, these investigators concluded that Heath-Carter's third component, derived from the inverse ponderal index, correlated more closely with performance scores than did the other components of somatotype. Mesomorphy and the second component were the least significant somatotype components. In general, it was observed that somatotype components had lower correlations with running and jumping variables than did body composition or body size variables such as height, weight, and percent of fat. Multiple regression analysis of somatotype components in combination with each other and with body size and body composition variables indicated little association with running performance but some association with jumping.

Skinfolds were used by Hensley et al. (1982) to assess body fatness of

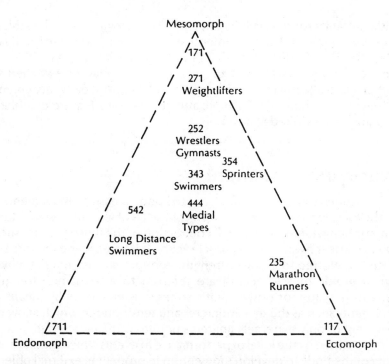

FIGURE 9.9. *Somatotypes of some Olympic performers. (Adapted from data by T. K. Cureton, Jr.,* Physical fitness of champion athletes. *Urbana: The University of Illinois Press, 1951.)*

preadolescent boys and girls to determine the effects of this variable upon performance scores in the vertical jump, standing broad jump, modified pull-up, 40-yard dash, and 400-yard run. The results indicated that the boys were slightly taller, heavier, and scored significantly better than girls on all the physical performance tests but there was no significant difference between the sexes on the sum of the two skinfold measures. With the exception of the modified pull-up, where body fat is inversely related to the ability to move total body weight, body fatness was only marginally related to performance. These investigators concluded that body fatness was of minimal importance in explaining performance differences between young boys and girls.

The prediction of growth rate and potential adult body build during the period of childhood has received considerable attention in terms of early recognition of potential athletes. The performances of Nadia Comaneci and Kornelia Ender in the 1976 Olympics focused attention upon the early selection of potential athletes. Nadia was selected for a special training program at 6 years of age (Deford, 1976) and Kornelia, at age 8, was sent to the Chemie Club, which specializes in rowers, swimmers, and middle distance runners (Mulligan, 1976). The growth rate of the athlete is carefully monitored in these intensive training programs and Mulligan (1976) cites Dr. Marder, formerly of the Chemie Club, as saying that "A swimmer who grows too fast or gets too heavy may be switched to another sport, like rowing." Such organized attempts at early recognition and selection of potential Olympic athletes are not a feature of athletic programs in the United States.

DEVELOPMENT OF STRENGTH

The contraction of the muscles of the body is basic to movement, so that the force with which muscles can contract is of vital interest in a study of motor behavior. If the force of contraction of the muscles is not sufficient to cause movement, the muscle action is **isometric** and the force so exerted is referred to as static strength; contractions resulting in movement (**isotonic** muscle action) are referred to as dynamic strength, strength-in-action, or power. Static strength is measured by means of instruments such as the **dynamometer** and **tensiometer**, which allow no movement or only extremely limited amounts. Dynamic strength is usually determined by the level of performance in events which measure the ability of the body to develop momentum in propelling external objects or the individual's own body.

Studies of the development of static strength in preschool and elementary school children have usually employed grip strength, as recorded by a hand dynamometer, because of its ease of administration. It is then inferred that such a measure is indicative of general body strength because grip strength has been found to be highly correlated with other static strength measures at older ages (Jones, 1949). Such an assumption may be open to question among younger children.

Metheny (1941a) found there was a rapid gain in grip strength of approximately 65 percent for both boys and girls between the ages of 3 and 6 years. Meredith (1935) noted that boys tend to double their grip strength between the ages of 6 and 11 and show an increase of 359 percent between 6 and 18 years of age. A similar study of the grip strength of girls revealed an increase of only 260 percent during the years of 6 to 18; the discrepancy was largely atttributed to their lessened increase in strength during the adolescent years (Metheny, 1941a). Peak torque measures for knee extension from 90 to 0 degrees were found to increase linearly for boys aged 13 to 17 years with a nonsignificant increase between 16 and 17 years. On the other hand, girls made significant knee extension peak torque gains only from 13 to 14 years with the peak torque remaining unchanged throughout 14 to 17 years (Miyashita & Kanehisa, 1979).

The correlations between grip strength and measures of physical growth such as weight, height, lung capacity, chest girth, and physical vigor for a group of primary and of fourth grade school children led Gates (1924) to conclude that increases in strength are a function of many aspects of growth. Grip and arm strength were measured in approximately 2500 males and 2000 females, aged 10 to 69, by Montoye et al. (1975). They found strength of the children to be clearly related to that of their parents with the relationship being stronger for younger children and probably indicating less influences of nonfamily environmental factors. Baldwin (1926) and Johnson (1925) have also noted that changes in strength are associated with general growth. Baldwin reports a correlation of .76 between grip strength and chronological age for boys between 7 and 15 years, while Johnson obtained a similar correlation between these same measures from 3 to 13 years. The parallel increases in grip strength and body size were found by Metheny (1941b) to be so close she concluded that the evaluation of grip strength in children should always be considered in the light of the child's body size. A study of the relationship between ankle extensor strength and roentgenographic measures of the leg muscles in 51 seven-year-old children produced correlations between these two measures ranging from .58 to .63 for the boys and from .22 to .52 for the girls (Rarick & Thompson, 1956).

Gains in body size reflect the gains made by the various body tissues during growth. Figure 9.10 indicates that the gains made in bone, muscle, skin, and subcutaneous tissue as recorded by roentgenographic measures at the maximum diameter of the calf are fairly consistent during the early part of later childhood. Both sexes show a peak in preadolescent fat increase followed by a negative velocity with the onset of a rapid increase in the development of bone and muscle tissue. In girls this increase and decrease is not as marked as it is in boys, however, and girls tend to maintain a higher level of subcutaneous fat and skin increases. Girls begin to make marked gains in bone and muscle between 9 and 10 years of age, and the boys begin their increased gains between 11 and 12 years of age.

When the mean gains in the various body tissues are compared with the isometric strength means of various muscle groups from ages 7 to 12 years (table 9.2), similarities in gains may be observed. The mean strength scores in table 9.2 are based upon the data of 115 boys and 101 girls who were tested in the Elementary School Growth Study conducted in Madison, Wisconsin, under the direction of members of the Department of Physical Education of the University of Wisconsin. It is interesting to note that the greatest gains in the strength made by the girls in four of the strength measures occur between 9 and 10 years while the boys make their greatest gains in strength in seven of the strength measures between 11 and 12 years of age.

It is possible that variations occur with respect to the onset of the

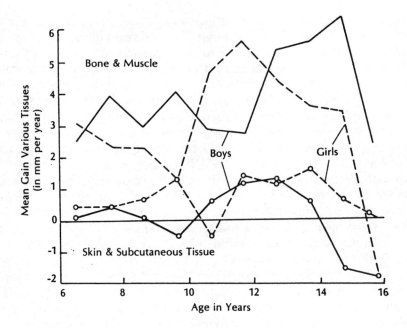

FIGURE 9.10. *Gains in breadth of bone, muscle, skin, and subcutaneous tissue. (Adapted from data by O. M. Lombard, Breadth of bone and muscle by age and sex in childhood. Child Developm., 1950, 21, 229–239.)*

greatest amount of gain in the various muscle groupings. Table 9.2 indicates both girls and boys make the greatest gain in wrist flexors between 11 and 12 years, whereas there is a difference of 2 years in the onset of gains in other muscle groupings for the sexes. In close association with wrist flexors, right grip strength shows its most marked gain for a group of California girls between the ages of 10 and 11 years to bring the mean right grip strength of the girls to the same value as that of the boys (Keogh, 1965). On the other hand, data for the sum of right and left grip strength analyzed by Montoye and Lamphiear (1977) indicates that boys are superior to girls at all age levels in this measure (figure 9.11). Additional data for arm strength scores studied by the same investigators reveals similar sex differences. The investigation of knee extension peak torque by Miyashita and Kanehisa (1979) reports significant sex differences in peak torque between the same age groups from 13 to 17 years for 569 boys and girls.

Although girls may equal, or even surpass, boys in strength at the peak of girls' strength gains, there is a definite sex difference in the strength of elementary school children (Metheny, 1941b; Rarick & Thompson, 1956; Keogh, 1965; Montoye & Lamphiear, 1977). Boys are found to be substantially stronger and, on the average, possess the

TABLE 9.2. Isometric strength means for various muscle groups (in pounds)*

Age (years)	7	8	9	10	11	12
Ankle Extensor						
Boys	60	67.5	83.5	89.5	96 †	123.5
Girls	56.5	66.5	75.5†	96.5	101.5	102
Knee Extensor						
Boys	63.5	75	96.5	107.5	110.5†	151.5
Girls	64.5	76.5	83.5†	116.5	127.5	139.5
Hip Extensors						
Boys	40.5	46.5	58	59.5	65.5†	87.5
Girls	34.5	44.5	47	57.5	63.5	73
Elbow Flexors						
Boys	31.5	41.5	45	50.5	56.5†	67.5
Girls	31	35.5	41 †	50.5	50.5	56.5
Shoulder Abductors						
Boys	37	49	53	53.5	64 †	81
Girls	33.5	43.5	43.5†	55.5	56	59
Shoulder Medial Rotators						
Boys	20	25.5	27.5	28	31.5†	37.5
Girls	16.5	21	22.5	25.5	28.5	29
Wrist Flexors						
Boys	23	25.5	29.5	32.5	33 †	42
Girls	20.5	22	25	28.5	29.5†	39

* The author is indebted to Professor G. L. Rarick, University of Wisconsin, for permission to use these data.
† Start of period of greatest gain

greater muscle size. The degree of sex difference in strength attributable to androgen production in the male during preadolescence would appear to be negligible, since equating boys and girls on the basis of muscle size reveals a superiority in strength for the boys which is significant only at the 30 percent level of confidence (Rarick & Thompson, 1956). However, on the basis of ratios of strength to body weight, boys are superior to girls in upper body strength measures to the extent that Montoye and Lamphiear (1977) consider pull-ups as not a good test for girls in that more than half of them cannot exert a force equal to their body weight. These investigators found that the mean ratios of the sum of grip strength to body weight for boys ranged from .65 at 10 years to 1.37 at 19 years, whereas those of the girls ranged from .53 to .85 for the same years. Similarly, the mean ratios for arm strength to body weight for boys ranged from 1.01 to 1.26 whereas those for girls ranged from .86 to .80 for the same age span.

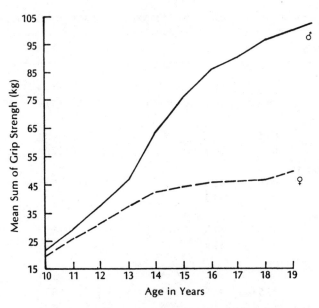

FIGURE 9.11. *Means of sum of right and left grip strength. (Adapted from data by H. J. Montoye and D. E. Lamphiear, Grip and arm strength in males and females, age 10 to 69. Research Quarterly, 1977, 48, 109–120.)*

Even though increases in strength accompany increases in body size, Meredith (1935) noted that the coefficient of variation in strength was, with the exception of weight, two to five times as great as any of the 18 anthropometric measures used in the University of Iowa Studies in Child Welfare. The greatest variabilities in strength were found to occur during periods of rapid developmental change, and growth in strength was noted to be less variable in childhood than during pubescence and post-pubescence. Similarly, the coefficient of variation for measurements of the breadth of bone and muscle tissue is around the level of 8 percent until 10 years of age, when the variation increases markedly for the girls in conjunction with the prepubertal growth spurt noted in figure 9.10. An increase in variation also occurs for the boys in association with the marked increases in bone and muscle tissue at 12 years (Lombard, 1950). The tendency for girls to be more variable in measurements of breadth of bone and muscle tissue even during the relatively stable period of child-hood, may, in part, account for the lower correlation coefficients obtained by Rarick and Thompson (1956) of the relationship between ankle extensor strength and muscle breadth in girls.

The development of muscular strength is symmetrical on both sides of the body, and strength is slightly greater on the dominant side of the body. Similarly, the percentage contributed to total strength by the arms and the legs tends to remain consistent between the ages of 5 and 18 years, with the legs contributing approximately 60 percent to total strength (Martin, 1918). Such findings are in keeping with a relatively symmetrical body structure and the greater muscle mass in the leg area in comparison with the musculature of the arms.

The relationship between static and dynamic strength has challenged a large number of investigators but, in general, little relationship has been obtained between static strength and motor performance in specific activities. Where relatively high relationships have been found, these have usually involved multiple correlations of a number of events. Carpenter's study (1942b) of the relationship between static dynamometric strength of the shoulder girdle muscles and certain motor performance events is typical of this type of approach. Using as subjects 217 primary grade boys and girls, this investigator obtained a multiple correlation of .50 for girls and .63 for boys when correlating "total shoulder girdle strength"—the sum of right grip, left grip, pull, and push—with weight and performance in the broad jump and shotput. On the basis of her results, she calculated the following regression equations as predictive of total strength for primary school children:

Boys' Strength=.1 broad jump + 2.3 shotput + weight
Girls' Strength=.5 broad jump + 3.0 shotput + weight

As a confirmation of her results, Carpenter (1942a) correlated the two dynamic strength measures in her regression equation with a composite score of the motor performance of primary school children in eight track and field events. The correlations between the motor performance total points score and the two dynamic strength measures were .70 for both the broad jump and the shotput for boys, and .74 for the broad jump and .61 for the shotput for the girls. Although these correlation coefficients indicate a substantial relationship between the dynamic strength measures as defined by Carpenter and a total points score of performance in events commonly engaged in by children of this age, it by no means indicates any relationship between static and dynamic strength. However, the shotput may be considered a good predictor of dynamic strength in the arms and the broad jump a good predictor of dynamic strength in the legs. Moreover, as the relative distribution of strength appears to have a consistent development (Martin, 1918), either one could be expected to be a reasonably good predictor of general dynamic strength.

Some significant correlations have been obtained between static strength and performance in specific activities, however. In relating the static strength of leg extensor muscle groups in 100 elementary school girls to the distance covered in the standing broad jump, Barsanti (1954) obtained significant correlations of .35 between the knee extensors and the standing broad jump and of .24 between the hip extensors and performance in the same activity. An exploration of the relationship between propulsive force and various leg extensor strengths in 10 boys at ages 8, 10, and 12 years resulted in correlation coefficients approaching the significance level at 10 and 12 years with only one value, of .64 for the hip strength at 10 years, actually being significant at the 5 percent level (Eckert, 1964).

Acceleration is a component of propulsive force so it is not surprising that correlations ranging from .52 to .73 were found for the relationship between static hip extensor strength and speed of angular movement in the hip joint (Eckert, 1964). Subsequently, higher values ranging from .74 to .79 have been found between static strength and speed of arm movement (Nelson & Fahrney, 1965). Eckert (1965) has proposed a force-energy concept which stresses the need to analyze motor performance tasks in terms of the amount of force or energy required for their execution. Using as a premise the fact that muscular action is the basis for all volitional body actions, it is hypothesized that there is a high positive relationship between maximal available strength and speed of movement in motor performance tasks where the range of movement and/or load, singly or in combination, provide the opportunity for the exertion of maximal force-energy.

Figure 9.12 depicts hypothetical maximal force curves for varying conditions of mass or resistance (load) and velocity of movement for three hypothetical subjects. Points B, C, and D illustrate that, for the same amount of mass, the stronger individual (III) is theoretically capable of moving that mass at a greater speed. Point A is indicative of a task which has mass-velocity requirements which can be readily achieved by all hypothetical subjects and level of strength would not be a determining feature of this task. These hypothetical curves are very similar to the strength-velocity curves generated using a Cybex (see figure 11.3).

Momentum is the product of the mass of an object and its velocity so that isometric (or static) strength can be considered to be a "pure" measure of strength of the muscles in the specific position in which the measurement is made. On the other hand, dynamic (or movement) strength is dependent upon the potential range of motion of the specific body segments involved in the development of angular velocity and on the mass of the body parts and/or that of any object which may be projected during the course of the physical action. The assessment of the relationship between strength and speed of movement is complicated by the fact that the lever action of the limbs results in variations in mechanical advantage depending upon the position of the limb and, therefore, results in variance in maximal isometric strength throughout the range of action of any one joint. In addition, the measurement of dynamic movement to determine the masses involved and the velocity of the various joint ac-

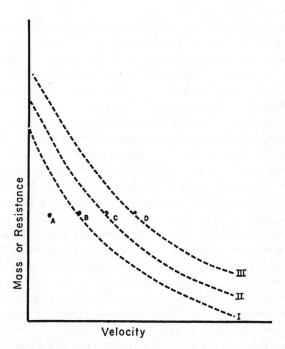

FIGURE 9.12. *Relationship between mass or resistance and velocity in muscular contraction. (Reprinted from Eckert, H. A Concept of Force-Energy in Human Movement. Journal of the American Physical Therapy Association. 1965, 45, 213–218. By permission of the American Physical Therapy Association.)*

tions and their contribution to the physical action is a tedious process but one which is becoming better and more easily analyzed with the development of computer programs for such purpose (Plagenhoef, 1973; McLaughlin et al., 1978). Despite these analytical problems, it is possible to make some assessment of the validity of the force-energy concept by examination of various research studies dealing with strength and limb momentum.

A study, by Whitley and Smith (1963), of static strength and velocity curves of an arm movement through an arc of 72 degrees resulted in a correlation of .37 between the unloaded limb speed and strength, whereas limb movement with a load of 11.730 kilograms resulted in a correlation of .73 for the same variables with the same subjects. Application of the force-energy concept to these results requires the calculation of the work loads for the unloaded and loaded arm action. For the unloaded arm action, the speed of .1530 second published by Whitley and Smith converts to 470.6 degrees per second for the 72 degree arc of the movement. When this angular velocity is multiplied by the limb mass of 1.199 kilograms estimated by Whitley and Smith, the resultant work load becomes 564.249

degree-kilograms. Similar computations using the loaded arm speed of .3341 published by Whitley and Smith results in an angular velocity of 215.5 degrees per second and a work load of 2450.235 degree-kilograms. Interpretation of the results of this study in terms of the force-energy hypothesis would lead to the conclusion that the loaded arm action required maximal available muscular force and hence shows a high relationship with speed. On the other hand, the unloaded arm movement does not require maximal force generation in terms of mass and is constrained in the angular velocity generation by the range of joint action and the viscosity of the muscles so that little or no relationship will exist between speed and maximal strength for this task.

A similar analysis of work load by Eckert and Day (1967) resulted in a **correlation coefficient** of .76 between calculated maximal strength and work load during push-ups. The subjects of this study, 15 well-conditioned college women who had been thoroughly trained in the correct technique for women's push-ups, were tested for the number of complete push-ups they were able to perform at a rate of 41 push-ups per minute. For statistical purposes, calculations of maximal strength for each individual were based on the average of the maximal arm strengths in the high and low push-up position and the weight supported in the high and low positions. The work load was calculated from the distance between the high and low positions, the average supported weight, and the number of push-ups the subject was able to perform until exhausted. It may be argued that performance to exhaustion is indicative of a fatigue orientation statistical design; however, the coefficient of determination (r^2) indicates that, in this instance, 58 percent of the variance in work load is accounted for by the relationship with maximal strength.

An isokinetic device (Cybex) was used by Miyashita and Kanehisa (1979) to measure peak torque of knee extension from 90 to 0 degrees at a velocity of 210 degrees per second. The peak torque measures for the 267 boys aged 13 to 17 years had a significant correlation of .688 with speed in meters per second for the 50-meter run. For the 281 girls in the same age groupings, the correlation coefficient was only .373 between peak torque and running speed in meters per second. The estimated proportions of the variance in running speed was 47.3 and 13.9 percent for the boys and girls, respectively. Thirty-five swimmers of both sexes, aged 11 to 21 years, were also measured for peak torque of arm pull muscles. Here, significant negative correlations of .728 and .515 were obtained between peak torque and best time in swimming the 100-meter front crawl for boys and girls, respectively. A significant negative correlation of .579 was obtained between knee extensor peak torque and best time for boy swimmers but no significant correlation was found between these measures for girl swimmers. Miyashita and Kanehisa (1979) also present graphs of the relationship curves between arm pull torque and knee extensor torque with swim time. The curves for significant correlations closely approximate the fast release curves of Fenn et al. (1931) used to illustrate the tension developed by human muscles at different velocities of shortening.

If the momentum aspects of the force-energy hypothesis are applicable to physical action, then in situations where maximal force-energy is expended it would be anticipated that changes in mass would result in accommodative changes in velocity and vice versa. Experimental design and logical analysis of human movement indicate that it is easier to experimentally change the mass of the body and then measure potential changes in velocity than it is to change velocity requirements and then look for any accommodations of body mass. The former experimental design was used by Eckert (1968) to assess the effect of added weights on joint actions in the vertical jump. The 17 well-conditioned male varsity basketball players used in this study were filmed doing vertical jumps under conditions of no additional weight and additions of a weighted belt containing weights of 6, 12, and 18 pounds. Analysis of the data indicated that for increasing amounts of weight there were decreases in maximal angular velocity from 649 to 592 degrees per second at the hip joint; from 915 to 859 at the knee; and from 1074 to 980 degrees per second at the ankle. Additional adjustments made to accommodate increases in weights were a very slight increase in the amount of time for each joint action from the point of deepest flexion to take-off. Changes in the speed with which the subjects attained maximal angular velocity are reflected in the maximal velocity-time ratios, which were found to decrease significantly at the hip and knee joints with increased weights, thus indicating a decrease in acceleration. In addition to supporting the momentum aspect of the force-energy hypothesis, this study indicates the complexity of the joint action adjustments made to accommodate increasing mass and points to our lack of precise knowledge of the adaptive mechanisms centering around optimal force production under changing conditions of mass or speed.

Studies which explore the relationship between strength and speed where statistical analysis is not based upon considerations of mass and angular velocity produce results that are more **equivocal**. Clarke (1974), in surveying strength and speed of movement studies, noted that most speed tests measured limited movements of an arm or leg, that is, forearm through 90 degrees or leg through 70 degrees. However, despite these very minimal movements, significant improvements in speed did occur as a consequence of strength training. Of the speed of movement experiments, isotonic exercises were the basis of weight training regimens in all but one study, and significant decreases in speed time were obtained in six of the 10 studies.

A more recent factor analysis of muscular strength by Jackson and Frankiewicz (1975) used 16 different tests to explore the viability of six conjectured factors of which the following four were supported: (1) Static-Force-Arms; (2) Static-Force-Legs; (3) Explosive-Power Arms; and (4) Dynamic-Work-Arms. In addition, the findings of the study led to the conclusion that arm work and arm force are independent constructs which may be due to a function of task specificity. These investigators state:

> One may argue that the basic differences between these factor findings may be traced to differences in type of muscular contraction. Eckert (1965) argues that the difference is not due to types of muscle contraction, but the task required. The factor analytic findings with leg variables tends to support Eckert's position. Cable tension leg strength tests loaded with leg power and leg work variables on three of the four solutions. Eckert's contention is further supported by the alpha residual scores solutions. Two factors (A-2′ and A-5′) were isolated with static leg strength tests and variables that involved moving the body through space. Since the residual scores transformations hold mass constant, force would equal acceleration and this relationship would be consistent with Newton's second law of motion. (p. 215)

Increasingly sophisticated statistical techniques are making it possible for the researcher of human movement and development to analyze collected data more precisely and minutely. However, there is still a marked tendency to use end-product data such as the speed of the run and the distance of a jump as indicative of either speed of movement or muscular power. Statistical techniques such as factor analysis are highly dependent upon the original input data for the identification of factors. Therefore, it is increasingly evident that the nature of the input data must become more minute and precise before it will be possible to resolve the equivocal nature of the relationship between strength and speed of movement. Hopefully, the development of computerized programs for analysis of segmental contributions to multi-jointed physical actions will provide the entry to more precise data collection and determination of critical momentum for the various joint actions (both agonistic to generate the required force and antagonistic to stop segmental momentum) so that generated force will not tear muscles, tendons, ligaments, and fascia, during maximal muscular performance tasks.

CHANGES IN MOTOR PERFORMANCE

With the steady increments that have been noted in body size and in strength, it is to be expected that there are also consistent increments in the basic skills of running, jumping, and throwing during later childhood. Similarly, the slight differences that have been noted favoring boys in these areas are duplicated in slightly better performances in running and jumping for boys. Distance throwing, however, shows an increasingly marked sex difference after the age of 5 years. Figures 9.13 through 9.16, based upon averages compiled from the data of a number of investigators, illustrate the changes with age in these activities for boys and girls from 5 to 17 years.

Running

The speed with which a person can run depends upon the length of the stride as well as its tempo. Figure 9.13 shows that there is a steady increase in running speed during the period of early childhood. This can easily be explained in terms of the steady increase in body size with its concomitant increases in lever length and strength providing increased length and tempo to the running stride. It is also, in part, a reflection of an increase in ability to run greater distances with increasing age. It is quite obvious that the start in the run has less effect on the total time of the dash in longer runs than in shorter runs. Therefore, in calculations based upon yards per second, the older age groupings, which tend to be based upon 50 and 60 yard dashes, have a lesser starting time influence in their yards-per-second averages than do the younger age groupings where the runs are usually 30 to 35 yards in length.

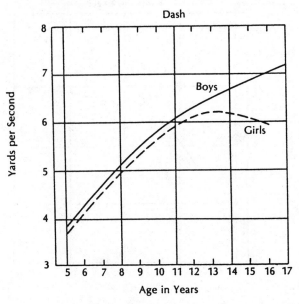

FIGURE 9.13. *Running. (From* Science and medicine of exercise and sports, *edited by Warren R. Johnson. Copyright © 1960 by Warren R. Johnson: "Motor Development" by Anna Espenschade. Reprinted by permission of Harper & Row, Publishers.)*

Jumping

The increases with age in both a vertical jump and a jump for distance are shown in figures 9.14 and 9.15, respectively. Increases in body size with age have both advantageous and detrimental effects upon performance in jumping. The increased body weight that occurs with increases in lever length and muscle mass must be overcome by proportionately greater gains accruing from these increments. Improvements in the mechanics involved in jumping would also appear to be a contributing factor to increases in performance.

An extensive investigation of the cinematographic records of six poor, average, and good jumpers of both sexes at each level from 6 to 12 years revealed that earlier thigh flexion appears as a sex difference after the age of 9 when the boys exhibit this characteristic sooner than the girls at all levels of performance (Clayton, 1936). A similar sex difference appears with respect to earlier trunk flexion for the boys at all performance levels from 9 through 12 years. Clayton concludes that there is some evidence of sequential development in the mechanics of the standing broad jump in children from 9 to 12 years of age, with boys in particular progressing toward a more mature and efficient manner of jumping.

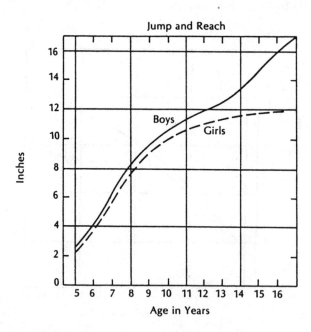

FIGURE 9.14. *Jump and reach. (From* Science and medicine of exercise and sports, *edited by Warren R. Johnson. Copyright © 1960 by Warren R. Johnson: "Motor Development" by Anna Espenschade. Reprinted by permission of Harper & Row, Publishers.)*

It is not surprising, therefore, that jumping has been considered a predictor of body strength (Carpenter, 1942b) and also a diagnostic test of motor coordination. Cowan and Pratt (1934) tested 540 children ranging in age from 3 to 12 years in their ability to hurdle jump and then plotted curves of growth in skill at successively higher age levels using median and Gesell "C" scores. Both these methods showed a continuous and relatively gradual improvement in hurdle jumping over the entire age range, with there being a slight indication of a sex difference in favor of girls below 7 years and of boys above this age level. Cowan and Pratt obtained no relationship between performance level at any age period and height or weight. They did, however, obtain a raw correlation of .77 between jumping performance and chronological age. As the correlation between age and the jump was .57 with height and weight partialed out, these investigators concluded that maturation was the determining factor influencing the height of the hurdle jump. As such, the hurdle jump is a true developmental test of motor coordination. However, another study of the relationship between the hurdle jump and performance in the standing broad jump, the jump and reach, the distance throw, and the 35-yard dash resulted in correlation coefficients ranging from .44 to

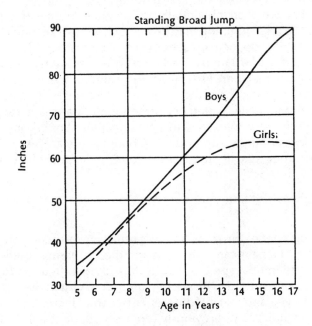

FIGURE 9.15. *Standing broad jump. (From* Science and medicine of exercise and sports, *edited by Warren R. Johnson. Copyright © 1960 by Warren R. Johnson: "Motor Development" by Anna Espenschade. Reprinted by permission of Harper & Row, Publishers.)*

.53 (Hartman, 1943). Since similar intercorrelations of the order of .50 among the comparative events were also obtained, it was concluded that the hurdle jump could be considered no better measure of general motor proficiency than any of the other measures.

In general, performance in jumping has been found to improve with advancing age, with the degree of improvement being greater for boys than for girls. However, there is a large variability in performance which results in considerable overlapping of performance scores between age groups and sexes. Kane and Meredith (1952) noted that the average jumpers at 7 years jumped approximately as far as the poorer 10 percent of 11-year-olds. Furthermore, the performances of the upper 10 percent of the 9-year-olds were equal or superior to the performance level of the middle 40 percent of the 11-year-olds. Since these findings are based upon cross-sectional data, one may speculate as to whether some of this variability may be caused by differential growth rates. However, Glassow and Kruse (1960), reporting on the motor performance of 123 girls aged 6 through 14 years and for whom data were available for at least three consecutive years, noted that individuals tended to remain in the same relative position within the group during the elementary school years; this being especially so in the run and the standing broad jump.

The maintenance of an individual's position in a group with respect to performance level in jumping may be as much a factor of mechanical execution as it would appear to be of body size. Cinematographical analyses of 10 skilled and 10 nonskilled performances in the standing broad jump indicate that there are characteristic differences in the angles of take-off and of landing and in the extent and duration of specific joint actions (Zimmerman, 1956). Skilled performers employ a greater range of movement in their performances with a greater amount of hip and knee flexion as the legs are drawn up under the body. There are also greater amounts of hip, knee, and ankle extension during the propulsive phase of the jump.

Throwing

The development of throwing ability is usually measured by the distance variously sized balls can be thrown and the increasing ability with chronological age in this type of throw is illustrated in figure 9.16. It is quite obvious that boys tend to be greatly superior to girls in the distance throw at all age levels and that this difference becomes increasingly great with increases in age. Wild's previously reported observations (1938) of the development of the overhand throwing pattern would indicate that some of this difference is caused by less mature throwing patterns on the part of girls. The larger forearm length and girth noted in boys also gives them a mechanical and strength advantage in the propulsion of an object

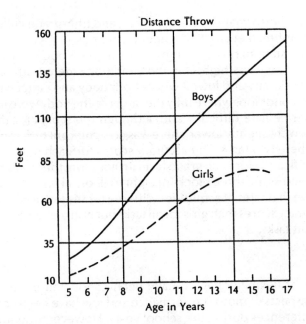

FIGURE 9.16. *Distance throw.* (*From* Science and medicine of exercise and sports, *edited by Warren R. Johnson. Copyright © 1960 by Warren R. Johnson: "Motor Development" by Anna Espenschade. Reprinted by permission of Harper & Row, Publishers.*)

for distance. Throws for accuracy, where production of force is not so demanding, since distance is confined along with the target area, do not produce such marked sex differences. However, such a difference does exist favoring the boys and here also there is improvement in performance with increasing age (Keogh, 1965).

The overarm throwing ability of seventh graders, who had previously been studied longitudinally from kindergarten through second grade, was examined by Halverson et al. (1982). When horizontal ball velocities were compared with annual rate of change predictions made when the subjects were in the second grade, the original estimate for the boys (5–8 ft/sec/yr) remained accurate but that of the girls had to be increased to 2–4.5 ft/sec/yr. Although the performance gap between the sexes increased throughout the elementary school years, it increased at a slower rate from second to seventh grade than it did during the primary years. The girls' rate of development was five to six years behind the boys' rate but the girls appeared more stable in their relative positions within their groups during the elementary years. Even by the seventh grade, few boys had reached an advanced level in all movement components although the self-reports suggested that the boys had participated in more overarm throwing than had the girls.

Throwing performance of first-, third-, and fifth-grade children was assessed by Hoffman et al. (1983) under task conditions which varied the motion states (stationary or moving) of the thrower's body and the target. Throwing accuracy was highest in the condition where both target and body were stationary and lowest where both body and target were moving. The task conditions where only the target or the body were in motion were of intermediate difficulty and, although the scores for the target moving task were slightly lower, there was no significant difference in the scores for these two tasks. The accuracy scores for each of the tasks improved significantly for each grade level. In addition, there was evidence of learning across the three blocks of eight trials on all tasks but there was no indication that rates of acquisition differed for the task types. Boys had higher accuracy scores than girls for all tasks but noticeably so for the two most difficult tasks.

Flexibility

Studies of flexibility have usually been conducted in conjunction with other aspects of motor performance and few have been concerned with age differences during the school years. However, one such study was undertaken by Hupprich and Sigerseth (1950) where 12 measures of flexibility were taken on 300 girls ranging in age from 6 to 18 years. There was a general increase in flexibility until the girls approached the age of 12 years, with a general decline thereafter. Exceptions to this trend were found in the shoulder, knee, and thigh where the girls showed a consistent decline in flexibility from 6 to 18 years. Eighteen-year-old girls were more flexible in certain aspects of five measurements than were girls 6 years of age. Of all the measures, ankle flexibility appeared to be the most constant throughout all the age groups and varied no more than 2.94 degrees at any age. Analysis of the results revealed low intercorrelations between the 12 measures of flexibility, which strongly suggests that a general flexibility factor does not exist and that each major joint appears to have its own specific flexibility. In this latter regard, it was noted that not a single girl was significantly above the average nor significantly below the average in all 12 measurements, while only six of the 300 girls reached their respective age-group averages in all 12 measurements.

Balance

From the previous discussions of the various large muscle activities, it is obvious that varying degrees of balance are required for successful performance. Two distinct types of balance have been identified as operating in most of our daily activities; namely, dynamic and static balance (Seashore, 1947; McCloy, 1945). The maintenance of a particular body position with a minimum of sway is referred to as static balance while dynamic balance is considered to be the maintenance of posture during the performance of a motor skill which tends to disturb the body's orientation. The distinct nature of these two types of balance is revealed by the low correlation of .34 obtained by Bass (1939) between measures of static and dynamic balance.

Walking board tests to measure dynamic balance were first standardized by Seashore (1947), and he reported steady improvements in boys from 5 to 11 years with a subsequent leveling off until 18 years. Similarly, steady improvement in both sexes of ages 5 through 11 is reported by Wallon et al. (1958) on the basis of different walking board tests. On the basis of railwalking tests given to over 700 Philadelphia children ranging in age from 6 to 14, continuing improvement for both sexes is reported over the entire age range studied, although there is some suggestion of a slackening in rate of gain from 12 to 14, especially for females (Heath, 1949). A repeat of this study over the age range of 8 to 16 years reports essentially the same results, including showing a slackening in rate of growth in females from 12 to 14 years (Goetzinger, 1961). Cron and Pronko (1957) used a 2x4 walking board that was 12 feet long to measure the dynamic balance of 322 boys and 179 girls. The scores for the task, which involved three trials of a round trip on the board, are illustrated in figure 9.17 and also indicate a leveling off of performance after 12 years, particularly for females.

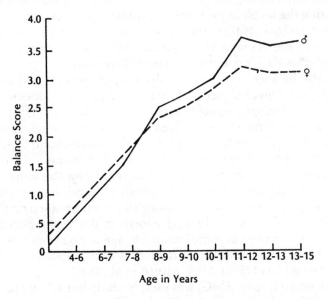

FIGURE 9.17. *Scores for walking length of balance board. (Adapted from data by G. W. Cron and N. H. Pronko, Development of the sense of balance in school children. J. Educ. Research, 1957, 51, 33–37.)*

However, Keogh (1965) claims there is rather clear indication that performance in beam walking does not increase steadily with age during childhood. He finds a consistent age change in boys except for a leveling off from 7 to 9, whereas girls have a marked increase from 7 to 8 followed by a leveling off from 8 to 10. An examination of the results of Seashore, Heath, Goetzinger, and his own led Keogh to the conclusion that mean age performance in beam walking remains stable for several years followed by a marked increase. Exact identification of the ages where the increases occur is not attempted, but it is suggested that they seem to be somewhere between 6 and 8 and between 9 and 11 with a plateau in performance between these increases. A comparison of these results with previously noted periods of rapid increments and plateaus in the development of bone and muscle tissue and of strength does not reveal a consistent patterning, but there is some suggestion that the plateaus in balance may coincide with the increments in bone and muscle tissue and in strength, with the reverse situation occurring with increments in balance. Certainly, a longitudinal study of all these factors would shed much more light on their interrelationships than the cross-sectional data that are currently available.

Sex differences in dynamic balance are reported by both Heath (1949) and Goetzinger (1961) favoring greater improvement in boys, whereas Keogh (1965) obtained sex differences during the periods of increase but none during the plateaus. Great variability has been found to exist among the levels of performance within a particular age group. For example, Seashore (1947) noted that some 7-year-olds were equal in performance to the average 15-year-olds, while the poorest 14-year-olds were at the level of the lowest quarter of 7-year-olds.

A static balance test in which the subjects were timed as to their ability to remain on a balance stick, 1" x 1" x 12", when the foot was placed lengthwise on the long axis of the stick was used by Seils (1951) to determine level of performance in children of the first three grades. Analysis of the data indicated a rather constant increase between 6 and 8 years. Static balance on a beam reveals age spurts for girls over the period 5 to 11 years whereas boys show a more consistent increase over the same age span (Keogh, 1965). Starting at the age of 6, steady increases are reported in the prepubescent years for both boys and girls in performance on the stabilometer (Bachman, 1961). Although Morris et al. (1982) report that girls were superior to boys in static balance at age 6, no sex differences are generally reported. However, variability is again reported to be great within one age level (Seils, 1951; Morris et al., 1982).

Electromyography (EMG) was used to study the activity patterns of four major muscles during a standard one foot balance test by 7- to 9-year-old boys (Layne and Abraham, 1987). The results showed that lateral shifts in balance were primarily mediated by the ankle musculature while hip muscles appeared to stabilize the pelvis. Action of the hip muscles was not consistently linked to ankle activity and the control of one-legged lateral balance does not rely on fixed hip-ankle synergies. Similarly, the task demands of one foot static balance on a stick were examined by Clark and Watkins (1984) using a test battery comprised of all combinations of body position, size of base of support, availability of visual cues, and leg used for support. The results from testing 6- to 9-year-old children indicated that body position, base of support, and visual cues significantly affected balance performance. The investigators concluded that the complex interaction between the dimensions tended to indicate that static balance ability in young children was a complex multidimensional construct.

Some investigators have suggested that the similarity in results between dynamic and static balance indicate a probability that growth in both may follow a similar course (Seils, 1951; Keogh, 1965). Furthermore, the wide range of proficiency in balancing activities at each age level seems to suggest that selective factors may be operating with respect to such proficiency and the choice of general motor activities made by children.

Coordination

Individuals are said to show good coordination when they move easily and the sequence and timing of their acts are well controlled. This essential element of motor performance is not readily measured objectively although high achievement in any event implies good coordination. Good general coordination should then be reflected in high achievement in a number of activities. A glance at the intercorrelations reported by various investigators of the relationships among the basic skills of running, jumping, and throwing indicates little communality (table 9.3). No consistent trends are evidenced, although there does seem to be a tendency for relationships between the dash and broad jump and between the broad jump and distance throw for boys to be slightly higher at the junior high school level than either before or after this time. In the case of girls, however, correlations are of approximately the same order at all age levels.

An investigation by Morris et al. (1978) of various motor performance tests administered to children aged 3 to 6 years indicated that the degree of interrelationship between test items may be a function of the test itself rather than reflecting the coordination of the individual. For example, the high correlation of .92 noted by Morris et al. (1978) between a distance throw using a softball and one using a tennis ball indicates a high degree of throwing consistency. However, the intercorrelations of the softball throw for distance with the run and the standing long jump were

TABLE 9.3. Intercorrelations reported by various investigators*

Age	Dash with Broad Jump		Dash with Distance Throw	
	Boys	Girls	Boys	Girls
49-78 months	.53		.36	
First 3 grades	.475	.576	.244	.442
10-14 years		.61		.43
10-13 years	.665		.502	
Junior High School	.642		.545	
	.787			
	.64	.61	.38	.51
	.67	.64	.48	.44
Senior High School	.44			
	.76			
	.58	.60		
	.48	.45	.38	.41
	.49		.24	.23
		.57		

Age	Broad Jump and Distance Throw		Broad Jump with Jump and Reach	
	Boys	Girls	Boys	Girls
49-78 months	.41		.53	
First 3 grades	.311	.441	.401	.547
8 years	.58	.35	.63	.62
10-13 years	.53			
10-14 years				.49
Junior High School	.721			
	.39	.45	.42	.30
	.60	.51	.45	.37
Senior High School	.46	.48	.65	.56
	.47	.42	.51	.64
			.604	

* From *Science and Medicine of Exercise and Sports,* edited by Warren R. Johnson. Copyright © 1960 by Warren R. Johnson: "Motor Development" by Anna Espenschade. Reprinted by permission of Harper & Row, Publishers.

only –.52 and +.64 respectively in comparison with intercorrelations between the tennis ball distance throw and the same run and jump where values were –.64 and +.74, respectively. The tennis ball throw for distance obviously resulted in higher intercorrelations between throwing and running and jumping. Similarly, the correlation of .33 between balance and the tennis throw is higher than the value of .08 between balance and the softball distance throw.

The intercorrelations for some of the basic skills tested in the Morris et al. (1978) study are presented in table 9.4. In addition, these investigators included a test of catching and balance in their test battery that are also listed in the correlation matrix. Here, as in table 9.3, the negative sign associated with correlations involving the run has been omitted. In general, the intercorrelations reported by Morris et al., for running, jumping, and throwing events are higher than those reported in table 9.3. Catching also has a substantial relationship with these test items, but balance, as measured in the Morris et al. study, has only a minor relationship with the other test items.

With such low intercorrelations being found between the basic motor activities, it is not surprising that attempts have been made to measure coordination with special coordination tests. The most commonly used test of coordination is the Brace test with its graded series of 20 stunts. Although an attempt was made to select events which measure control, balance, agility, and flexibility, and to provide for even steps in difficulty, these aims have been imperfectly met. One of its drawbacks is the scoring of all items on a pass or fail basis. As some individuals can pass all tests in the battery, the range is also inadequate for all abilities. However, the test is fairly objective and reliable and has been shown to measure abilities which are only slightly, if at all, related to strength and height or weight.

Both sexes perform equally well and consistently improve in total performance in the Brace test until the age of 11 years, after which there is an increasingly greater sex difference, with girls leveling off while boys continue to improve at a relatively consistent rate (figure 9.18). The percentage of both sexes passing the items designated as measuring "control" and "agility" is approximately equal between 10.5 and 13 years (Espenschade, 1947). The most striking sex difference at all ages is item five

TABLE 9.4. Motor performance intercorrelations: Boys and girls, aged 3–6 years*

	Catching	Speed Run	Standing Long Jump	Tennis Ball Distance Throw
Catching				
Speed run	.63			
Standing long jump	.70	.79		
Tennis ball distance throw	.59	.64	.74	
Balance	.38	.36	.44	.33

* Adapted from data from A. M. Morris; A. E. Atwater; J. M Williams; and J. H. Wilmore. *Preliminary report on the motor performance test battery for preschool children.* Western Society for Physical Education of College Women Conference, November, 1978.

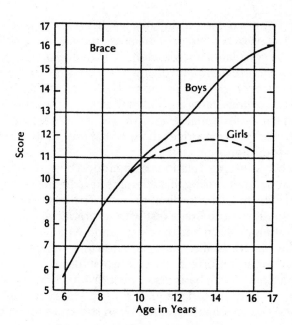

FIGURE 9.18. *Brace test. (From* Science and medicine of exercise and sports, *edited by Warren R. Johnson. Copyright © 1960 by Warren R. Johnson: "Motor Development" by Anna Espenschade. Reprinted by permission of Harper & Row, Publishers.)*

of the Brace test consisting of three push-ups, while the greatest similarity is in item 7 where the individual sits down and then stands again with the arms folded and the feet crossed.

When various test items of motor coordination are subjected to factor analysis, there would seem to be a considerable amount of interrelationship between balance, speed, ability, and control which tends to be task-specific. For example, administration of 23 items that had been used to measure some phase of motor coordination to 92 third-and fourth-grade girls produced, when the data were subjected to the multiple-group method of factoring, nine factors (Cumbee et al., 1957). Five of the nine factors extracted were identified as:

1. Balancing objects
2. Total body quick change of direction
3. Speed of change of direction of arms and hands
4. Body balance
5. Vertical total body quick change of direction

The results obtained in this study were compared with a similar factor analysis of motor coordinations of women at the college level (Cumbee,

1954) with the variable findings suggesting that consideration should be given to a different definition of motor coordination for different age levels.

More recently, research studies that have explored the development and functioning of coordinated action systems have tended to emphasize the fine structure of coordinated action sequences. For example, Southard (1985) analyzed reaction and movement times of single- and two-hand movements in his investigation of how children (age range 5 to 14 years) coordinate and control interlimb movements. His data indicated that similar changes occurred in both times for all conditions with the movement times for the hand moving the easy target in the two-hand (left easy-right difficult) condition being significantly elevated over the corresponding single-hand (left easy) condition. Further, nonsignificant reaction and movement times between hands for two-hand conditions were considered to support the concept of a systematic linkage of muscles (coordinative structures) which made two-handed movements unitary in nature. Southard concluded that coordinative structures represent an invariant mode of interlimb control across changes in age.

Fentress (1984), in his review of the development of coordination, indicates that, during development, processes of differentiation and integration are combined to make coordinated action possible. He offers the perspective that it is valuable to seek relative degrees of continuity-discontinuity and change-stability from several complementary perspectives to understand the development of coordinated action. He considers that coordinated action results from a dynamic interplay between events intrinsic to one system and the broader surround in which the system operates. In a similar review, Lee (1984) explored research associated with neurally based units of action (neuromotor synergies) as a possible basis for coordinated intentional as well as automatic actions. Computerized models for parallel computation for controlling an arm have been presented by Hinton (1984) and Abbs et al. (1984). These researchers have presented hypotheses concerning multimovement coordination with emphasis upon the sensorimotor mechanisms in speech motor programming. These types of studies of coordination (or motor control) have marked potential for defining fine structure of coordination of movement especially when combined with noninvasive techniques such as electroencephalograms (EEGs) and positron emission tomography (PET).

General

Innumerable studies have been undertaken of various specific motor performances, while others have attempted to develop some index based upon performance in specific activities which would give an overall rating or predict general motor ability, educability, agility, or coordination. In addition to the motor activities already mentioned, these have included such things as grasping, striking, relaying objects, catching, kicking, hopping, and various quick changes in body position. These activities have all been found to show increased performance with age in varying degrees of increment for boys and girls.

In general, boys have been found to excel in those activities requiring strength and in grosser movements, whereas girls tend to excel in the finer coordination activities such as exactness in walking, speed in grasping, exactness of grasping, and lying down (Yarmolenko, 1933). Boys are superior in throws for distance at all ages and gender differences of lesser magnitude are found for speed run and standing long jump with boys generally being superior to girls even in pre-school years (Morris et al., 1982). Girls have been found to be better than boys in performance in the 50-foot hop in one instance (Jenkins, 1930), whereas in other instances mean performance in the same test has been found to be almost identical for both sexes during childhood (Meyer, 1951; Keogh, 1965). In all of the studies, however, a greater percentage of boys failed to complete the entire 50-foot distance of the test and, in controlled hopping, girls were found to be superior to boys at ages 6 through 9 (Keogh, 1965). In the latter instance, girls were more graceful and hopped on the balls of their feet, whereas boys hopped in a very flatfooted manner. Differences were also noted in the technique of good and poor performers. The less able children held their nonhopping foot in a high position with the knee and foot in front of the body rather than down and behind the body in a lower position as is done by more able performers (Keogh, 1965).

Boys have been found to be superior to girls in kicking a ball for distance, and the superiority of the boys increased with advancing age as it does in the distance throw (Jenkins, 1930; Yarmolenko, 1933).

In the majority of activities at all age levels, however, there is a great deal of variability in performance, so that there is a considerable overlapping of the sexes in performance within a given age level (Jenkins, 1930). Children are still perfecting their skills and some of the variability is undoubtedly due to the propensity to avoid repetition of combinations of movements that have produced unsuccessful results (Victors, 1961).

OTHER DEVELOPMENTAL ASPECTS

It is to be expected that there will be varying degrees of interest in motor activity among children as there is among adults. The free play of children may be considered an adequate method for assessing the attitudes, interest, and skill level of young children in physical activities. When the videotaped free play of 6- and 8-year-old children was analyzed, at 15-second intervals, in terms of activity organization, activity orientation, size and sex of play group, and motor skill competency, the data revealed sex differences at 8 years for all performance parameters except skill competency (table 9.5). However, it should be noted that there was a sex difference in activity organization (activity complexity) at 8 years and the combined interpretation of activity organization and skill competency is that the boys were equally as competent in higher level activity complexity as the girls were in lower level skills. In addition, there was a marked increase in the size of the play group for boys at 8 years. Activity orientation refers to gender preferred activities with girls tending to select feminine-categorized activities (low score) and males increasing their selection of masculine-preferred activities (higher score) with increasing age. At both ages, same sex children were the preferred playmates (Crum & Eckert, 1985).

The increasing participation of males in masculine-preferred activities may be considered indicative of cultural influences. East and Hensley (1985) report that the social-cultural variables of influence of mother and father, hours of television watched, and extracurricular play experiences consistently loaded high on the regression analysis of the relative contribution to overhand throwing performance of boys and girls in grades kindergarten to third. However, they also found that as a child grows

TABLE 9.5. Means and Standard Deviations of Various Measures

Variable	6 Years		8 Years	
	M	SD	M	SD
Activity organization				
Boys	3.64	1.11	6.28[a,b]	1.85
Girls	3.57	0.53	3.56	0.89
Activity orientation				
Boys	4.41[a]	1.09	5.53[a,b]	0.88
Girls	2.89	0.82	2.65	0.77
Size of play group				
Boys	2.91	1.34	7.81[a,b]	4.69
Girls	2.44	1.26	3.35[b]	1.47
Skill competency				
Boys	4.26	1.40	5.47[b]	0.60
Girls	4.52	1.47	5.03	1.04

[a] Significant difference between the sexes for one age grouping
[b] Significant difference between age grouping for one sex

(Reprinted from Crum J. F., & Eckert, H. M. Play Patterns of Primary School Children. In J. E. Clark & J. H. Humphrey (Eds.), *Motor Development. Current Selected Research.* Princeton, NJ: Princeton Book Company, Publishers, 1985. By permission of the publisher.)

older, factors other than sociocultural determinants become relatively more important in the explanation of overhand throwing performance. As overhand throwing is a skill in which there are sex differences at an early age, these results suggest that skill competency may be an important factor in physical participation. Ulrich (1987) found that children's reported perceptions of physical competence were significantly related to their demonstrated motor competence. In addition, the motor competence of those children in kindergarten through the fourth grade was significantly related to participation, i.e., participants in organized sports programs performed selected gross motor tasks better than did nonparticipants.

In their study, East and Hensley (1985) noted that active sports-minded fathers had active sons who performed well on the overhand throw for distance. On the other hand, for the girls, over 25 percent of the variance for overhand throwing performance was attributable to the stereotype father-figure who socialized the daughter away from sports and physically competitive situations. Therefore, interest in physical activity will depend, to a large extent, upon the opportunities for motor activity and the interest that is expressed in such activity by the persons with whom the child identifies during the growing years. Interest has been found to increase in motor activities through childhood to adolescence, with a marked increase during the latter part of childhood and early adolescence for both boys and girls (figures 9.19 and 9.20). This is, of course, the period in which the child wants to be a member of the "gang" and motor activities offer an excellent opportunity for such association.

After 9 years of age children begin to perfect an increasing number of activities which will enable them to take part in adult sports and games with only body size limiting the level of performance. Such emulation of adult activities undoubtedly is a factor in increasing interest. Conversely, however, lack of ability will also be a deterrent at this peer-conscious age and will result in withdrawal from unproficient areas and an expressed decline in interest.

More proficient children have been found to come from homes where the parents have been highly active in sports and have provided the children with greater opportunity and provision for play. These opportunities included a wider variety of play materials at an earlier age which allowed for the use of large muscle activity and more frequent visitations to playgrounds so that the child acquired a wider range of interests and activity in play (Rarick & McKee, 1949). Opportunities for participation in good physical education programs in school also contribute to proficiency. A comparison of 81 12-year-old boys who had participated in a good physical education program for at least three years was made with 81 boys of the same age who had had little or no physical education in the elementary school. Although the two groups were sim-

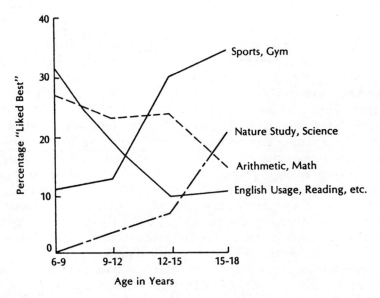

FIGURE 9.19. *Expressed interests of boys. (From data by A. T. Jersild and R. Tasch,* Children's interests and what they suggest for education. *New York: Bureau of Publications, Teachers College, Columbia University, 1949. By permission of the publisher.)*

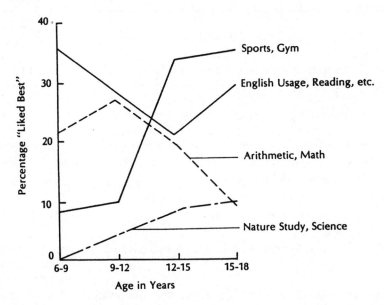

FIGURE 9.20. *Expressed interests of girls. (From data by A. T. Jersild and R. Tasch,* Children's interests and what they suggest for education. *New York: Bureau of Publications, Teachers College, Columbia University, 1949. By permission of the publisher.)*

ilar with respect to chronological age, weight, height, skeletal age, and Wetzel grid developmental level, the boys in the good program surpassed the boys in the poor program in the Rogers Physical Fitness Index, the Metheny-Johnson Test of Motor Educability, the Indiana Fitness Test, the vertical jump, and back, leg, and arm strength (Whittle, 1961).

According to Godin and Shepard (1986) attitudes, current physical activity habit, and prior experience of exercise all contribute significantly to explaining the variance in exercise. In addition, more variance of exercise intentions can be explained in students who had personal experience of physical activity early in childhood and the investigators concluded their results supported the value of early socialization towards physical activity. Similarly, a meta-analysis by Gruber (1986) led to the conclusion that participation in directed play and/or physical education programs contributes to the self-esteem of children.

Opportunities for perfecting the skills that have been developed during infancy and early childhood remain of considerable importance in later childhood if the child is to maintain a level of performance similar to his age-mates. In addition, the health related aspects of physical activity, in particular as they relate to obesity (Williams, 1986), are of considerable concern. Haskell, Montoye, and Orenstein (1985) recommend the following health-fitness goals for youth (1–14 years):

a) Optimal physical growth and development
b) Good psychological adjustment
c) Development of interest and skills for active lifestyle as adult
d) Reduction of coronary heart disease risk factors

The recommended physical activity plan includes:

- Type of exercise: Emphasis on large muscle, dynamic exercise; moving body over distance against gravity; some heavy resistive activity and flexibility exercise.
- Intensity: Moderate to vigorous intensity.
- Duration: Total of more than 30 minutes per day in one or more sessions.
- Frequency: Every day. The goal is increased activity to and from school.

The general developmental characteristics associated with later childhood listed in table 9.6 reemphasize the relationship between physical structure and function. In addition, the expanding intellectual and social capabilities of the child must receive attention for the optimal development of the individual.

TABLE 9.6. Summary of general developmental characteristics during late childhood

Characteristics
1. Relative stability in growth
2. Limbs continue to grow more rapidly in proportion to the rest of the body
3. Some preadolescent changes in the shoulder/hip ratio for the sexes
4. Preadolescent fat spurt for some individuals, particularly males
5. Differential growth rates become more marked at end of period as early maturers begin adolescent growth spurt
6. Balance becomes well developed
7. Basic motor patterns are more refined and adapted to structural differences
8. Better coordination and body control
9. Continued increase in strength and endurance
10. Eye-hand coordination improved; increased proficiency in manipulative skills
11. Increased attention span
12. Sees need to practice skills for improvement, to gain social status and to develop endurance
13. Spirit of adventure high
14. More socially mature; interested in group welfare
15. Intellectually curious
16. Greater interest in proficiency and competitive spirit—hero worship of athletes
17. Some sex differences in performance and some antagonism towards opposite sex

Needs	Experiences
Use of skill for specific purposes; opportunity to take part in a wide variety of activities to gain knowledge of proficiencies	Introduction to sports skills; lead-up games; self-testing activities; use of apparatus; drills and self-testing practice situations; low organization games requiring courage
Opportunity for group activities	Team activities; dance composition; folk and square dance
Opportunities to explore; learn mechanical principles; physiology, kinesiology of movement	Self-testing and problem-solving activities related to own skill; creative dance; developmental exercise programs
Ability grouping for some individual activities and team games, particularly those involving strength and endurance components	Self-testing activities; relaxation techniques; developmental exercises and interval training; combatives

SUMMARY

1. Indices of growth and maturation include: chronological age, height, weight, indices using combinations of these, skeletal age, dental age, and biological indices (secondary sex characteristics). School grade has also been used to indicate level of maturity but is not as precise as the others.

2. The limbs, especially the legs, grow more than the trunk so there is a gradual decrease in the sitting height/standing height ratio during childhood.

3. During late childhood, growth in shoulder width in boys becomes more than that of girls and girls grow more in hip width so that the hip/shoulder ratio begins to become greater for girls.

4. Body build has been assessed by different types of anthropometric indices most of which include height and weight. In addition, somatotype techniques have been developed such as the Sheldon system (endomorphy, mesomorphy, and ectomorphy). The Heath-Carter modification of somatotyping includes anthropometric measures in the assessment of body type.

5. Increases in strength are associated with increases in muscle mass and are usually measured as isometric strength (static; no movement) and isotonic strength (dynamic; movement of joint). Measures of maximal strength at different speed (isokinetic strength using a Cybex) indicate that higher strength values are attained at low speeds than at high speed in keeping with the physical law $F = MxA$ where the F (maximal strength) is fixed.

6. Boys tend to be superior to girls in activities requiring strength and in performance tasks such as running and jumping and are significantly so in distance throwing and kicking a ball for distance. Girls are somewhat better than boys in fine motor skills and in some locomotor activities such as hopping and skipping.

7. Intercorrelations between gross motor tasks tend to be low to moderate during late childhood but higher for boys than girls. In multi-item tests of coordination, such as the Brace test, boys tend to score higher than girls but such differences may be a feature of item selection.

8. Little or no relationship has been found between static and dynamic balance and a great deal of variability in both these types of balance exists at any one age level. Although increases in performance are reported with increasing age, there appear to be plateaus, or slower gain periods, which may be associated with growth and maturational changes.

9. Interest in physical activity is associated with past participation experience, level of competency, opportunities for participation, and sociocultural factors.

10

Adolescent Development

Adolescence is usually said to begin with the physical changes relating to puberty and to continue until growth is complete and the individual thus is mature, in a physical sense. The biologically most important of these is the development of the reproductive system into its mature state in both sexes. Figure 10.1, illustrating the growth in weight of the **testes**, prostate, ovaries, and uterus, shows that the development of the reproductive organs begins earlier in females than in males. The onset of puberty is difficult to assess in males and is usually based upon the development of the secondary sex characteristics and the growth of the genitalia. In females, the menarche, or first menstrual period, is usually taken as the onset of puberty, although Ashley Montagu (1946) has pointed out that the adolescent girl may be sterile for some months after the onset of menstruation.

In boys, the first sign of impending puberty is usually an acceleration in the growth of the testes and scrotum with, perhaps, slight growth in pubic hair beginning at the same time. Pubic hair growth tends to proceed slowly until the beginning of the general growth spurt, after which it increases rapidly to its mature distribution. In general, the spurts in height and penis growth begin about a year after the onset of testicular acceleration. Although this sequence of events tends to be relatively consistent in the development of boys, the times at which they occur is extremely variable so that it is possible to have boys at the ages of 13 and 14 years who may vary in development from childhood through all stages to almost complete maturity. Figure 10.2, developed by Tanner (1955) from the data presented in numerous studies of adolescent males, indicates the timing of these developmental events for an average boy and also the range of ages at which each event may begin and reach its termination.

For girls, the first sign of approaching puberty is usually the appearance of the breast bud, although the appearance of pubic hair may sometimes precede it. Figure 10.3, also developed by Tanner (1955) from the

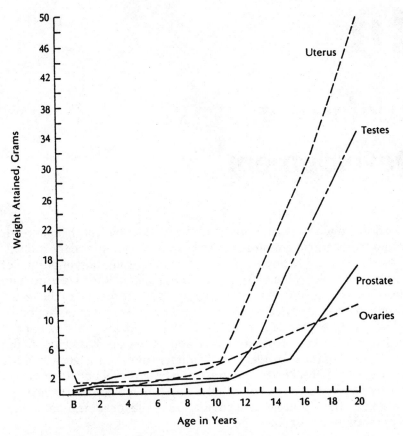

FIGURE 10.1. *Growth in weight of the reproductive organs. (From J. M. Tanner, Growth at adolescence. Oxford, Eng.: Blackwell Scientific Publications, 1955. By permission of the publisher.)*

data presented in a number of studies of adolescent girls, shows the sequence of events for the average girl with the range in times for the appearance of breast bud, beginning of pubic hair growth, menarche, and peak velocity in height being indicated directly under each event. It may be noted that the range and duration of the events associated with adolescence in females appears to be less than those characteristic of males during adolescence.

A number of scales are available for rating genital developmental stages, breast development stages, and pubic hair stages. Typical of the first is the following five stage rating of genitalia maturation in males:

1. Infantile;
2. Enlargement of scrotum, first reddening and texture change;

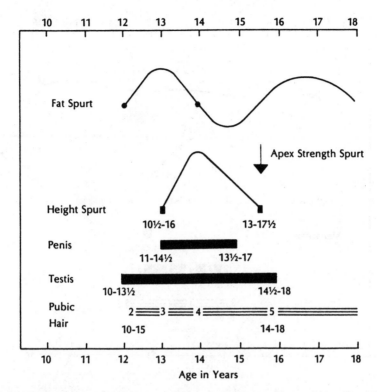

FIGURE 10.2 *Diagram of sequence of events at adolescence in boys. An average boy is represented: the range of ages within which each event charted may begin and end is given by the figures placed directly below its start and finish. (From J. M. Tanner,* Growth at adolescence. *Oxford, Eng.: Blackwell Scientific Publications, 1955. By permission of the publisher.)*

3. First "sculpturing" and enlargement of penis;
4. Pronounced sculpturing and darkening;
5. Essentially adult, reddish brown color, loose penile skin, loss of sharp sculpturing.*

A five stage rating scale for female breast development is as follows:

1. The infantile form: elevation of papilla only;
2. The bud stage: elevation of the breast and papilla as a small mound;
3. Intermediate state: elevation of breast and areola with no distinct separation of their contours;

---

* From E. L. Reynolds & J. V. Wines, Physical changes associated with adolescence in boys. *Amer. J. Dis. Child.*, 1951, *82*, 529–547. By permission of the authors and publisher.

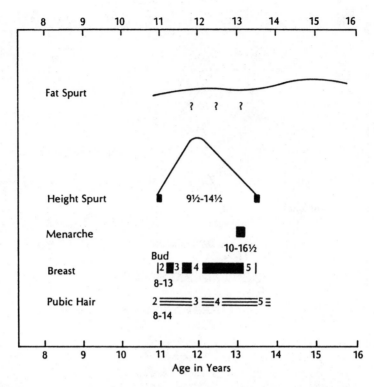

FIGURE 10.3. *Diagram of sequence of events at adolescence in girls. An average girl is represented: the range of ages within which some of the events may occur is given by the figures placed directly below them. (From J. M. Tanner, Growth at adolescence. Oxford, Eng.: Blackwell Scientific Publications, 1955. By permission of the publisher.)*

4. Primary mamma stage: areola and papilla form a secondary mound above the level of the breast;

5. Mature stage: the papilla only projects, owing to the recession of the areola to the general contour of the breast.*

The development of pubic hair in boys has also been classified into five stages, namely:

1. Infantile;

2. First appearance, pigmented, usually straight, sparse;

3. Slight curl, slight spread, usually darker;

---

* From E. L. Reynolds & J. V. Wines, Individual differences in physical changes associated with adolescence in girls. *Amer. J. Dis. Child.*, 75, 329–350, 1948. By permission of the authors and publisher.

4. Curled, moderate amount and spread, not yet extended to thighs;
5. "Adult" in type, profuse, forming an inverse triangle extending to thighs.*

Although pubic hair rating stages differ from those of genitalia and breast development, they are the most frequently used to assess sexual development, since they are most reliably observed. **Axillary** hair generally appears about two years after the beginning of pubic hair growth, which places it at approximately the end of pubic hair stage 3. In boys, facial hair begins to grow at about the time that axillary hair first appears and its development is usually not completed until stage 5 is reached in both pubic hair and genitalia development. The remainder of the body hair in males starts to appear at this time also and continues to do so for a considerable time afterwards, with the hair on the thigh, calf, abdomen, and forearm usually preceding that on the chest and upper arms.

Other secondary sex changes include the enlargement of the larynx in boys, which tends to coincide with the spurt in sitting height, and the deepening of the voice. Both sexes have an increase in axillary sweating, which is believed to be due to an enlargement of the apocrine sweat glands of the axilla that begins at approximately the time of axillary hair growth (Tanner, 1955). Intercorrelations which have been calculated to determine the relationships between the various criteria of maturity produce correlation coefficients ranging from .71 to .95 (Nicholson & Hanley, 1953), indicating there is a unity in the adolescent spurt with respect to bodily growth, physiologicial changes, and growth of the reproductive organs.

FACTORS AFFECTING THE ONSET OF PUBERTY

Since the menarche in girls is an easily ascertained event, its occurrence is usually used to study trends in the onset of puberty. A marked secular trend of lowering in the age of menarche has been noted (Mills, 1950). Figure 10.4 indicates the average ages at menarche from 1850 to 1970 in Norway and over segments of this period for girls in Sweden, Finland, England, and the United States. The trend towards earlier onset of menarche is very similar in all countries from 1850 until 1950, and Tanner (1955) indicates an earlier occurrence of $\frac{1}{3}$ to $\frac{1}{2}$ year per decade.

The patterning of the secular trend for menarche is not as consistent after 1950. A comparison of data collected in 1950 and similar data col-

---

* From E. L. Reynolds & J. V. Wines, Physical changes associated with adolescence in boys. *Amer. J. Dis. Child.*, 82, 529–547, 1951. By permission of the authors and publisher.

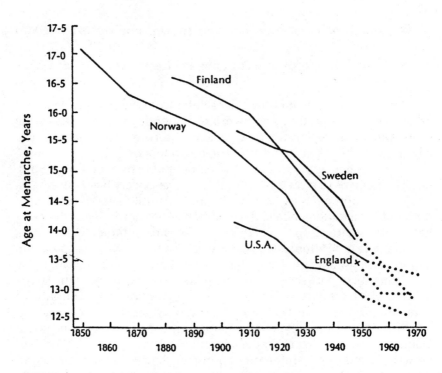

FIGURE 10.4 *Secular trend in age at menarche. (1850 to 1950 from J. M. Tanner,
Growth at adolescence. Oxford, Eng.: Blackwell Scientific Publications. By per-
mission of the publisher. English data for 1959 and 1966–1967 from J. M. Tanner,
Trend towards earlier menarche in London, Oslo, Copenhagen, the Netherlands
and Hungary. Nature, 1973, 243, 95–96. Swedish data for 1968 from B.-O. Ljung; A.
Bergsten-Brucefors, and G. Lindgren, The secular trend in physical growth in
Sweden, Annals of Hum. Biol., 1974, 1(3), 245–256. Norwegian data for 1970 from
G. H. Brundtland and L. Walloe, Menarcheal age in Norway: Halt in the trend
towards earlier maturation. Nature, 1973, 241, 478–479. American data for
1964–1965 from L. Zacharias; R. J. Wurtman; and M. Schatzoff, Sexual maturation
in contemporary American girls. Amer. J. Obstet. Gynec., 1970, 108 (5), 833–846.)*

lected in 1968 by Ljung et al. (1974) indicates a continuation of the
downward trend with menarche tending to occur approximately 4.5
months earlier per decade in Sweden. A similar downward trend was
noted by Zacharias et al. (1970) who reported that the age of menarche
was 4.5 months earlier for 6217 American student nurses than for their
mothers. The mean menarcheal age for the students who were surveyed
in 1964–1965 was 12.65 years. However, the trend seems to have stopped
in Norway. Recalculations of previously published 1952 data place the
mean age of menarche at 13.27 years, which is slightly earlier than the
previously listed mean of 13.44 years. Brundtland and Walloe (1973) used

similar calculation procedures to determine that the mean age of menarche in Oslo in 1970 was 13.24 years. Figure 10.4 shows the mean menarcheal age reported by Brundtland and Walloe in conjunction with the previously reported 13.44 age in 1952 so that a slight decline would seem to have occcured. However, if the recalculated mean menarcheal age for 1952 is accepted, then there has been no change in the menarchael onset in Norway between 1952 and 1970 indicating that the secular trend towards earlier occurrence may have stopped. A similar leveling off of the mean menarcheal age at 13.02 from 1959 to 1966–1967 has been reported for London girls (Tanner, 1973). It should be noted that the countries in which the leveling off appears to be occurring were those in which the mean menarcheal age was 13.5 years or less in 1950.

Figure 10.4 also indicates that there are age differences in the onset of menarche in the various countries. On the basis of a number of studies, it would appear that these regional variations in the menarche tend to be caused by climatic, nutritional, and racial differences. A survey of the average age at first menstruation for girls in the Americas, Europe, and Asia indicates that the menarche occurs consistently earlier in the central temperate areas and tends to be delayed in the colder northern and southern regions. The menarche also appears earlier in girls in the United States than in any other country (Shuttleworth, 1949). Mills (1950) found that prolonged heat tended to retard growth in girls and delay the onset of menarche, whereas boys did not show as great a susceptibility to heat. Similar results were obtained by Ellis (1950) in comparing a group of Nigerian school children with a control group of school children in Great Britain.

Seasonal variations in the onset of menarche also exist, but apparent relationships are more equivocal. Bojlen and Bentzon (1974) report the highest incidence of menarche onset in January for Japan and Northern Europe with the greatest variability for onset occurring in summer in these regions. On the other hand, Zacharias et al. (1970) found that the peak incidence of menarche was in June and July in the United States. In this study, the lowest incidence occurred in October and March so that there was a secondary peak in December and January. Zacharias et al. (1970) cite the amount of light as a potential factor mediating the seasonal variation in the onset of menarche. However, in a subsequent examination of seasonal variation, Marshall (1975) concluded that seasonal variations in light and temperature exert, at most, only a small effect on growth rates and perhaps none at all.

It is possible that the seasonal variation in the onset of menarche is associated with the seasonal variations in weight gain which are discussed later in this chapter. Zacharias et al. (1970) report that menarche tended to occur earlier for obese girls and this earlier occurrence was proportional to the degree of obesity in the 10 to 30 percent above standard weight range. Therefore, the seasonally greater gain of weight in fall may account for the higher incidence of menarcheal onset in January reported by Bojlen and Bentzon and for the secondary peak in the data of Zacharias et al. Regional differences in menarcheal age have also been attributed to altitude with girls in Denver reportedly having a tendency to mature somewhat later than girls in San Francisco. The significantly earlier menarche in Northeastern United States in comparison with the rest of the country that was noted by Zacharias et al. (1970) was considered to be due to urbanization or the presence in that population of a greater proportion of ethnic groups that exhibit earlier menarche.

Little or no difference between the average ages of sexual maturity in Negro and white boys is reported (Ramsey, 1950). Ito (1942), however, reports varying ages of menarche for girls of different racial origin who were attending Los Angeles City College. Those girls of Mexican origin had an average menarcheal age of 12.5; for Europeans it was 12.9; while for Japanese and Negroes it was 13.1; and for Chinese 13.9 years. Conversely, no difference is reported in the age of menarche between whites and Negroes of similar economic circumstances in New York (Michelson, 1944). Certainly racial differences do exist as indicated by the survey of menarcheal onset based on climatic regions by Shuttleworth (1949) and based upon regional differences in Europe by Krogman (1955).

Differences within racial groupings also exist either as natural variation or on a nutritional basis. Bolk (1926) and Ley (1938) noted that in both Amsterdam and Mainz, Germany, darker-haired children tended to have a later menarche, whereas the reverse situation might be expected on the grounds that the hair tends to darken somewhat with age. The menarche was found to occur 1.6 years sooner in school girls in Columbo, Ceylon, than in girls of rural areas of the same country (Wilson & Sutherland, 1953). The influence of nutrition is pointed up by Ito's data (1942) which shows that Japanese girls born and reared in California mature 1½ years earlier than those born in California but reared in Japan.

The observation of Barker and Stone (1936) that menarche occurs in obese girls approximately eight months earlier than in thin girls is supported by Pryor's findings (1936) that girls with a broad build achieve menarche sooner than those of a slender build. The strong hereditary component noted by Parnell (1958) with children having similar physiques to those of their parents suggests that menarcheal onset is a factor of genetics rather than nutrition in this instance. In his survey of genetic control of menarche, Tanner (1955) concludes that there is a fairly high correlation between onset of menarche of mothers and daughters and cites Popenoe's report of a correlation of .40 for 200 mothers and 351 daughters and one of .39 for sisters.

Activity level may also influence the onset of menarche. Frisch and McArthur (1974) reported that a minimum weight for height (representing a critical lean/fat ratio) was necessary for menarche and the maintenance of regular ovulatory cycles. Since then Frisch et al. (1980) has reported delayed menarche and amenorrhea in ballet dancers. In addition, Frisch et al. (1981) have reported similar results for pre-menarche trained college swimmers (menarche mean 15.0 years) and runners (menarche mean 15.2 years) in comparison with postmenarcheal trained teammates in swimming (menarche mean 12.6 years) and runners (menarche mean 12.9 years). For all the pre-menarche trained athletes, menarche was delayed about 0.4 years for each year of training. Amenorrhea was also found more frequently in the pre-menarche trained athletes and increased during training for both groups and decreased after the training season.

FACTORS AFFECTING PUBERAL GROWTH SPURT

A comparison of the appearance of the puberal height spurt in both boys and girls of Sweden as measured in 1883 and in 1938 reveals a trend toward acceleration of the growth spurt in keeping with the previously reported earlier appearance of the menarche (Broman et al., 1942). Figure 10.5 illustrates this secular trend in the adolescent growth spurt. Boys have a large displacement in the peak of gain, and the amount of growth

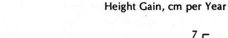

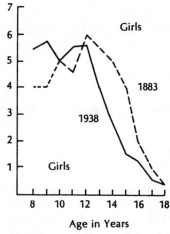
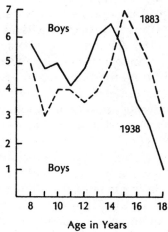

FIGURE 10.5 *Secular trend in time of adolescent spurt. Velocity curves of height for Swedish girls and boys measured in 1883 and 1938–1939. (From J. M. Tanner, Growth at adolescence. Oxford, Eng.: Blackwell Scientific Publications, 1955. By permission of the publisher.)*

in height is greater for both sexes during preadolescence in 1938 children. Other data indicate that the peak height gain occurred as late as age 17 in males in the year 1800 (Kiil, 1939) in comparison with more current data which places the peak gain in height between 14 and 15 years in boys.

The marked tendency for puberty to occur earlier as indicated by the foregoing studies of the menarche and of the growth spurt has led to speculation as to causative influences. Mills (1949) has theorized that the acceleration in growth is due to a gradual change in world temperature conditions and cites as evidence work with experimental animals indicating that conditions which create difficulty of heat loss tend to retard growth. Most investigators, however, usually credit better nutrition and generally improved environmental circumstances for the secular trend toward earlier maturation and cite the slowing down of growth and the retardation of puberty during malnutrition. The data of Howe and Schiller (1952) indicate a uniform increase in the heights and weights of school children of all ages in Stuttgart, Germany, for the period from 1920 to 1940, with a reversal during the latter part of the 1939–1945 war period when the food intake of the children was considerably restricted. From additional data collected in France by Douady and Tremolières (1947) and in Belgium by Ellis (1945), it appears that war-time privation may be more effective in retarding puberty than in slowing down earlier growth.

Numerous studies indicate that during short periods of malnutrition the organism's growth is slowed up as if to wait for better times. When conditions improve, growth takes place unusually rapidly until the animal has returned to its genetically determined growth curve and growth again proceeds at its normal rate (Clarke & Smith, 1938; Barnes et al., 1947). On the basis of data collected by Engle et al. (1937) on rats, it would appear that, under adverse nutritional conditions puberty simply waits until the body has grown, however slowly, to approximately its normal puberal size or to its genetically determined maturity. In addition to adverse nutritional conditions, other environmental factors such as disease or radiation exposure may affect physical growth and maturity. In the latter regard, Greulich and Turner (1953) found some retardation in height, weight, and skeletal maturity for children exposed to A-bomb radiation at Hiroshima and Nagasaki.

In the light of the secular trend in menarche and puberal growth spurt and the advances in nutrition and generally improved environmental conditions, it is not surprising, then, that there has also been a marked increase in body size at all age levels. Figure 10.6 illustrates this secular trend in heights and weights of Swedish school children with a separate recording of the age ranges of 7 to 14 years from the elementary schools and of 10 to 18 from the secondary schools. It also indicates that differences between these two school populations were greater in both height

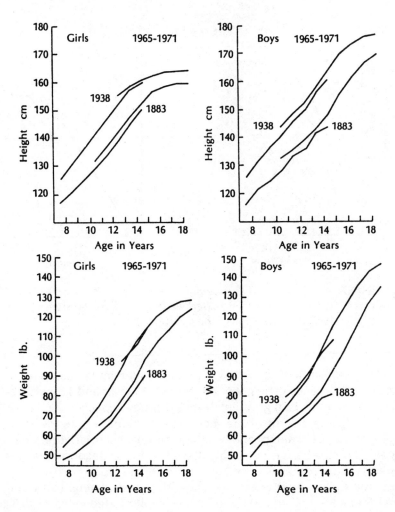

FIGURE 10.6. *Secular trend in growth in height and weight. Height (above) and weight (below) of Swedish girls and boys. (Data in 1883 and 1938–1939; elementary schools age 7 to 14, secondary schools 10 to 18. From J. M. Tanner,* Growth at adolescence. *Oxford, Eng.: Blackwell Scientific Publications, 1955. By permission of the publisher. Data for 1965–1971 adapted from B.-O. Ljung; A. Bergsten-Brucefors; and G. Lindgren, The secular trend in physical growth in Sweden.* Annals of Hum. Biol., *1974, 1 (3), 245–256.)*

and weight for both sexes in 1883 than in 1938. This is undoubtedly a reflection of greater socioeconomic differences between the groups in 1883.

A similar secular trend of increased body size and weight in American children has been noted over a 40-year period. Figure 10.7 illustrates

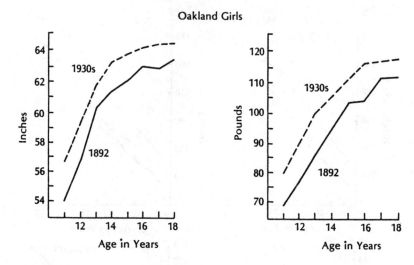

FIGURE 10.7. *A secular trend as shown in growth curves for girls. (From H. E. Jones and M. C. Jones, Adolescence. Berkeley: University Extension, University of California, 1957. By permission of the publisher.)*

the changes from 1892 to the 1930's for girls while similar results for boys indicate a difference in height of 2.3 inches at 11 years and 3.3 inches at 16 years favoring the 1930 grouping (Jones & Jones, 1957).

As with the advent of the menarche, regional variations are also noted in growth in height and weight. Although such variations may be expected on the basis of regional differences in socioeconomic status, it appears that, in some instances, these differences are so great as to overcome the socioeconomic factors. The differences in height and weight for girls in Kansas, California, and Tennessee illustrated in figure 10.8 are such an example. Here the lower of two social groups in California was on the average taller and heavier at each age than the higher social group in Tennessee (Jones & Jones, 1957).

A similar comparison of boys measured at the University of Iowa Child Welfare Station with boys in the Oakland Growth Study indicates that the California boys acieved greater growth in height even though the social status of the Iowa boys' parents was somewhat superior (Jones & Jones, 1957). Figure 10.9 gives the growth curves of these two groups and also the amount of gain in height. It clearly indicates that the growth of the Iowa and California boys was similar in childhood but that the California group grew more rapidly during adolescence. This more rapid growth spurt on the part of the California boys at puberty may be, in part, an explanation of their greater height in subsequent years.

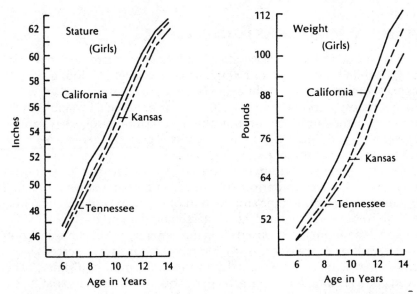

FIGURE 10.8. *Growth in height and weight: regional comparisons. (From H. E. Jones and M. C. Jones,* Adolescence. *Berkeley: University Extension, University of California, 1957. By permission of the publisher.)*

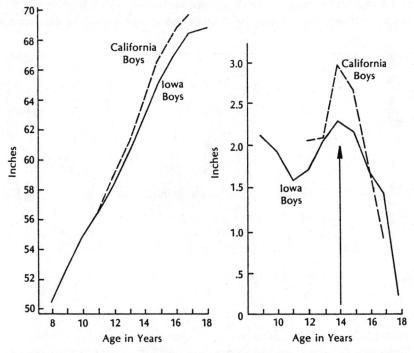

FIGURE 10.9. *Growth in height: Iowa and California boys. (From H. E. Jones and M. C. Jones,* Adolescence. *Berkeley: University Extension, University of California, 1957. By permission of the publisher.)*

SEASONAL VARIATIONS IN GROWTH

Well-defined seasonal variations have been found to exist in the rate of growth in both height and weight at all age levels, including adolescence, with growth in weight being fastest in the autumn and growth in height fastest in spring. Figure 10.10 shows the seasonal variations in the rate of weight gain of children in the northern hemisphere. October, November, and December are the months of greatest increase, with this weight increment sometimes being five or six times the amount of gain during the minimal increment months of April, May, and June. In general, over a six-month period, two-thirds of the annual weight gain is made between September and the end of February and the remaining one-third between the months of March and the end of August. These seasonal variations are imposed upon the general growth curve and, during periods of low rate of growth, it is possible for a small percentage of children to actually lose weight during the spring months (Palmer, 1933). Even upon termination of the growth period, such seasonal variation exists; adults show weight gains averaging about one pound in the fall and loss of the corresponding amount in the spring (Kemsley, 1953).

The maximum height gains in childhood and adolescence are made at the same time minimal increases are recorded in weight. The majority of data indicate that 55 to 57 percent of the annual gain in height is made

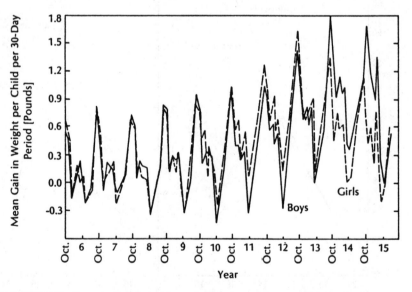

FIGURE 10.10. *Seasonal variation in weight gain, as observed in yearly age groups of elementary school children, Hagerstown, Md. (From C. E. Palmer, Seasonal variations of average growth in weight of elementary school children. Pbl. Hlth. Rep., Wash., 1933, 48, 211–233.)*

between the beginning of April and the end of September, with the average rate of gain during the months of April, May, and June being 2 to 2½ times that during the months of October, November, and December. More new ossification centers appear in the spring than in the fall, so that seasonal variation in skeletal maturity tends to coincide with seasonal variations in height gain (Reynolds & Sontag, 1944).

Since strength is more highly correlated with weight than with height, it might be expected that seasonal variations in strength should resemble the weight pattern. Such is not the case, however, for seasonal increments in stength and height gains coincide, with the greatest gains in strength being made in April while the smallest gains or, in the case of the girls, the greatest losses, are made in October. Although the seasonal variations are similar in both sexes, the absolute increments for boys are greater, as they would have to be to account for their greater increase in strength, but, even with the lesser increments, the seasonal differences are more marked in girls (Jones, 1949). The apparent seasonal discrepancy between weight and strength gains may be attributed to a lag between increases in muscular mass, as represented by weight, and gains in muscular functioning as indicated in strength measurements. Furthermore, total weight includes an element of "dead weight" which is uncorrelated with strength, and it is possible that this "dead weight" gain is minimal during periods of rapid gain in height.

CHANGES IN BODY PROPORTIONS

The physical changes associated with sexual maturation of the individual reach their peak during the period of adolescence. One of the earliest manifestations of such maturation is the puberal growth spurt which, as with previously mentioned indices of maturation, appears first in female children. In girls, this growth spurt lasts from about 11 to 13½ years of age during which time the peak height gain averages 3¼ inches per year. In boys the growth spurt begins about two years later, from 13 to 15½ years, and has a peak gain in height growth of about four inches per year. Figure 10.11, based on data by Shuttleworth (1939), illustrates this earlier growth spurt in girls and points up the fact that it is of a lesser magnitude for girls than for boys.

Figure 10.11 also indicates that there is a marked difference in the height increments for early as compared with late maturing boys and girls. This difference, coupled with differential growth rates of the various segments of the body, tends to sculpture the body configuration of the adolescent and postadolescent. The peak period of growth of the various parts of the skeleton and the body tissues tends to coincide with the peak period of the puberal growth spurt. Figure 10.12 indicates this general

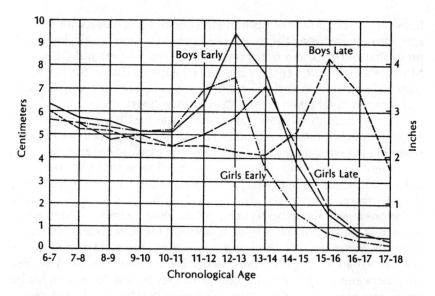

FIGURE 10.11. *Average yearly increments of growth in standing height for early-as compared to late-maturing boys and girls (late and early categories determined by age of maximum growth). (From J. E. Horrocks, The adolescent. In L. Carmichael (Ed.),* Manual of child psychology. *New York: John Wiley & Sons, Inc., 1954. By permission of the publisher.)*

coincidence in three body measures with gain in height and weight in males and also points up the variations in rates of increase between these body areas. For example, the slight spurt in hand length prior to the spurt in height undoubtedly accounts for the early adolescent appearing to be "all hands and feet."

Reynolds and Schoen (1947), using longitudinal data of males, found that leg length tends to reach its peak first and is followed four months later by hip width and chest breadth. A few months after the peak of hip width and chest breadth gain, shoulder breadth reaches its peak, with trunk length and chest depth being the last of the skeletal measurements to achieve their peak gain. Since approximately one year separates the peaks of leg length and trunk length gains, the peak gain in stature consequently lies between the two. However, as more of the gain in height can be attributed to increases in trunk length than to leg length during this time, the peak in stature gain tends to be closer to the peak of trunk length gain. These differential growth rates of the various body segments from birth to adult conformation involve a doubling of head size; a trebling of trunk length; a quadrupling of the upper limbs; and a quintupling of the lower limbs (Krogman, 1955).

A quick glance at figure 10.11 would seem to indicate that early ma-

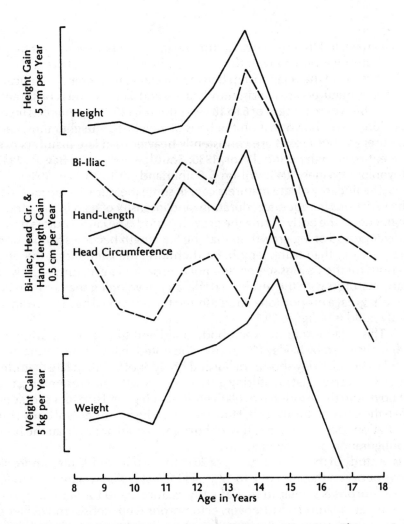

FIGURE 10.12. *Adolescent spurts in various body measurements. The curves are arranged one beneath the other without regard to zero on the vertical scale. Average figures for 3 monovular triplets, each measured at each age. (From J. M. Tanner,* Growth at adolescence. *Oxford, Eng.: Blackwell Scientific Publications, 1955. By permission of the publisher.)*

turing girls and boys grow taller than the late maturers on the basis of a lesser gain of the latter in peak height increments. However, such is not the case, since the late maturers grow over a longer period of time and, although they may be shorter during the early part of the adolescent period, they tend to be as tall or taller during adulthood. Measurement of 188 cadet officers at the Royal Military Academy in Sandhurst by Tanner

(1955) revealed that there was a strict relationship between adult height and maturity grouping with the latest maturers being the tallest.

A study of the relationship between weight and menarche indicates that early maturers are consistently heavier and late maturers consistently lighter between the ages of 6 to 18 years (Richey, 1937). Numerous investigations have shown that on the basis of weight-for-height ratios, early maturers of both sexes are consistently heavier than late maturers over the entire growth period (Pryor, 1936; Shuttleworth, 1939; Bayley, 1943; Reynolds & Wines, 1948; Wilson & Sutherland, 1950; Tanner, 1955).

The linearity of late maturers can, in some measure, be attributed to the variations in sequence, duration, and intensity of gain in the various segments of the body during the growth period. The late maturers have a longer period of leg growth so that the leg length becomes proportionately greater than trunk length. Furthermore, the gain during the peak periods for the various segments is not as great for late maturers as it is for early maturers with the results that the later developing segments do not have as great a proportional increase and the individual has a more linear body build (see figure 10.11).

This relationship between body build and timing of maturing has been observed by Bayley (1943) also. She noted that early maturing boys tend to be relatively shorter of leg and broader of hip than late maturing boys. Conversely, late maturing girls have a growth spurt resembling that of boys, and these girls have relatively longer legs and broader shoulders than the early maturing girls. However, even here the general body configuration only approaches that of boys and would not overlap the body configuration of the average boy.

A study of the growth curves of 26 ectomorphic and 28 mesomorphic boys between the ages of 2 to 17 years indicates that weight growth for mesomorphs is similar to that of early maturers and for ectomorphs to that of late maturers. Moreover, ectomorphs were consistently taller at all ages after four years. Peaks in the puberal height spurt occurred about one year later in the ectomorphs (Dupertuis & Michael, 1953). Similarly, a significantly greater percentage of endomesomorphic boys are advanced than retarded in skeletal maturity (Clarke, Irving, & Heath, 1961), and slow skeletal maturers are predominantly ectomorphic (Acheson & Dupertuis, 1957).

Studies of the relationship between somatotype and the menarche by Barker and Stone (1936), who used the Kretschmerian body typing, revealed that pyknic (obese) women have their first menstruation approximately eight months earlier than leptosomic (thin) women. Similarly, girls with a slender body build tend to menstruate later than girls with a broad build (Pryor, 1936).

Sex differences in body build become noteworthy after puberty. In general, the chief skeletal differences between adult men and women are in overall size and in greater shoulder width and limb length in men and broader hips in women. The relatively longer arm of the male when the sexes are equated for size is due mainly to a sex difference in the development of the forearm (Dupertuis & Hadden, 1951). This difference is already established at 2 years and is increased during the period from 2 years to adolescence by the continuously greater relative growth rate of the forearm to the upper arm in boys (Maresh, 1943). The data of Meredith and Boynton (1937) indicate that this sex difference also extends to the circumference of the forearm as well as the length of the segment.

Variations between the sexes in hip and shoulder width may be attributed to differential sex hormone secretions. Figure 10.13 indicates that the rate of gain in hip width tends to be the same for both sexes but continues slightly longer for girls so that they will, on this basis alone, have slightly larger relative hip widths than boys. In shoulder width, however, girls have a relatively low gain in comparison with the marked gain for boys (figure 10.14). It is this latter low segmental growth that accounts for the relatively larger hipped, narrower shouldered configuration of women (Simmons, 1944).

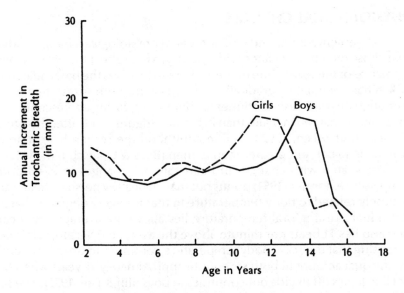

FIGURE 10.13. *Annual increments in trochantric (hip) breadth. (Adapted from data by K. Simmons, The Brush Foundation Study of child growth and development. II. Physical growth and development. Monogr. Soc. Res. Child Develpm., 1944, 9 (1), 1–87.)*

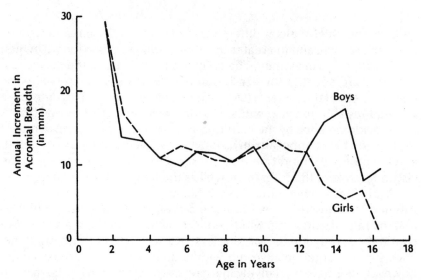

FIGURE 10.14. *Annual increments in acromial (shoulder) breadth. (Adapted from data by K. Simmons, The Brush Foundation Study of child growth and development. II Physical growth and development. Monogr. Soc. Res. Child Develpm., 1944, 9 (1), 1–87.)*

PHYSIOLOGICAL CHANGES

Adolescence is marked by a number of physiological changes, other than those directly associated with puberty, which affect the physical performance of the sexes. One of these changes involves the basal heart rate which has been falling gradually and equally for both sexes since birth. Although this decrease continues for both sexes during adolescence, it is much more marked in males than in females (figure 10.15) after the age of 12 years (Iliff & Lee, 1952), until in adulthood the resting heart rate of women is 10 percent greater than in men (Boas & Goldschmidt, 1932).

Associated with changes in heart rate are changes in basal body temperature. Tanner (1951) points out that, in healthy persons, heart rate is closely related to body temperature in that for every degree F that an individual's resting oral temperature lies above the average, the heart rate also lies 11 beats per minute above the average. Therefore, it is not surprising that the basal body temperature continues to drop from birth by an equal amount in both sexes until approximately 12 years when the decline levels off in girls but continues in boys (Iliff & Lee, 1952). The sex difference of about one-half degree in body temperature that results persists into adult life (Cullumbine, 1949).

Systolic blood pressure has been found to rise steadily during childhood with a much more rapid increase during adolescence until adult

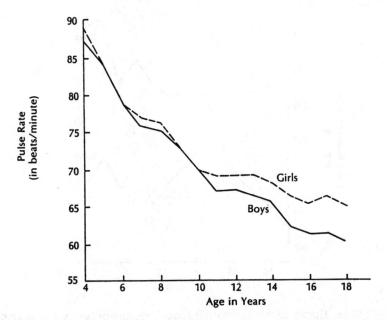

FIGURE 10.15. *Curves of average basal heart rates for boys and girls. (Adapted from data by A. Iliff and V. A. Lee, Pulse rate, respiratory rate, and body temperature of children between 2 months and 18 years of age. Child Developm., 1952, 23, 237–245.)*

values are reached (Richey, 1931; Downing, 1947). As with other measures, the changes occur first in girls, but the boys' adolescent rise, when it appears, is greater than the girls' increase, with the resultant difference accounting for the higher resting systolic pressure in young adult males (figure 10.16).

Adolescence brings only a very slight change in the diastolic blood pressure with no statistically significant differences between the sexes (Shock, 1944). Therefore, the changes in pulse pressure parallel those in systolic blood pressure (figure 10.17). It has been suggested that the greater increase in heart size in males during adolescence results in the establishment of a greater basal stroke volume which accounts for the increased pulse pressure and systolic blood pressure (Nylin, 1935).

An additional cause for the higher systolic blood pressure in males may be their increased blood volume (Tanner, 1955). Although there is no sex difference with respect to blood volume before puberty in relation to the height or weight of the individual, a greater increase in boys has been noted during adolescence, which results in a higher male adult value (Sjöstrand, 1953). This higher blood volume in the young male adult also reflects a large increase in red blood cells for boys during adolescence.

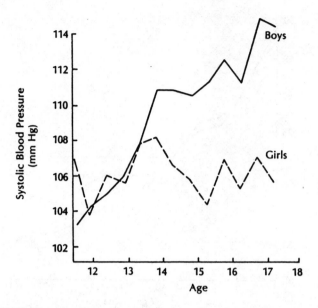

FIGURE 10.16. *Curves of average systolic blood pressure of boys and girls. (From N. W. Shock, Basal blood pressure and pulse rate in adolescents. Amer. J. Dis. Child., 1944, 68, 16–22. By permission of the author and publisher.)*

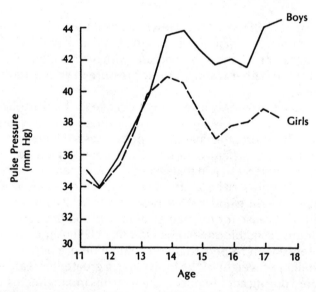

FIGURE 10.17. *Curves of average pulse pressures of boys and girls. (From N. W. Shock, Basal blood pressure and pulse rate in adolescents. Amer. J. Dis. Child., 1944, 68, 16–22. By permission of the author and publisher.)*

Mugrage and Andresen (1936, 1938) report a greater rise in the number of red blood corpuscles in boys and a consequent increase in the hemoglobin of the blood in comparison with girls (figures 10.18 and 10.19). These increases are accomplished with little or no changes in mean corpuscular volume, mean corpuscular hemoglobin, or mean corpuscular hemoglobin concentration (Mugrage & Andresen, 1936, 1938; Berry et al., 1952). Girls do not exhibit this increase in red blood cells and consequent increase in hemoglobin during adolescence, nor do well-trained women athletes achieve sufficient increases in both areas to eliminate this sex difference (Marloff, 1949).

An increase in red blood cells and in hemoglobin volume requires a complementary increase in available oxygen for its effective use in the body. During adolescence, basal respiratory rate shows no sex difference nor any variation in the consistent fall noted from birth (Iliff & Lee, 1952). However, there are changes in the respiratory volume, vital capacity, and maximum breathing capacity. The resting respiratory volume, both on a per minute and per breath basis, increases considerably in boys but very little in girls (Shock, 1946). Similarly, the maximum breathing capacity, which is the volume breathed during a 15-second period in which the subject breathes as deeply and rapidly as possible, and the vital capacity, namely, the maximal expiration following a maximal inspiration, have been found to show a considerable adolescent increase for boys but not

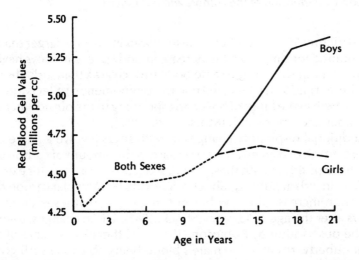

FIGURE 10.18. *Mean red blood cell values in boys and girls. (From data by E. R. Mugrage and M. I. Andresen, Values for red blood cells of average infants and children.* Amer. J. Dis. Child., *1936, 51, 775–791. E. R. Mugrage and M. I. Andresen, Red blood cell values in adolescence.* Amer. J. Dis. Child., *1938, 56, 997–1003. By permission of the authors and publisher.)*

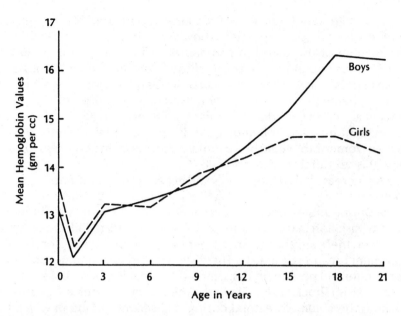

FIGURE 10.19 *Mean hemoglobin values in boys and girls. (From data by E. R. Mugrage and M. I. Andresen, Values for red blood cells of average infants and children. Amer. J. Dis. Child., 1936, 51, 775–791. E. R. Mugrage and M. I. Andresen, Red blood cell values in adolescence. Amer. J. Dis. Child., 1938, 56, 997–1003. By permission of the authors and publisher.)*

for girls (figures 10.20 and 10.21). The increases in boys are larger than can be accounted for simply by the increase in body size, with boys having a greater vital capacity for the same body surface area than girls after puberty (Tanner, 1955). It is believed that this phenomenon reflects a greater inside growth in the lungs of boys corresponding to the outside increases in shoulder and chest width (Morse et al., 1952).

Additional respiratory changes in both sexes involve a decrease in the percentage of oxygen and an increase in the amount of carbon dioxide in the expired air, with these changes occurring to a greater extent in boys than in girls at puberty (Shock & Soley, 1939). Alveolar carbon dioxide tension increases in boys but not in girls, so that a sex difference appears after the age of 13 years (Shock, 1941). These changes, together with the observation by Robinson (1938) that the alkali reserve of boys rises at puberty, result in the male's blood being able to absorb greater quantities of lactic acid and other muscular metabolites during muscular exercise than can a woman's blood without a change in the pH of the blood. Such an adjustment would seem to be a necessity due to the relatively greater development of muscular bulk in males during the adolescent growth spurt.

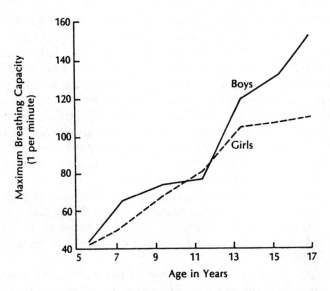

FIGURE 10.20. Curves of average maximum breathing capacity in boys and girls. (From data by B. G. Ferris; J. L. Whittenberger; and J. R. Gallagher, Maximum breathing capacity and vital capacity of male children and adolescents. Pediatrics, 1952, 9, 659–670. B. G. Ferris and C. W. Smith, Maximum breathing capacity and vital capacity in female children and adolescents. Pediatrics, 1953, 12, 341–352. By permission of the authors and publisher.)

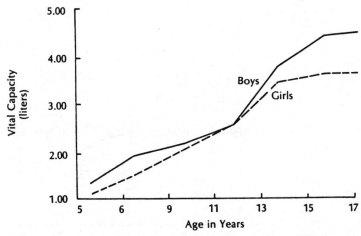

FIGURE 10.21. Curves of average vital capacity in boys and girls. (From data by B. G. Ferris; J. L. Whittenberger; and J. R. Gallagher, Maximum breathing capacity and vital capacity of male children and adolescents. Pediatrics, 1952, 9, 659–670. B. G. Ferris and C. W. Smith, Maximum breathing capacity and vital capacity in female children and adolescents. Pediatrics, 1953, 12, 341–352. By permission of the authors and publisher.)

The increase in respiratory volume and decrease in the percentage of oxygen in expired air of boys reflects the increased oxygen consumption that has been noted in males at puberty (Garn & Clark, 1953). This increase is closely associated with changes in basal metabolism rate during adolescence. The basal metabolic rate, which is the amount of heat produced per square meter of body surface under resting conditions, falls continuously from birth to old age. However, the data of Lewis et al. (1943) indicate that the basal metabolic rate is consistently higher in boys than for girls and that this difference becomes greater during the period of adolescence when the decline in rate for boys is arrested to a greater extent than it is in girls (figures 10.22 and 10.23). This relative increase, or slowing down of the declining rate, coincides with the adolescent growth spurt and is indicative of the extra heat production that would appear to be inseparable from the building of new tissue, although there may also be some contributions from the hormonal effects of the thyroid or of androgens in the male.

The greater metabolic rate and oxygen consumption relative to surface area of boys in comparison with girls at all age levels has been attributed to the greater mesomorphy of boys (Garn et al., 1953). Muscle tissue is known to have a greater resting oxygen consumption than fat tissue,

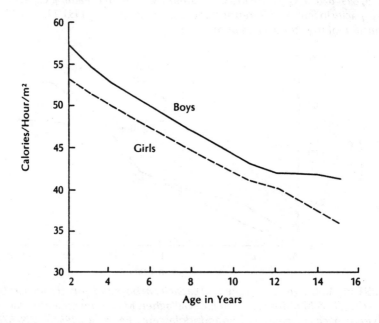

FIGURE 10.22. *Curves of average basal metabolic rate in boys and girls. (Adapted from data by R. C. Lewis; A. M. Duval; and A. Iliff, Standards for the basal metabolism of children from 2 to 15 years of age, inclusive. J. Pediat., 1943, 23, 1–18.)*

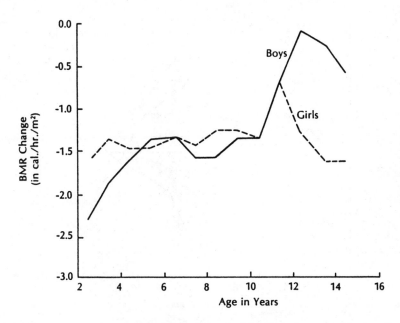

FIGURE 10.23. Curves of average change in basal metabolic rate in boys and girls. (Adapted from data by R. C. Lewis; A. M. Duval; and A. Iliff, Standards for the basal metabolism of children from 2 to 15 years of age, inclusive. J. Pediat., 1943, 23, 1–18.)

and muscular children have also been found to have a greater oxygen consumption than fat ones. However, the differences noted in body size and muscle mass would not seem to be great enough to account for the amount of sex difference, nor of the increase in the sex difference, during adolescence. A comparison of boys and girls with the same muscular bulk as measured by x-rays of the calf revealed that boys had a higher oxygen consumption per kilogram of body weight. A difference has also been found to exist between the strength of males and females with the same muscular bulk (Rarick & Thompson, 1956; Morris, 1948). It is possible that male hormone secretions account for such differences and their heightened production during adolescence and adulthood increases sex differences in muscular metabolism.

CHANGES IN BODY TISSUES

Marked proportional changes occur in the bone, muscle, and fat tissues at adolescence. As may be expected, gains in bone and muscle parallel increments in height and weight. Figure 10.24, based upon the longitudinal data collected on three **monovular** triplets (Reynolds &

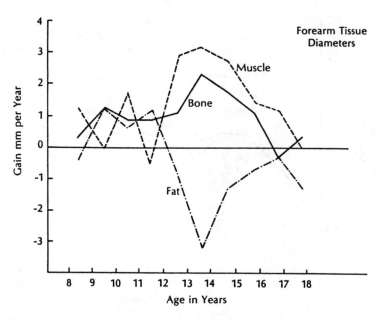

FIGURE 10.24. *Adolescent spurt in bone, muscle, and subcutaneous fat diameters of the forearm, taken at right angles to long axis of limb one-third of way up forearm from distal end of radial disphysis, by x-ray. Average of three monovular male triplets. (From J. M. Tanner,* Growth at adolescence. *Oxford, Eng.: Blackwell Scientific Publications, 1955. By permission of the publisher.)*

Schoen, 1947), gives a very clear picture of the spurt in bone and muscle. It also indicates the inverse relationship between these two measures and fat deposition during the peak growth period. While this decrement in fat gain is very marked in boys, it has a much lesser magnitude in girls (see figure 9.10). Here fat gains are also consistently higher at all ages. In general, girls appear to have an equally intense gain in bone and muscle growth as boys but do not have the same duration of gain nor as pronounced a reduction in fat gain during adolescence. Malina and Johnston (1967) have indicated that the preadolescent muscle/bone ratio, which is the same for both sexes at 2.6:1, remains the same for females after puberty at 15.5 years of age, whereas that of the males indicates only a slightly relatively greater amount of muscle with a ratio of 2.7:1. On the other hand, the muscle/fat ratio which remains fairly consistent for the females, with a ratio of 2.3:1 during preadolescence and 2.4:1 at postadolescence, increases markedly for males from a slightly higher preadolescent muscular component ratio of 2.5:1 to 5.6:1 at 15.5 years and is attributed primarily to a loss of fat in males.

A study by Reynolds (1944) of 48 girls and 30 boys between the ages of 7½ and 12½ years points up the differences in bone, muscle, and fat development for early and late maturers. The data indicate that early maturing girls are significantly larger than late maturers in the following measures:

- Total calf breadth, 8½ through 12½ years
- Breadth of fat, all ages
- Breadth of muscle, 10½ through 12 years
- Breadth of bone, 8½ through 12½ years

During the period from 7½ to 12½ years, early maturing girls show a mean increase in total calf breadth of 26.5 millimeters while the late maturing increase only 11.9 millimeters. The boys' data indicate early maturers are larger than the late maturers in mean calf breadth and in fat, muscle, and bone from 9½ through 12½ years, although the differences are not as great as in girls. The main differential in boys appears to be the faster rate of growth in fat breadth in late maturers, although early maturing boys are, as are early maturing girls, consistently larger in fat breadth at every age. Malina and Johnston (1967) observed that faster maturing children had larger upper arms, but relatively less muscle, before the growth spurt than slower maturers. At all ages from 6 through 16 years, the males had greater absolute values for all measures except fat.

STRENGTH INCREMENTS

The marked physiological and structural changes of the adolescent growth spurt are reflected in large increments and sex differences in strength development. Jones (1949) has reported the results from a longitudinal study of static muscular strength development undertaken at the University of California Institute of Child Welfare with approximately 90 subjects of each sex from 11 through 17½ years of age. Development of strength in hand grip, arm pull, and arm thrust is nearly the same for both boys and girls until after 13 years when the boys increase in strength much more rapidly than the girls. A comparison of changes relative to initial status indicates the total amount of change in gripping strength for boys is almost twice as great as for girls (see figures 10.26 and 10.27), while for pulling and thrusting strength the total amount of change is approximately four times as great.

Previously reported studies of strength during childhood indicated the great variability of strength within the sexes, so that there is considerable overlapping of the strength measures of stronger girls with those of boys. Figure 10.25 shows that such overlapping is greatly reduced after the adolescent growth spurt, with no girls exceeding the average strength of the boys in the measures tested by Jones (1949). There is, however, still a great deal of variability in strength within the sexes and

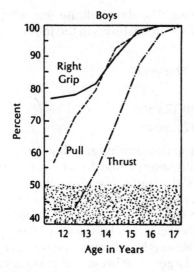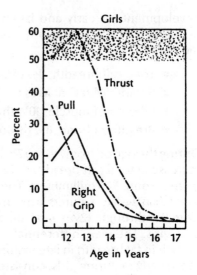

FIGURE 10.25. *Percentage of boys and girls surpassing the mean of the opposite sex in various strength measures. (From H. E. Jones,* Motor performance and growth. *Berkeley: University of California Press, 1949. By permission of the publisher.)*

the strongest girls may still equal or slightly surpass the weakest boys in strength.

Maturity indices have a decided relationship to strength development. When classified as early, average, and late maturers according to age at menarche, the growth curves in strength of the late maturing girls lag behind the average at all ages. The early maturers exhibit a tendency towards more rapid growth in strength from 11 to 13 years, but their growth is retarded relatively soon thereafter and they reach a terminal position below the group mean (Jones, 1949). Figure 10.26, illustrating the growth curve of right hand grip strength, shows the tendency for both early and late maturers to be weaker than average maturing girls after 13½ years of age.

The differences in strength growth curves of early, average, and late maturing boys, assessed on the basis of skeletal age, are illustrated in figure 10.27. The early maturers exhibit a growth curve that is not far from linear, with acceleration usually falling between 12 and 13½ years and a tendency to level off after the 16th and 17th year. The late maturing boys, on the other hand, reveal two phases of growth, namely, a slow increase in each function followed by an acceleration at 14 years or later. There is also a marked relationship between strength and skeletal maturity, in that the early maturing boys are above the group mean in strength from age 13 through 16, while the late maturers tend to fall below the norm at these

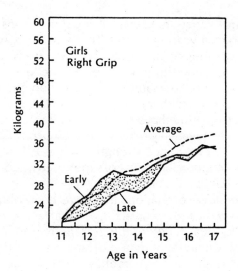

FIGURE 10.26. *Growth curves (right grip) for early, average, and late maturing girls, classified on the basis of age at menarche. (From H. E. Jones,* Motor performance and growth. *Berkeley: University of California Press, 1949. By permission of the publisher.)*

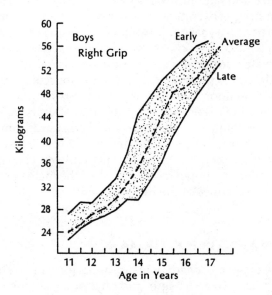

FIGURE 10.27. *Growth curves (right grip) for early, average, and late maturing boys, classified on the basis of skeletal ages. (From H. E. Jones,* Motor performance and growth. *Berkeley: University of California Press, 1949. By permission of the publisher.)*

ages. Within minor variation, each individual maintains approximately the same position relative to age mates. Those boys who were superior in strength at the beginning of the Oakland Growth Study remained superior at its termination, and those who were in the lower percentile also tended to remain in about the same relative position. Since early maturity has also been associated with mesomorphy and late maturity with ectomorphy, it is not surprising that strength is moderately related to mesomorphy and slightly negatively related to ectomorphy (Jones, 1949). On the other hand, for endurance strength such as is exemplified by the flexed arm hang, ectomorphic boys are superior to mesomorphs from 10 through 16 years (Ellis et al., 1975).

However, the low correlations that have been obtained between either height or weight and strength suggest that factors other than gross body size are influential in determining strength in adolescence (Jones, 1949). Additional longitudinal data indicate that the peak in strength spurt in boys occurs about 11½ years after the peak height increases and about one year after the peak weight gains (Dimock, 1935; Stolz & Stolz, 1951). Although there are no clear cut data available on the growth of muscles alone, it has been suggested that the peak gain of muscular growth coincides with, or even precedes, the peak weight gain (Tanner, 1955). Such discrepancy in peak gains seems to indicate that muscles grow first in size and later in strength.

Data on androgen excretion approximates the growth in strength for it continues to rise for a year or more after growth in height has practically ceased (Tanner, 1955). A close association may be made between strength and male hormonal secretions on the basis of studies by Simonson et al. (1941), which show an increase in the muscular strength of **eunuchs** and **castrates** upon injection of **methyl testosterone**, and of Burke et al. (1953), showing a decline in grip strength after the age of 30 years which generally resembles the decline in 17–**ketosteroid** output in males. In general, then, there is a period of about one year between achievement of full body size and the development of full muscular power in the male which may be attributed to the effects of the male hormones upon the proteins and enzymes of the muscle fibers.

CHANGES IN MOTOR PERFORMANCE

As may be expected, changes in motor performance tend to parallel the changes in body size, strength, and physiological functioning at puberty. Sex differences in basic motor skill performances become increasingly marked with boys showing continued improvement, whereas performance increments for girls are negligible or, in some instances, decline after menarche. Figures 9.13 and 10.31 illustrate these changes in running; figures 9.15 and 10.32 in the standing broad jump; and figures 9.16 and 10.33 in the throw for distance. In the study cited, girls reached their maximum in running at 13 years and showed little change in distance throwing and jumping after this age (Espenschade, 1960). More recent cross-sectional studies which coincide with an emphasis on physical fitness suggest a somewhat different trend. In California, for example, slight improvement in running and jumping was noted for girls from 13 to 16 years.

In an age-grade comparison undertaken in Georgia (Vincent, 1968), tenth grade girls (mean = 15.3 years) had the best scores in accuracy throw, ball bounce, wall ball, and distance throw. For the base run and jump for height items, the ninth grade girls (mean = 14.4 years) were the best performers, whereas college freshmen women (mean = 18.4 years) attained the highest scores in the side step and jump rope. Thus some improvement in performance for females does occur after puberty, and it would appear that the general failure of girls to improve in physical performance after puberty is strongly influenced by the cultural milieu.

Skeletal or menarcheal age correlates substantially with chronological age and such a relationship must be recognized when motor performances are related to skeletal age or menarcheal age. When motor performance of girls is graphed in relation to skeletal maturity (figures 10.28

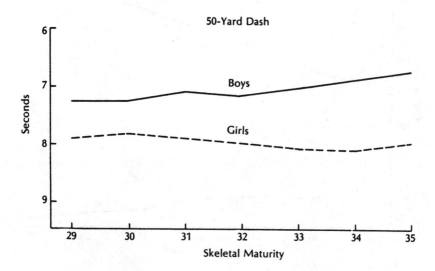

FIGURE 10.28. *Curves of skeletal maturity and performance in the 50-yard dash for boys and girls. (From Anna S. Espenschade, Motor performance in adolescence including the study of relationships with measures of physical growth and maturity. Monogr. Soc. Res. Child Develpm., 1940, 5 (1), 1–126. By permission of the publisher.)*

and 10.29), motor performance has either leveled off, as in the dash, or has been declining steadily, as in the distance throw, with increased skeletal maturity. Treatment of these same data on the basis of age of deviation from menarche reveals similar results. However, in this instance, there were very few cases more than .5 years before the menarche. In general, motor performance of girls in basic skills tends to level off shortly before the achievement of biological maturity, which is reached approximately three years prior to skeletal maturity (Espenschade, 1940).

Conversely, boys continue to improve in motor performance with increasing skeletal maturity. However, the skeletal rating range in figures 10.28 and 10.29 does not include the rating of 37, which signifies skeletal maturity in boys, and it is possible that the graphed relationship may, to some extent, be a function of the interrelationships between skeletal maturity and other physical maturity measures such as chronological age, height, and weight (Espenschade, 1940). Partial correlation techniques have produced results indicating that skeletal age accounts for less than 9 percent of the variance in motor performance (Rarick & Oyster, 1964).

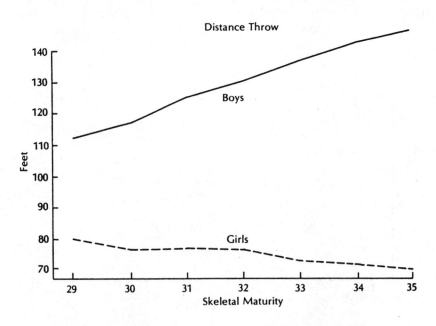

FIGURE 10.29. *Curves of skeletal maturity and performance in the distance throw for boys and girls. (From Anna S. Espenschade, Motor performance in adolescence including the study of relationships with measures of physical growth and maturity. Monogr. Soc. Res. Child Developm., 1940, 5 (1), 1–126. By permission of the publisher.)*

Variation in the rate of skeletal development does, however, bear some relationship to motor performance in boys as was noted in the preceding chapter. When boys at 9, 12, and 15 years from the Medford, Oregon, Boys' Growth Project were categorized into retarded, normal, and advanced maturers, the advanced maturers had higher performance means in strength measures and in the standing broad jump than retarded maturers. In general, it was found that the highest and most significant differences between maturity groupings were obtained at 15 years with those at 12 and 9 years being of decreasing order with chronological age. Furthermore, a comparison of the chronological ages within similar maturity groupings indicated that the chronologically older boys were taller and stronger (Clarke & Harrison, 1962).

Studies of the relationship between motor performance and pubescence reveal a similar slight relationship for boys and little relationship for girls. The few records that are available for girls do not present a parallel picture with previously reported strength development where the average maturers eventually exceeded both the early and late developers (Jones, 1949). Atkinson (1925) grouped 9000 Philadelphia high school girls on the basis of deviation from menarche and found no marked differences in comparison with arrangement by chronological age. A study of the best performances in each event, however, revealed that the very late maturing girls tended to excel in jumping, the distance throw, and basketball goal shooting while the early maturing girls were more proficient in rope climbing and the running events. Similarly, correlations between deviations from the menarche and performance events in the longitudinal Oakland Growth Study were negligible (Espenschade, 1940). It would appear then, that the advent of the menarche marks the peak of steady increase in motor performances in girls but does not necessarily signal the end of all growth.

The rate of biological maturation for boys, on the other hand, has shown some relationship to motor performance. Low correlations ranging from .06 to .37 were obtained between performance in the various events in the Oakland Growth study and pubescent zone, or stage, but some differences were noted in the percentage of change in performance in the various groupings. In general, the pubescent boy gains steadily in running whereas relative improvement increases early in jumping and somewhat later in throwing during pubescence (Espenschade, 1940). These results are in accord with studies of physical growth sequence indicating that the legs lengthen and the hips widen prior to shoulder girdle development.

A similar longitudinal study was carried out in Saskatchewan on the standing broad jump, flexed arm hang, and bent knee sit-ups performance of 106 boys tested annually from 10 through 16 years (Ellis et al., 1975). The largest percentage increase in performance occurred between

14 and 15 years in the standing broad jump and between 11 and 12 years for flexed arm hang and bent knee sit-ups. When increments in performance were related to peak height velocity, it was noted that maximum increment for the standing broad jump and flexed arm hang coincided with peak height velocity, whereas maximum increment for bent knee sit-ups occurred one year prior to peak height velocity. These results reflect the earlier increments in limb length which would be mechanically advantageous to performance in the bent knee sit-ups in that the trunk would be relatively shorter. The increased leg length is also advantageous for jumping, but gains in muscle strength tend to lag behind growth in size and Ellis et al. (1975) report that early maturers were superior to late maturers in standing broad jump performance.

When a combined motor performance score for five track events, including runs, jumps, and the shot put, was graphed against McCloy's Classification Index scores for each of three pubescent groupings, the pre- and postpubescent boys improved steadily in each classification grouping while pubescent boys of all classes scored approximately the same number of motor performance points. The prepubescent boys tended to be slightly better in performance than the pubescents at the higher classification index ranges for these groups, but the rate of gain and the actual motor performance scores were greater for the postpubescents at all overlapping indices (Nevers, 1948).

Similarly, the participants in the 1955 Little League World Series, who ranged in age from 10 to 12 years, were found to be mainly pubescent and postpubescent (Hale, 1956). At 13 and 16 years, boys in the Medford, Oregon Boys' Growth Study who were advanced in pubescent development had higher mean scores on various motor ability tests with the most effective differentiation by pubescent assessment occurring at 13 years. As with skeletal age, differences between various pubescent groupings are also partially conditioned by chronological age. Boys who are older chronologically, but with the same pubescent rating, generally have significantly higher mean performance scores (Clarke & Degutis, 1962).

An age-wise increase in static force production was reported for boys aged 6 through 12 years by Teeple and Massey (1976). However, controlling the age-related increase in physical growth through covariance indicated that the rate function, as well as peak force function, for elbow flexion and grip squeezing were closely associated with body size and composition. The survey of body physique, maturity, and motor performance by Malina and Rarick (1973) stresses the genetic component associated with physique and maturity. Hence, the early maturing boy, in relation to his peers, has decided advantages in terms of body size and build, strength, and possibly physiological functioning which allow him to excel in physical performance during adolescence.

MOTOR COORDINATION AND BALANCE

Although the total scores on the Brace test indicate that there is a steady increase with chronological age for boys, whereas girls show no improvement after 14 years (figure 9.18), these total scores are a composite of 20 items, each of which is scored on a pass or fail basis. An analysis of performance in the individual items reveals growth patterns which are masked in the total score. In several of the items sex differences are not as great as the total scores would imply, while in others the differences are greater. For example, the stunt which requires the subject to "fold arms across the chest, cross the feet and sit down crosslegged, then stand again without unfolding the arms and moving the feet from the floor" shows the least amount of sex difference and the least amount of variation over the entire age range for both sexes. Events in which boys are especially superior are those agility items requiring rapid change of direction of the body or its parts such as jumping full turns with the position held at the finish and jumping through a loop made by grasping a foot in the opposite hand. These agility measures present a greater problem for older girls than for younger ones, but in stunts requiring control or static balance older girls are able to maintain their position (Espenschade, 1947).

It is possible that the decline in agility in girls after 14 years—whereas little change is shown in control, fexibility, and balance items—may be attributed to lack of interest rather than to actual decline in capacity. Longitudinal data from the Oakland Growth Study, where the subjects had practice during the process of being tested every six months, indicates a slight increase for the total scores of the Brace test up to 16 years (Espenschade, 1940). However, when these same data are analyzed in terms of skeletal maturity (figure 10.30), a decline is noted with increasing skeletal age. This decline may reflect increased puberal weight with its negative effect on motor performance in girls as much as the changed interests and attitudes which accompany biological maturity.

Figure 10.30 also indicates that boys show increased performance with skeletal age except for a slight decline between the skeletal maturity ratings of 32 and 33. When these longitudinal data were supplemented with additional cross-sectional data, little gain was found in total test scores between 12½ and 14 years. An analysis of the items of the Brace test shows increased ability to perform in events of all the subcategories, with amount of gain being greater after 14 years than before this age. Furthermore, gains are more rapid in agility than in control events. On the other hand, test items in which dynamic balance can be considered a factor show a marked adolescent lag. It is possible that these items play the largest role in the reduction of increases in the composite Brace score during the period from 12½ to 14 years (Espenschade, 1947).

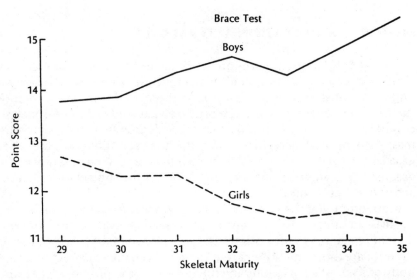

FIGURE 10.30. *Curves of skeletal maturity and performance in the Brace test for boys and girls. (From Anna S. Espenschade, Motor performance in adolescence including the study of relationships with measures of physical growth and maturity. Monogr. Soc. Res. Child Developm., 1940, 5 (1), 1–126. By permission of the publisher.)*

Although higher mean scores are reported from 13 to 16 years for prepubescent boys, an analysis of the rate of gain over a two year period revealed a pattern of increase before puberty, a slackening in the rate of increase during the months around the time when a boy reaches pubescence, and further increase after puberty (Dimock, 1935). Reorganization of the Brace test data from the Oakland Growth Study with respect to pubescent status does not indicate any superiority of prepubescent boys, but does reveal each advancing state of maturity to be superior to that preceding except for the few cases which mark the earliest appearance of a stage or level (Espenschade et al., 1953). Such results indicate that motor coordination or ability, as measured by the Brace test, tends to increase less rapidly during the period of onset of puberty.

Various studies of dynamic balance during adolescence indicate a slackening in the rate of gain for both sexes. When measured on the walking board, this plateau in the rate of gain for girls appears from 12 through 14 years (Heath, 1949; Goetzinger, 1961; Cron & Pronko, 1957). In some instances, steady improvement in performance on walking beams has been reported in boys up to 14 and 16 years (Heath, 1949; Goetzinger, 1961) while, in others, steady improvement was noted until 11 years with a subsequent decline in gain (Seashore, 1947) or greater variability (Wallon et al., 1958). Another study of boys aged 11½ to 16½ years shows consistent gains in beam walking with chronological age, although the rate of change is much less from 13 to 15 years than occurs earlier or later. Classification of the boys in this study into puberal groupings reveals similar results, with the pre- and postpubescent group curves both rising sharply, while the intermediate pubescent groups show little gain (Espenschade et al., 1953).

Similarly, there is an apparent adverse effect during adolescence which occurs earlier in females than in males for balance as measured by the stabilometer. Conversely, however, this same group was superior in performance in a ladder-balancing task during adolescence in comparison with other periods (Bachman, 1961). This latter task may involve factors other than balance to a considerable extent, however. On the basis of a correlation coefficient of .62, it may be assumed that there is a substantial relationship between dynamic balance and ratings in physical ability of junior high school boys (Espenschade et al., 1953). Therefore, some indications should also be found of slight puberal lag in other motor activities. Previously cited studies by Hale (1956), found only 17 percent of Little League participants to be pubescent, while 37.5 and 45.5 percent were pre- and postpubescent respectively. Nevers (1948) reports pubescent boys as being poorer in achievement in track events at upper classification indices than were prepubescent boys. Both studies tend to suggest a slight adolescent lag in motor ability. It seems logical that rapid changes in physique, strength, and body proportions will require some readjustment of sensory-motor functioning, and it is possible the decreased rate of gain in balancing and motor ability noted by a number of investigators at puberty may be associated with such adjustments.

SECULAR TRENDS AND GEOGRAPHIC VARIATION
IN MOTOR PERFORMANCE

The reported secular trend in increased height and weight at all ages gives rise to the potential that such a trend should also exist for motor performance. Figures 10.31 through 10.33 indicate increased performance for both boys and girls in running, jumping, and distance throwing over a period of seven years from 1958 to 1965. However, a similar sampling of children in 1975 indicates that only the girls improved in performance in the 50-yard dash and in the broad jump in comparison with previous performance levels. The performance of boys in 1975 was slightly below that of the previous years at all age levels for the same two measures. Although the distance throw was not repeated in 1975, it is probable that the results for this test would have been similar to those of the dash and jump. The distance throw utilizes upper arm strength, and in the 1975 tests for upper arm strength, namely, boys' pull-ups and girls'

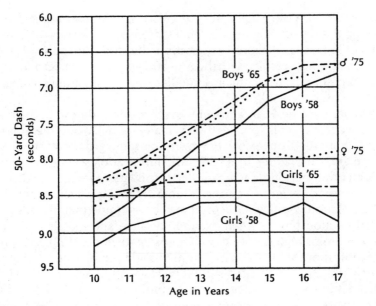

FIGURE 10.31. *Youth fitness test norms for 50-yard dash. (Data for 1958 and 1965 from P. A. Hunsicker and G. G. Reiff, A survey and comparison of youth fitness 1958–1965. J. Health P. E. Rec., 1966, 37, 23–25. By permission of the publisher. Data for 1975 adapted from P. Hunsicker and G. Reiff, Youth fitness report: 1958–1965–1975. JOPER, 1977, 48 (1), 31–32.)*

flexed-arm hang, boys' performance tended to be slightly below that in 1965, whereas girls' performance was superior in 1975.

Other test items included in the 1975 AAHPER Youth Fitness test battery are the 600-yard run, shuttle run, and bent knee sit-up. Hunsicker and Reiff (1977) report that, while significant gains occurred in almost all cases between 1958 and 1965, there were no gains among all 40 comparisons on the boys' data between 1965 and 1975. The only difference was the lower score for 14-year-old boys in the long jump. Of the 48 comparisons made between 1958 and 1965 performance levels, girls had significantly better scores in 39 instances in 1965. Although girls did as well or better in 1975 than in previous years, in only seven out of the 40 comparisons were the girls significantly superior in performance. The greatest number of significant improvements occurred for 14-year-old girls who showed significantly better scores in three of the five items; namely, 600-yard run, long jump, and flexed-arm hang.

The improvement in performance from 1958 to 1965 would seem to be in keeping with a structure-function relationship of increases in height and weight resulting in increases in performance. However, the lack of improvement, and in some instances decline, in performance from 1965 to 1975 indicates that other factors are more influential in the

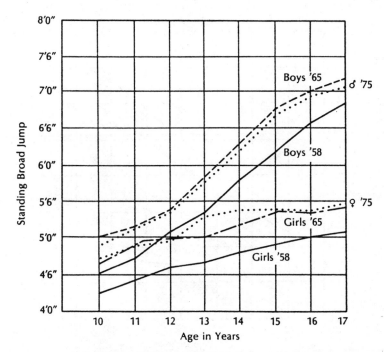

FIGURE 10.32. *Youth Fitness Test norms for standing broad jump. (1958 and 1965 data from P. A. Hunsicker, and G. G. Reiff, A survey and comparison of youth fitness 1958–1965. J. Health P. E. Rec., 1966, 37, 23–25. By permission of the publisher. Data for 1975 adapted from P. Hunsicker and G. Reiff, Youth fitness report: 1958–1965–1975. JOPER, 1977, 48 (1), 31–32.)*

establishment of nationwide norms. The period between 1958 and 1965 was marked by considerable interest and attention to the level of fitness in children. Subsequently, the emphasis has been less marked and considerable discussion has centered around improved physical performance opportunities for girls in compliance with Title IX, which prohibits discrimination on the basis of sex. The improved performance levels of 14-year-old girls in 1975 may reflect a change in social-cultural expectations so that girls are now encouraged to develop optimally.

A comparative study of motor performance of 13-year-old girls and 13½-year-old boys in the same region and with similar socioeconomic backgrounds does not show improved performance in all test items over a 24-year period. Significant increases are noted in height and weight for both sexes and conform with studies reporting such increases over a much longer period of time. Such increases in weight appear to be more advantageous for boys than girls, however. Boys register significant increases in performance in the distance throw, jump and reach, Brace test, grip, and pull, whereas girls improve significantly only in the jump and

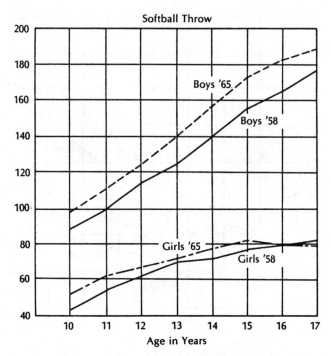

FIGURE 10.33. *Youth fitness test norms of 1958 and 1965 for the softball throw for distance. (From P. A. Hunsicker and G. G. Reiff, A survey and comparison of youth fitness 1958–1965. J. Health P. E. Rec., 1966, 37, 23–25. By permission of the publisher.)*

reach and pull. The increase in height and weight appears to have had a detrimental effect on performance in the dash and standing broad jump for both sexes, with significant decrements occurring in performance levels. Girls also were significantly weaker in the push in 1958 in comparison with their 1934 counterparts (Espenschade & Meleney, 1961). Norms for large groups of California children tested in 1960 were also lower in dash and broad jump than those reported in California children in the 1930s.

Previously reported studies generally tend to indicate a low, but positive, correlation between height and weight and performance in the run and jump. Therefore, it is possible that the significant decrease registered by both sexes in the dash and standing broad jump is a reflection of decreased interest and opportunity for the achievement of individual optimal performance in these activities for the average boy and girl. This conclusion would seem to have considerable merit on the basis of data reported by Montpetit et al. (1967) for the grip strength of children in Michigan in 1899 and 1964. During the comparative ages of 10 through 17, the mean grip strength of the children in 1964 was greater than it was 65 years previously at all age levels except for boys below age 13. In general, the 1964 Saginaw boys were advanced by about one year in comparison with the 1899 boys, with similar comparisons for the girls indicating an advancement of about one and a half years. Additional data collected from 1892–1894 in St. Louis on 16,527 girls and 15,686 boys produced similar comparative results with the grip strength of boys in 1964 being advanced by about one and a half years and that of the girls by two years. The 1964 Saginaw children were greater in size than the 1892–1894 St. Louis children but, when the mean grip strength at each age is divided by the mean weight for that age, the resultant indices indicate no difference between the groups. It appears, therefore, that the secular trends in increased weight account for the secular trend in increased grip strength.

The observed secular trends in increases in body size and strength have been reflected in increased proficiency of performance by outstanding athletes in athletic events such as the Olympics. However, the average child does not seem to be benefiting from the increased secular increments in body size and strength and may, in fact, be becoming less adept in motoric activities. The fact that potential does exist for improved performance for the average child is indicated by increased performance in the basic motor skills for both sexes over the seven-year period between the nationwide Physical Fitness Test surveys (Hunsicker & Reiff, 1966).

It may be argued that regional differences account for decrements over a period of time in one area while nationwide norms are increasing. This, however, is not a valid explanation of the decreases noted in the 24-year comparative study since, on the basis of scores made by over 200,000 children, California had higher state norms in running, jumping, and distance throwing for both sexes at all age levels in 1958 than those of the nationwide Physical Fitness Test.

It is undoubtedly a truism that geographic variations in motor performance are conditioned by cultural patterns. To a certain extent, however, basic motor skills also reflect noted geographic variations in onset of puberty. A comparison of performance in running, jumping, and throwing of 19,000 Bulgarian students between the ages of 8 and 20 years conducted in 1951 (Mangarov, 1964) with performance in the same events by American children as reported in numerous studies (Espenschade, 1960) illustrates both these types of variations.

The jumps used in the two sets of data are of different types and are, therefore, not numerically comparable. However, an examination of the growth curves shows a consistent increase in all types of jumps for the males of both countries until the later adolescent years when there is a slight leveling off. In the American data for jumps, a marked leveling off occurs after the 13th year for girls, while similar leveling off does not occur in the Bulgarian girls until the 16th year. Data for the run and distance throw are comparable upon conversion of the metric system to yards and feet. Table 10.1 gives the average performance scores in the distance throw for boys and girls of both countries in the overlapping age ranges and figure 10.34 illustrates similar averages for the run.

An examination of table 10.1 indicates that the American boys and girls have preadolescent increments in performance which enable them to exceed their Bulgarian counterparts, whereas performances for the two groups were either comparable or slightly better for the Bulgarians before and after these increments. Ages in which performances of the American girls exceed the Bulgarian are 9 and 10 years, and performances of the American boys exceed the Bulgarian at 10, 11, and 12 years. It may be recalled that menarche occurs sooner in American girls than in European girls (Shuttleworth, 1949) and earlier increments in performance may reflect this difference. Table 10.1 also indicates that the performance of American girls declines after the age of 15, whereas the Bulgarian girls' performance is still increasing.

Similarly, figure 10.34 indicates faster running scores for American boys until 17 years of age when Bulgarian boys equal their performance, and for American girls until 15 years when Bulgarian girls equal and subsequently surpass their performance level. The Bulgarian performance curves for the run are complicated by different distances from ages 8 to 11 inclusive and from 12 to 18 years. At the younger ages, the 40-meter dash

TABLE 10.1. Comparison of Bulgarian* and American† performance scores in distance throw in feet

	Boys		Girls	
Age	Bulgarian	American	Bulgarian	American
8	65.0	57.4	32.5	30.0
9	72.8	66.6	36.8	38.7
10	81.3	83.0	42.3	47.0
11	90.5	95.0	55.8	54.0
12	101.0	104.0	61.7	61.0
13	114.5	114.0	68.2	70.0
14	123.4	123.0	75.1	74.5
15	131.6	135.0	82.0	75.7
16	145.7	144.0	86.3	74.0
17	162.4	153.0		

* Based on data from Ivan Mangarov, Physical development and capacity of Bulgarian students. Bulletin d'Information, Bulgarian Olympic Committee, Year IX, 1964, 5, 22–28.
† From Science and medicine of exercise and sports, edited by Warren R. Johnson. Copyright © 1960 by Warren R. Johnson: Motor development by Anna Espenschade. Reprinted by permission of Harper & Row, Publishers.

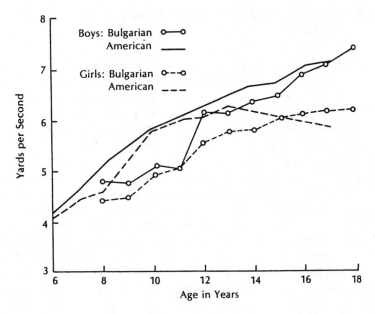

FIGURE 10.34. *Curves of running performance for Bulgarian and American boys and girls. (Adapted from Bulgarian data by Ivan Mangarov, Physical development and capacity of Bulgarian students.* Bulletin d'Information, Bulgarian Olympic Committee, Year IX, 1964, 5, 22–28. Adapted from American data by Anna Espenschade, Motor development. *In Warren R. Johnson (Ed.),* Science and medicine of exercise and sports. *New York: Harper & Row, Publishers, 1960. Used by permission.)*

was used; the 60-meter dash was standard for the remaining ages. This discrepancy in distance may account for the lower scores of the Bulgarian children, in comparison with the American, from 9 to 11 years, and for the sharp increase in yards per second between 11 and 12 years, since the relative weighting of the start will have less effect on the time in the longer run. Even with approximately comparable distances in the run, however, American girls equal the performance of Bulgarian boys at 12 and 13 years, following which time the American girls decline steadily.

It would appear, then, that regional variation in performance of basic motor skills is conditioned by some of the same factors that influence growth until the age of puberty, after which time cultural influences play an increasingly prominent role in motor performance.

In summary, changes in body size and physique and in biological and physiological functioning are very marked in boys during adolescence. The increased leverage, strength, and endurance associated with these changes result in large improvements in performance in all motor activities. Although girls have equally as marked changes in body physique and biological functioning, the changes associated with body size and physiological functioning are not as great as in boys. Furthermore, increments in leverage, strength, and endurance are less than for boys, and some of the changes in body physique may actually be detrimental to performance in some activities. Therefore, performances in girls tend to level off, and in some instances decline, with the advent of the menarche.

The American culture has, in the past, encouraged participation in sporting and athletic events for males but not for females, especially during adolescence and adulthood. Therefore, performance scores for males were obtained in a culturally-approving environment, whereas the average performance scores for females tended to be based upon culturally indifferent, or discouraged, performance. However, increasing emphasis and opportunities for females to participate at high performance levels has stimulated interest in female performance at all age levels. For example, Thorland et al. (1987) have reported on the strength and anaerobic responses of elite female sprint and distance runners aged 9.58 to 17.67 years. In addition, emphasis on health-related aspects of physical activity appear to be stimulating more females to participate in physical activity.

Haskell, Montoye, and Orenstein (1985) have identified the following health-fitness goals for young adults aged 15 to 24 years:

a) Optimal physical growth and development
b) Good psychological adjustment
c) Reduction of coronary heart disease risk factors
d) Development of interest and skills for active lifestyle as adult

The recommended physical activity plan includes:

- Type of exercise: Emphasis on large muscle, dynamic strength and flexibility exercise.
- Intensity: Moderate to vigorous intensity (more than 50 percent maximum oxygen uptake).
- Duration: Total of more than 30 minutes per session (more than four kilocalories per kg of body weight).
- Frequency: At least every other day. The recommended goal is increased activity to and from school or regular physical activity participation.

SUMMARY

1. The adolescent growth spurt marks the final growth period to attain adult stature (Table 10-2).

2. Factors affecting onset of puberty and the puberal growth spurt are: genetic, sex, race, geographic (climate), altitude, seasonal variations, nutrition, socioeconomic, secular trend, health, and intensity of training.

3. Variability in growth rate of the various body parts is the method which constructs the adult body build. The sequence in rate of growth prior to adolescence is: limbs, especially the legs, grow most, followed by the trunk, and growth of the head is least. During the adolescent growth spurt the sequence of peak growth is a) leg length; b) hip width and chest breadth; c) shoulder breadth; d) trunk length and chest depth.

4. The degree to which growth occurs in the various segments is influenced by the rate of maturation. Early maturers tend to have less leg growth and relatively more growth during the adolescent growth sequence. Therefore, early maturers tend to be mesomorphic and/or endomorphic and late maturers tend to be ectomorphic (longer leg growth period).

5. Growth changes in body tissues in adolescence result in increased muscle mass for males and less fat tissue, and for females smaller increases in muscle mass with the same or increased fat deposition. These changes result in marked increases of strength for males and also increases in speed in most activities.

6. Sex differences resulting from anatomical changes during adolescence include:

a) height and weight: males taller and heavier
b) shoulder width: males wider, more rotation torque
c) forearm length: males longer, more lever torque
d) hip shape: insertion of femur more oblique in females
e) elbow and knee joints: males parallel; females)(shaped
f) leg length: relatively longer in males
g) chest girth: males greater thoracic cavity
h) center of gravity: males higher, females lower
i) fat free weight: males more muscle, bigger bones

7. Sex differences in physiological functioning after adolescence include:

a) resting heart rate: slightly higher in females
b) maximal heart rate: slightly higher in females
c) heart volume: higher in males
d) red blood cells: greater number in males
e) hemoglobin (total body): greater in males
f) vital capacity: greater in males
g) ventilation volume: greater in males
h) maximal oxygen uptake: greater in males
i) oxygen content in blood: greater in males

TABLE 10.2. Summary of developmental characteristics during adolescence

Characteristics

1. Development of secondary sex characteristics and biological maturity due to increased hormone secretion; estrogen for females and androgen for males
2. Rapid growth spurt resulting in marked gains in height and weight
3. Differential growth rates of body parts during growth spurt
4. Greater shoulder width gain for males raises center of gravity; greater hip width gain for females lowers center of gravity
5. Proportionately longer limb length growth for males
6. Changes in physiological systems (e.g., cardiovascular and respiratory) result in higher levels of physical activity tolerance for males than females
7. Increased sex differences in body tissue composition: males more muscle and females more fat
8. Increased limb length increases leverage for speed
9. Rapid and very marked gain in strength for males
10. May be some plateauing in balance, coordination, eye-hand coordination, and/or endurance activities during growth spurt
11. Attention span high
12. Very peer oriented
13. Great interest in proficiency
14. Competitive spirit high, especially in males
15. Interest in opposite sex increases
16. Increase in social maturity
17. Greater between individual variability due to differences in maturation rates, that is, early and late maturers

Need	Experience
Increased experience in variety of activities, especially those suitable for adult years	Team games and self-testing activities at high skill levels; individual and dual sports
Increased opportunities for group activities, especially with opposite sex	Developmental exercise programs
	Rhythmic activities in social context
Increased opportunities to explore	Separate activities for sexes in contact activities; high strength and/or body-build related activities also separate at high skill levels, e.g., basketball

j) body temperature: slightly higher in females

k) basal metabolic rate: higher in males than females

8. The changes resulting from anatomical growth and physiological changes during adolescence place males at a decided advantage in all physical performances in which body size and strength are major determinants.

11

Performance in Adulthood

Following the period of rapid adolescent development, there is a period of gradual increase in size and capacity and finally a leveling off or plateauing in adulthood when few growth changes occur. Increments in physical performance are now due mainly to practice, training, experience, and interest. The differential maturity rates of the adolescent period are no longer a dominant feature of physical performance, but the changes in physique associated with differential growth rates become of prime importance as does, to a lesser degree, the enhanced experiential opportunities of the early maturing male. In addition, sexual maturity peaks during the adult years so that changes in physique and physiological functioning associated with sex differences are maximized. Although the period of adulthood is marked by the closure of the epiphysis and stability in physical growth and physiological functioning for each individual, the genetic endowment and environmental influences for different individuals make the period of adulthood one which exhibits the greatest variation in performance parameters within each sex and between the sexes.

PHYSIQUE AND MOTOR PERFORMANCE

The extent of such variation is illustrated in figure 11.1 where the mean and standard deviation of strength index scores are plotted against Bayley's androgeny ratings of 17- to 18-year-old males and females (Bayley, 1951). The calculated strength index is, in this instance, based upon the best of three trials for the sum of right grip, left grip, thrust, and pull which is divided by the height in centimeters times the weight in kilograms. Such division has the effect of ruling out, or minimizing, differences in body size, whereas the categorization in terms of androgeny ratings tends to maximize the effect of the shoulder-hip ratio which is a

329

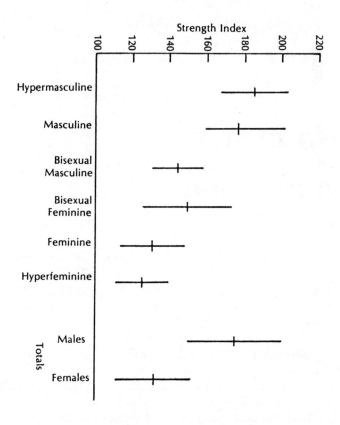

FIGURE 11.1. *Means and standard deviations of strength index scores for androgeny groupings. Strength index: sum of right and left grip, thrust, and pull divided by height and weight. (Adapted from data by Nancy Bayley, Some psychological correlates of somatic androgeny. Child Develpm., 1951, 22(1), 45–60.)*

dominant feature of the Bayley and Bayer somatic androgeny classification. The strength tests used in this study are all upper limb measures with the higher index scores associated with androgeny ratings having relatively broader shoulders in relation to hip width for each sex. The higher mean value and larger standard deviation for the bisexual feminine than in the masculine category cannot, in this instance, be attributed to differences in sample size as the same number of subjects, 10, are recorded in both classifications. The difference may be accounted for, in part, by varying maturation rates as some of the late maturing boys may not have achieved optimal strength at 18 years of age. The data do, however, indicate the possibility that observed sex differences in strength may be more closely associated with sex differences in body size and physique than to marked qualitative differences in muscular structure and composition.

If an association is made between androgeny rating and the relative proportion of androgens and estrogens within the individual rather than in terms of the overtly observable shoulder-hip ratio, then the association between androgeny categories and strength index scores shown in figure 11.1 could be interpreted as indicating that individuals with a higher androgen/estrogen ratio within any one sex would have greater strength. No studies appear to have been made in this regard, but it is well known that the chromosomal array of female athletes is determined prior to Olympic competition.

On the basis of a study by Montoye and Lamphiear (1977) of the relative strength for both sexes at all age levels from 10 through 59 years, it would appear that body size and physique are the major contributing factors to differences in strength between the sexes. In this instance, the relative strength scores—which were calculated from the sum of right grip, left grip, and arm strength adjusted for age and sex specific regression equations based upon height, weight, biacromial diameter, triceps skinfold, and arm girth—were very similar for both sexes at all age levels with mean ranges from 97.0 to 103.0 for the males and 97.5 to 102.1 for the females. However, these investigators point out that the statistical manipulation of data, which rules out the effects of body size and fatness, is valuable for statistical analytical purposes but may often have little or no bearing upon physical activities where the individual must be able to lift his own body weight.

When Montoye and Lamphiear (1977) calculated the ratios of the summed grip strengths to body weight, they noted that the ratios were consistently higher for males, being above 1.00 at 14 years and thereafter, whereas those of females never were higher than .86. Similarly, the ratios of arm strength to body weight were above 1.00 at all ages for males whereas those of females had a maximum value of .86. These results led to the conclusion that pull-ups is not a good test for girls because more than half of the girls cannot exert a force equal to their own body weight. The ratios of the combined sum of grip strengths and arm strength to body weight illustrated in figure 11.2 show that females have markedly less upper limb strength in comparison to body weight than do males at all age levels.

In a similar comparison of upper and lower body strength as a function of lean body weight, Heyward and associates (1986) found that women were about one-half (54 percent) as strong as men in shoulder flexion strength and two-thirds (68 percent) as strong as men in knee extension strength. When measures of lean body weight, arm girth, thigh girth, triceps and thigh skinfolds were held statistically constant, the shoulder flexion and knee extension strengths of the men and women did not differ significantly. However, multiple regression analysis indicated that a substantial portion of the variance in shoulder flexion and

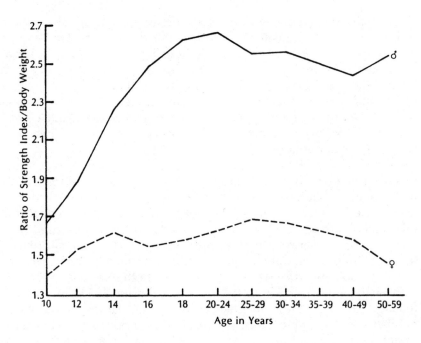

FIGURE 11.2. *Means of ratio of strength index to body weight. (Adapted from data by H. J. Montoye and D. E. Lamphiear, Grip and arm strength in males and females, age 10 to 69.* Research Quarterly, *1977, 48, 109–120.)*

knee extension was explained by lean body weight only. On the other hand, higher shoulder flexion strength in females was associated with more lean body weight, and a lesser amount of subcutaneous fat on the thigh was associated with higher knee extension strength. As a result of their findings, the investigators concluded that gender differences in upper and lower body strength are a function of differences in lean body weight and distribution of muscle and subcutaneous fat in the body segments.

The fact that body fat was associated with strength in women and not in men in the Heyward et al. study (1986) may have been a function of the low (9.4%) body fat of the males in comparison with females (16.11%). Percentage of body fat is associated with performance in both males and females as is illustrated by the report of Cureton et al. (1979) that the linear regression equations predicting performance scores from percent of fat within groups of males and females are significantly different with the exception of modified pull-ups where the detrimental effect of fat was significantly greater in males than females. The higher percentages of body fat in women account, in part, for poorer performance in types of activities where total body weight must be moved. When muscular force is calculated in terms of body weight, sex differences in strength are reduced. In their study of elite volleyball players, Puhl et al. (1982) reported changes in torque production of knee extension and flexion at varying velocities in terms of absolute measures (figure 11.3) and as expressed on the basis of body weight. The marked sex difference in absolute torque at low speeds was reduced at higher velocities and calculations in terms of force per body weight resulted in reduced differences at all velocities. The investigators suggested that the relative strength/power differences would not account for the sex differences in jumping ability and pointed out that hip extension and limb segment length also play a role in force production.

These strength studies all support the recognized fact that muscle groups differ in strength and figure 11.3 clearly indicates that even antagonistic muscle groups (i.e., flexors and extensors) around the same joint do not have the same maximal strength. Similarly, Hoshizaki and Massey (1986) noted that, for the five muscle groups studied, muscular endurance was specific to the muscle group and that endurance was specific to the task being performed. In addition, continuous contraction resulted in significantly greater fatigue than did intermittent contraction with the

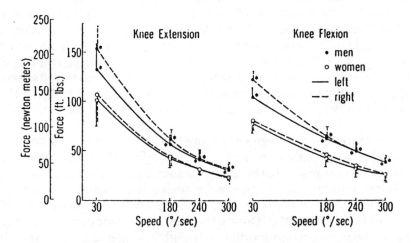

FIGURE 11.3. *Peak isokinetic (Cybex II) torque production for knee extension and flexion at velocities of 30, 180, 240 and 300 degrees per second. Values are group means ± the standard deviation. Sex differences tend to be reduced with increasing velocity. (From Puhl, J.; Case, S.; Fleck, S.; & Van Handel. Physical and Physiological Characteristics of Elite Volleyball Players.* **Research Quarterly for Exercise and Sport**, *1982, 53, 257–262. Reprinted by permission of the American Alliance for Health, Physical Education, Recreation and Dance, 1900 Association Drive, Reston, Virginia 22091.)*

fatigue curves effectively described by single and double component polynomial regression curves. Sex differences in absolute endurance were reported by Clarke (1986) who also noted that females fatigued at a faster rate than did males throughout most of the hand-grip fatigue exercise. As with previously reported maximal strength values, the females were also significantly lower in initial and final strength with the fatigue curves being two-component exponentials (i.e., similar to the curves in figure 11.3).

Sex differences in body size and composition occur at birth. Palti and Adler (1975) report males to be bigger than females in weight, crown-heel and crown-rump length, and head and upper arm circumference. On the other hand, the fat content of females was higher on the basis of the triceps subcutaneous fat/weight ratio. With the exception of the earlier growth spurt of females which results in earlier gains in height and weight and, hence, in taller and heavier girls at about 11 through 13 years of age (Krogman, 1955), males tend to be taller and heavier at all other age levels and become markedly so with the gains made during adolescence. Females, on the other hand, maintain a consistently higher subcutaneous fat level at all ages with the sex differential becoming much more marked during adolescence when there is a decrease in fat level for males, whereas females maintain, or may even increase, the percentage of fat. In this regard, Behnke and Wilmore (1974) report fat levels of 17.9, 14.6, and 9.0 percent for males at ages 5, 10, and 16, respectively, whereas the percentages are 22.3, 21.3, and 24.5 for females at the same age levels. These data were similar to that presented by Parizkova (1973) who also reports increases in the amount of subcutaneous fat for both sexes after 30 years of age. The weight increases with increasing age (illustrated in figure 11.5) tend to coincide with these increased percentages of fat in the adult years.

Sex differences in segmental growth rates also produce variations in physique which influence motor performance. The longer length of forearm for the males that becomes obvious during early childhood persists into adulthood as does the larger girth of the forearm and the larger thoracic circumference (Boynton, 1936; Meredith & Boynton, 1937; Dupertuis & Hadden, 1951). During the period of infancy and early childhood, the female has proportionately slightly longer legs than the male, but increased leg growth by the males during adolescence results in proportionately longer legs for males in relation to stature and also in longer absolute leg length as the adult male is taller than the female (Bayer & Bayley, 1959). The greater absolute height of the mature male gives him a longer chest cavity which, in association with a larger thoracic circumference, results in a greater vital capacity for the male (figure 10.21). The greater limb lengths of the males provide greater leverage advantage in speed events and it would appear that the increased respiratory functioning, associated with the noted anatomical differences in the chest cavity, together with the sex differences that occur in the cardiovascular system during adolescence provide the mature male with an enhanced physiological endurance component.

The broader shoulders of the male (figure 10.14) also contribute to the leverage system for throwing events and provide the framework for more massive musculature. The larger inner measures of the pelvis of the female (Reynolds, 1945, 1947) result in a more U-shaped pelvis so that the angle of insertion of the femur into the **acetabulum** of the pelvis is different for the female and tends to produce more hip sway during bipedal locomotion. The relatively broader hips of the female (figure 10.13) in association with relatively shorter legs results in a lower center of gravity for the female and potentially greater stability. It apparently does not result in greater balance for the female as indicated by railwalking studies (figure 9.17). The joint angle of the knee and elbow also tend to slant inwards in the female as opposed to the straighter or outward slant of the male. This apparent adaptation of the limb joints to the relatively narrower shoulder width and broader hip width of the female results in a tendency for the feet to move outwards in the run and for the arm to hyperextend in such activities as archery.

Any observer of the various Olympic athletic events easily discerns that the physique of the weight lifters is markedly different from that of the marathon runners, and that of gymnasts is considerably different from that of basketball players. The somatotypic differences for athletes participating in the various Olympic events has been well documented by Cureton (1951) and by de Garay et al. (1974). Figure 11.4 clearly shows that, for similar events, males tend to be more mesomorphic and females more endomorphic. The somatotypes for about 370 non-athletes from Mexico who volunteered to serve as a reference group were also reported by de Garay et al. (1974). For both males and females, these reference groups had lower mesomorphy and higher endormorphy components. A survey of the body composition of female athletes by Wyrick (1974) indicates that gymnasts are markedly below normal in fat content with runners and swimmers slightly lower, whereas throwers and basketball players are average or slightly above. In a study of female distance runners and champions in field events by Behnke and Wilmore (1974), the nine runners had a mean fat content of 12.6 percent, whereas the eight throwers had a mean fat content of 24.6 percent.

Similar body composition analyses of male athletes indicates that football backs and receivers have 8.1 percent mean fat content whereas the linemen and linebackers have a mean of 17.4 percent fat content. A male channel swimmer was found to have a relative fat content of 26.37 percent; assessment of the body composition of four weight lifters indicated a mean of 13.8 excess muscle, that is, that above the normal devel-

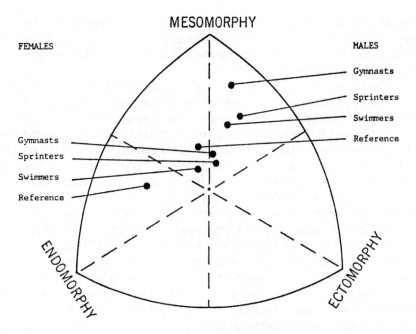

FIGURE 11.4. *Mean somatotypes for Olympic female and male athletes in various sports and reference groups. (Adapted from data by A. L. de Garay; L. Levine; & J. E. L. Carter (Eds.),* Genetic and Anthropological Studies of Olympic Athletes. *New York: Academic Press, 1974.)*

opment of the individual (Behnke & Wilmore, 1974). An examination of the body composition of marathon runners by Aloia and associates (1978a) indicated that the runners were slightly taller and lighter than the contrast group and had more lean body mass. In addition, although the bone width of the radius was essentially the same for both groups, the bone mineral content was somewhat elevated in the marathon runners. The close association between body physique and physiological functioning parameters to performance levels is shown by the similarity in these parameters in males and females who were matched for performance on the 15-mile run. Although the males were taller, heavier, and had higher hemoglobin concentration, Pate and associates (1985) found very similar metabolic and cardiorespiratory responses for the sexes and the percent of body fat of the runners was similar (males = 16.3 percent; females = 17.8 percent).

For most physical performance events, with the notable exception of swimming where it provides buoyancy, fat content is considered to be dead weight that contributes little to or handicaps performance. It is not surprising, then, that the survey of physique and strength by Malina and Rarick (1973) indicates strength to be greater for mesomorphic males than for either endomorphic or ectomorphic males in both absolute and relative measures. They concluded that, in terms of strength per pound of body weight, mesomorphic boys as a group were stronger on the average than ectomorphs and endomorphs at 11 years of age and older. Results for females are more equivocal, but data from Espenschade (1940) report that girls with the best motor performances are taller, lighter in weight, and have less subcutaneous tissue than the low performing group. In addition, the high performers had slightly superior manual and shoulder girdle strength suggesting to Malina and Rarick (1973) that the differences in strength between extreme categories were not great but that the girl of ectomesomorphic body build tended to be stronger than the endomorph in spite of the fact that her body weight was substantially less.

SECULAR TRENDS IN SIZE AND PERFORMANCE

The secular trend of increased height and weight during childhood and adolescence is reflected in increased stature and weight during adulthood. The trend towards increased weight from 1820 to 1955 for adults in various countries has been noted by Garn (1960). For males, this weight trend persisted in 1974, but for females there is some indication that increased medical and cultural emphasis on weight control is resulting in a change in weight patterning after 35 years of age. (See figure 11.5).

Data on Norwegian adults show little height gain from 1760 to 1830, but hereafter gains of about 1.5 centimeters (0.3 centimeter/decade) from 1830 to 1875 and approximately 4 centimeters (0.6 centimeter/decade) between 1876 and 1935 (Kiil, 1939). Similarly, the average height of American enlisted men increased from 67.5 inches to 68.1 inches from World War I to World War II (Jones & Jones, 1957). Between 1960–1962 and 1971–1974, the average heights of men in the United States increased by .7 inches and that of women increased .5 inches (Metropolitan Life Insurance Co., 1977). The secular trend towards increased height in the United States is illustrated in figure 11.6. For this cross-sectional data, the downward trend in heights with increasing age should not be interpreted only as showing a loss in stature with increasing age but rather also as indicative of the fact that older people never were as tall as younger people.

The secular trend towards increased body size in adulthood may be expected to have some effect upon motor performance. Long range data for average adult performance is limited but the comparison of grip strength data from 1884 collected in England with 1976 data collected in Tecumseh, Michigan, indicates that the Tecumseh males are both heavier and stronger than males in 1884. Montoye (1985) also compared the

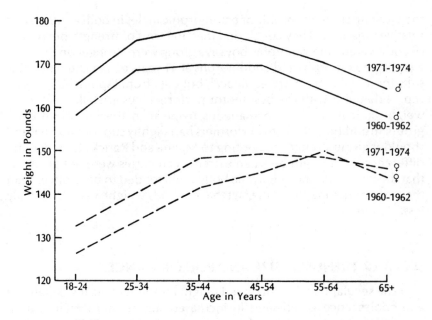

FIGURE 11.5. *Weight at various age levels in 1960–1962 and 1971–1974. (Adapted from data by Metropolitan Life Insurance Co. Trends in average weights and heights among insured men and women.* Statistical Bulletin, *October, 1977, 58, 2–6.)*

strength-to-body-weight ratios and noted that the difference in body size accounted for the difference in grip strength for the two populations until about the age of 25 after which the Tecumseh males had a higher strength ratio than the males in 1884. When maximum mean strength which occurred at about age 25 was designated as 100 percent and calculations made on the basis of percent of maximum, a higher percentage of absolute strength was preserved into later life in the 1884 males but the strength/weight ratio was better preserved in the Tecumseh males. The difference in these percentages of maximum calculations was due mainly to different trends in secular weight gain for the two populations. The Tecumseh males had a weight gain of approximately five kilograms between the ages of 25 and 60 years whereas the weight gain for the English males was approximately 10 kilograms during the same period starting from a much lower level at age 25.

The limited data on adolescents indicates that cultural influences may play a larger role in average performances (Espenschade & Meleney, 1961). The data for the AAHPER Fitness Test (Hunsicker & Reiff, 1966, 1977) illustrated in figures 10.31, 10.32, and 10.33 indicate variations in the secular trend for average performance levels from 1958 to 1976. In a com-

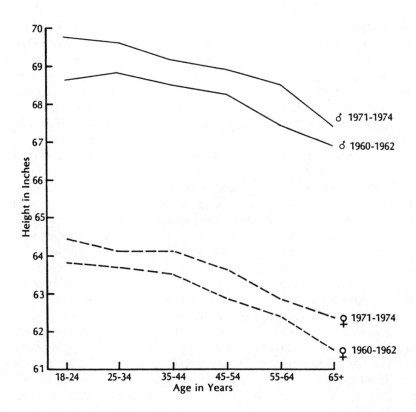

FIGURE 11.6. *Height at various age levels in 1960–1962 and 1971–1974. (Adapted from data by Metropolitan Life Insurance Co. Trends in average weights and heights among insured men and women. Statistical Bulletin, October, 1977, 58, 2–6.)*

parison of the motor performance of fathers and sons on the same test items, Cratty (1960) reports that the fathers had significantly better mean performance scores in chin-ups, the 100-yard run, and the standing fence vault. As there were also substantial correlations of .86 between father and son performance in the broad jump and of .59 in the 100-yard run, the poorer performance of the sons may be attributed to sociocultural changes from 1925 to 1959 rather than marked deviations in genetic components. Previous investigations of a secular trend for these performance items indicated a general decline in chin-ups and total performance scores. However, the constant improvement in world records by champion athletes over the years would certainly indicate that body size is important, in addition to advances that have been made in training methods, performance techniques, and equipment.

A survey of male and female records of Olympic performance in running and swimming events undertaken by Wyrick (1974) indicates improved performance for both sexes over the 48-year span from 1924 to 1972. The males remain consistently superior to the females in all events. During recent Olympiads, females have exceeded males in distance in the shot put and discus throw but these performances were achieved with weights that were one-half (shot put) and almost one-half (discus) of those used by males. In the javelin throw where the weight differential is not so great, female performance is well below male levels. The winning times for the 100-meter and the 400-meter freestyle swimming events during the 1948 to 1984 Olympics reflect the secular trends in improved performance and also encompass the period of most marked change in the sex differential (figure 11.7). Sex difference is least in the longer distance swimming events where a 7 percent difference favors the males as opposed to a 13 and 14 percent difference for the 100-meter freestyle and backstroke respectively. Wyrick attributes the reduced sex differential in the 400-meter freestyle to greater buoyancy of the female which reduces energy expenditure and to the coolant factor of water dissipating body heat so that the female disadvantage of greater heat stress is minimized. The female physique would seem to be advantageous in events such as channel swimming as the most recent record for this event was set by 23-year-old Penny Dean of Santa Clara who crossed the English Channel from Dover's Shakespeare Beach to Cap Gris Nez near Calais in 7 hours and 42 minutes, thereby bettering the previous record—8 hours and 45 minutes set by Nasser El Shazli—by one hour and three minutes (*This World*, 1978c).

Secular trends in increased body size as well as increased understanding of female biomechanics and improved coaching are attributed by Wyrick (1974) as accounting for the more marked increases in the discus and shot put throwing events in comparison with the secular increments of the male performances from 1948 to 1972. While recognizing the secular trends towards improved performance, Wyrick (1974) concludes that:

> The overall shape of the regression lines of performance over Olympic years is ample evidence that male and female physical performance in events of running, throwing, jumping, and swimming are in different performance classifications. (p. 413)

FACTORS INFLUENCING MOTOR PERFORMANCE

In the previous chapters, emphasis was placed upon the strong genetic component influencing the body build of the individual and reviews of research such as those by Sinning (1985) and Carter (1985) as well as overt observation have shown that specific types of body build are more suited to some types of physical activities. In addition, the physiological

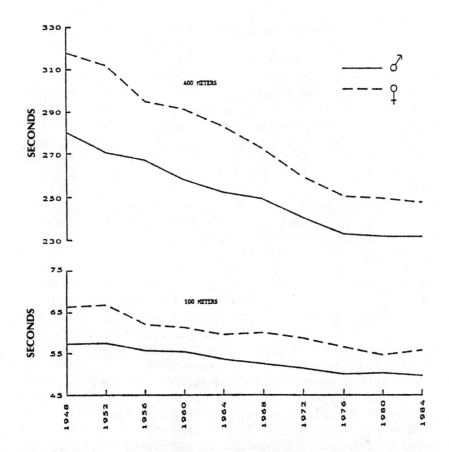

FIGURE 11.7. *Winning times in 100-meter and 400-meter freestyle swimming from 1948 to 1984. (Adapted from data for 1948 to 1980 in N. McWhirter,* Guiness Book of Olympic Records. *New York: Sterling Publishing Co. Inc., 1983. Data for 1984 from* Games of the XXIIIrd Olympiad Los Angeles 1984 Commemorative Book. *International Sports Publications, Inc., 1984.)*

capabilities of the individual are also genetically mediated. For example, the results of the Tecumseh Community Health Study of approximately 2500 males and 2000 females, ages 10 through 69, indicate a clear relationship between strength, skinfolds, height, and heart rate response to exercise of children and similar measures of their parents. Such a relationship was stronger for young children, and this was considered as probably indicating less influence of nonfamily environmental factors during the early years. The genetic component of motor performance related parameters is further illustrated by relationships of height, strength, heart rate response to exercise, and body fatness in siblings (Montoye et al., 1975).

Reviews of physiological functioning such as metabolic requirements of distance runners (Nagle & Bassett, 1985), parameters of anaerobic performance (Skinner & Morgan, 1985), and performance parameters of females (Wells, 1985) provide information regarding physiological requirements for optimal performance levels. In addition, such genetically mediated psychomotor tasks as reaction and movement times, balance, kinesthesis perception, and motor coordination also influence optimal performance levels (Spirduso, 1984, 1985). Such reviews clearly indicate that body build and physiological functioning are primary factors influencing the individual's potential for outstanding motor achievement.

Emphasis, in previous chapters, has also been placed upon the importance of environmental influences in enabling each individual to attain optimal genetic potential. Familial environmental influences on motor performance parameters are also indicated by the observation of Montoye et al. (1975) that husbands and wives were similar in strength, body fatness, and height. Rarick and McGee (1949) noted that individuals receiving parental encouragement during the formative years of basic skill development tended to participate more actively and to be better performers. Nonfamilial environmental encouragement such as good physical education programs also resulted in improved performance (Whittle, 1961). Moreover, different types of physical education programs vary in effectiveness with Slava et al. (1984) reporting that a lecture-laboratory (concepts) course resulted in attitude-knowledge-activity profiles that differed from those of undergraduates who had previously received traditional physical education programs (transfer group). The investigators noted that knowledge was consistently the greatest contributor of differences between the transfer and concepts groups over the two years studied and suggested that a college-level conceptual physical education class can have positive long-term effects. In a strength training program for young (mean age = 21.5 years) and mature (mean age = 44.4 years) women, both groups improved significantly in strength during the 12 weeks of training and both groups also showed significant improvements in self-satisfaction, physical self, and global self-concept scores in comparison with control groups of similar age (Brown & Harrison, 1986). It appears, then, that positive environmental influences and active participation tend to reinforce each other.

The emphasis placed upon outstanding performance by the news media, and its potential ramifications, have resulted in different types of social and environmental influences in different countries. For example, Buskirk (1985) cites the Bulgarian organization and training systems for weight lifters. The Russian organizational and training systems for gymnasts have been dramatically illustrated by the performance of Nadia Comaneci (Deford, 1976) and Kornelia Ender was a participant in the East

German organizational and training programs (Kirshenbaum, 1976). In comparison to these highly structured and highly supportive organizational systems for all phases of selection and preparation of outstanding athletes, the U.S. Olympic Committee with its U.S. Olympic Training Center at Colorado Springs is a final selection committee and training organization. Within this type of organizational system, athletes such as Bruce Jenner, Greg Louganis, and Mary Meagher must have non-governmental support systems and tremendous personal commitment to achieve outstanding performance levels.

Increasing knowledge of the biomechanics of movement and application of these principles to our increasing knowledge of body build and composition together with increased understanding of physiological and neurological processes and functioning have contributed to the development of better training programs. Because of secular trends in changes in body size, it is difficult to determine to what degree the secular increases in optimal performance levels are due to body size or to improved training techniques. However, in one sport, namely weight lifting, there are body weight categories that can be related to the amount of weight lifted. Croucher (1984) has analyzed world weight lifting records for the snatch and the clean and jerk events and for both these events there are consistent increments for all weight classes from 1956 to 1982. When the lifted weight is plotted against the body weight of the competitor, there is a marked linear increase in the lifted weight for all body weights up to 110 kilograms after which there is a leveling off to 155 kilograms. In his report, Croucher points out that it would be unwise to state definitely that the peak is close to being achieved in any weight division with the exception of the super-heavy class where increments have been small since 1976.

The psychological factors associated with training and performance of athletes has been extensively studied by Morgan (1985) who proposes a mental health model with the basic thesis underlying the model being that positive mental health is directly correlated with success in sport. For example, this model predicts that anxious, depressed, neurotic, or schizoid athletes will be less successful in sport than will individuals scoring in the normal range. When the Profile of Mood States was administered to runners, wrestlers, and rowers, these successful athletes possessed comparable psychological profiles and tended to be below average in measures of negative effect (i.e., tension, depression, fatigue, and confusion) but above average on the single positive measure of vigor. Morgan points out that the use of selected psychological states and traits provides predictive rates which exceed chance but the accuracy of the prediction is not acceptable for selection purposes.

Interest and ability are strong factors in continuing participation in various physical activities. However, over the years there is a change in interests which reflects reduced physical capacity. A decline in interest is noted in such activities as driving an automobile, tennis, and being pitted against another in politics or athletics. Increasing interest is expressed in visiting museums, observing birds, and gardening (Pressey & Kuhlen, 1957). In general, decreased interest is expressed in those activities requiring a high degree of physical capacity and stress, whereas there is an increased liking for those activities which are more sedentary and less stressful. However, there is also a decreased liking for continual changing of activities as the individual grows older (Pressey & Kuhlen, 1957). A survey of 2340 men, ranging in age from 20 to 59 years, indicates that the change in proportion of likes and dislikes was only 7.5 percent during this time with most of the changes taking place between 25 and 35 years (Strong, 1931). In general, an individual's activity participation tends to remain fairly stable (Desroches & Kaiman, 1964) but there are very definite differences in activity patternings within various socioeconomic groupings (Heyman & Jeffers, 1964).

Interest in an activity would appear to be strongly conditioned by one's facility in the particular activity. Reduction of interest in driving an automobile may, in part, be attributed to decreased skill on the basis of bad records and blame for accidents on the part of drivers over 60 years of age (McFarland et al., 1964). Furthermore, aging athletes have a significantly lower participation record in athletic activities than do older non-athletes (Montoye et al., 1957). In this instance, although the athlete may still have a slightly higher level of performance at all ages than the non-athlete, his decline in proficiency is obviously greater in comparison to his peak performance and, consequently, satisfaction may not be obtained from what, to him, is an inferior performance. However, increasing emphasis on physical fitness and opportunities to participate in masters programs encourages more athletes to remain active. Increasing social emphasis and medical endorsements for physical activity as a maintenance and/or preventive health measure is a key to changing the attitude of individuals with regard to participation in physical activities during the adult years.

PERFORMANCE TRENDS

In adulthood, the basic motor activities of childhood, such as running, jumping, and throwing, are no longer commonly engaged in by large numbers of individuals. Moreover, for those individuals who still partake of these activities there is no central organizing structure such as the school where data comparable to that of the growing years may be collected.

However, the AAHPER Youth Fitness Test Manual gives norms,

based upon scores from thousands of individuals, for various events from the age of 10 years to college level. A comparison of the 50th percentile scores of 17-year-old boys and girls with college men and women indicates a general superiority of the college groupings over the 17-year-olds. Table 11.1 shows that college women are superior in performance in sit-ups, shuttle run, standing broad jump, 50-yard dash, and 600-yard run-walk, whereas performance in modified pull-ups and softball throw is slightly lower. Similarly, table 11.2 lists college men as being superior in all items except pull-ups and 50-yard dash, but even here the norms are identical.

A study of physical fitness of Army Air Force personnel indicates a decline in performance for various test items after the age of 21 years (Larson, 1946). Here a steady decline was noted in 60-yard dash, sit-ups, chinning, standing broad jump, squat-thrust (Burpee) test, and 360-yard

TABLE 11.1. 50th percentile scores for women in various fitness test items*

Age	17 Years	College
Modified pull-ups	21	20
Sit-ups	16	20
Shuttle run (seconds)	11.8	11.6
Standing broad jump	5' 0"	5' 4"
50-yard dash (seconds)	8.6	8.4
Softball throw (feet)	79	70
600-yard run-walk (minutes)	3:11	2:58

* Adapted from *AAHPER Youth Fitness Test Manual*. Washington, D.C.: American Association for Health, Physical Education and Recreation, 1961. By permission of the publisher.

TABLE 11.2. 50th percentile scores for men in various fitness test items*

Age	17 Years	College
Pull-ups	6	6
Sit-ups	44	47
Shuttle run (seconds)	10.3	9.7
Standing broad jump	6' 11"	7' 3"
50-yard dash (seconds)	6.8	6.8
Softball throw (feet)	176	184
600-yard run-walk (minutes)	2:04	1:52

* Adapted from *AAHPER Youth Fitness Test Manual*. Washington, D.C.: American Association for Health, Physical Education and Recreation, 1961. By permission of the publisher.

run for men from 21 to 48 years with the physical fitness rating, based upon all test items, showing a similar decline. Men in this study were highly motivated and without doubt represented a selected sample of the total population. Thus the decrease in scores should be thought of as representative of adult males in good physical condition.

This steady decline in motor performance from 21 to 48 years is in accord with the data of Montoye and Lamphiear (1977) showing a similar decline in the strength index/weight ratio (figure 11.2). As absolute strength (figure 11.8) shows little decline over the same age span, it would appear that this decline in motor performance is due to the increased weight gain (figure 11.5) which would appear to be mainly fat and, therefore, impede performance in the test items. In a study of anthropometric changes of longshoremen who exhibit the predominant characteristic of massive musculature, Behnke and Wilmore (1974) noted that weight increased from before 45 years of age through the grouping of 45 to 54 years of age, after which there was a decline. There is also a redistribution of weight in that the abdomen enlarges and the muscular masses in the extremities are reduced with age. This cross-sectional study also indicated slight decreases in height with age but these may, in part, be an arti-

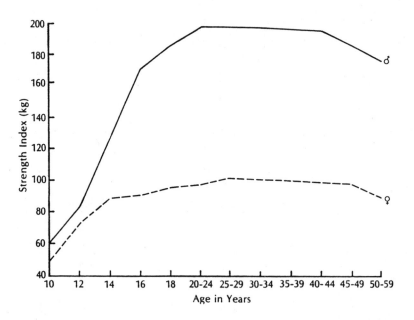

FIGURE 11.8. *Means of strength index (sum of right and left grip and arm strength). (Adapted from data by J. H. Montoye and D. E. Lamphiear, Grip and arm strength in males and females, age 10 to 69. Research Quarterly, 1977, 48, 109–120.)*

fact of the secular trend to increases in height, so that the younger groupings were taller than the older groupings, as well as a feature of the slight loss in height that occurs with aging.

PEAK PERFORMANCE

Although there is considerable variability in maximal performance levels within and between the sexes, it appears that the peak in maximal strength is achieved by both sexes from 25 to 29 years of age (figure 11.8) and that peak work performance also occurs within this age grouping (figure 12.6). The idiosyncratic nature of various types of physical activities places different demands on physical performance parameters and, if one regards championship performance as indicative of peak proficiency in an activity, then, according to table 11.3, the range of such performance is 22 to 35 years. However, a survey of the ages of athletes in the 1968 Olympics indicates that outstanding performance occurs in the age rage of 14 to 49 years for males and from 12 to 38 years for females. It is possible that the age range could be extended in either direction as the data in table 11.4 are not based upon all Olympic competitors but on 31.4 percent of the men and 22.4 percent of the women in the listed sports (de Garay et al., 1974). For men, the youngest mean ages occur in swimming and diving and the oldest in weight lifting and wrestling. Swimmers and gymnasts have the youngest mean ages for women, and divers and canoeists the oldest. In general, peak proficiency is attained at an earlier age in those activities requiring strength, speed, and endurance, whereas championship performance is more common at the later ages in relatively less vigorous activities where experience is also a factor.

Lehman (1953) compared the results in table 11.3 with the ages at which 1359 superior contributions were made by 933 individuals in the fields of science, mathematics, and practical invention. In each instance, to reduce the curves to a comparable basis, proper allowance is made for the mortality rate, and the age at which the greatest number of contributions are made is set at 100 percent. The contributions at other ages are proportionally adjusted to this standard. Figure 11.9 indicates that the age of maximum proficiency in all 17 physical skills listed in table 11.3 occurs approximately four years before the age of maximal number of superior contributions in the scientific fields. Furthermore, the curve of championship contributions in physical achievement falls away much more abruptly from the optimal age at 30 years than does that for the contributions in the scientific fields.

However, when a comparison is made with age of maximal proficiency in five physical activities involving fine neuromuscular coordination and precision of movement rather than vigorous performance, the

TABLE 11.3. Ages at which individuals have exhibited proficiency at "physical" skills*

Type of Skill	No. of Cases	Median Age	Mean Age	Years of Maximum Proficiency
U.S.A. outdoor tennis champions	89	26.35	27.12	22-26
Runs batted in: annual champions of the two major baseball leagues	49	27.10	27.97	25-29
U.S.A. indoor tennis champions	64	28.00	27.45	25-29
World champion heavyweight pugilists	77	29.19	29.51	26-30
Base stealers: annual champions of the two major baseball leagues	31	29.21	28.85	26-30
Indianapolis Speedway racers and national auto-racing champions	82	29.56	30.18	27-30
Best hitters: annual champions of the two major baseball leagues	53	29.70	29.56	27-31
Best pitchers: annual champions of the two major baseball leagues	51	30.10	30.03	28-32
Open golf champions of England and of the U.S.A.	127	30.72	31.29	28-32
National individual rifle-shooting champions	84	31.33	31.45	32-34
State cornhusking champions of the U.S.A.	103	31.50	30.66	28-31
World, national, and state pistol-shooting champions	47	31.90	30.63	31-34
National amateur bowling champions	58	32.33	32.78	30-34
National amateur duckpin bowling champions	91	32.35	32.19	30-34
Professional golf champions of England and of the U.S.A.	53	32.44	32.14	29-33
World record-breakers at billiards	42	35.00	35.67	30-34
World champion billiardists	74	35.75	34.38	31-35

* From Harvey C. Lehman, *Age and Achievement*. Published for the American Philosophical Society by Princeton University Press, Princeton, 1953, p. 256. By permission of the American Philosophical Society.

TABLE 11.4. Ages of performers in various events in the 1968 Olympics*

Event	Men			Females		
	N.	Mean	Min—Max	N.	Mean	Min—Max
Track	246	24.3	16-42	82	20.8	15-29
Field	71	25.2	17-43			
Swimming	67	19.2	14-25	32	16.3	12-23
Diving	16	21.3	16-30	7	21.1	16-38
Water polo	71	22.9	16-37			
Basketball	63	24.0	18-38			
Canoeing	49	24.2	18-38	4	22.0	18-25
Cycling	104	23.6	17-32			
Gymnastics	28	23.6	18-31	21	17.8	13-26
Rowing	86	24.3	18-40			
Weight lifting	59	26.7	17-49			
Boxing	142	22.9	17-35			
Wrestling	90	25.8	17-37			

* Adapted from data by A. L. de Garay; L. Levine; and J. E. L. Carter. *Genetic and anthropological studies of olympic athletes.* New York: Academic Press, 1974.

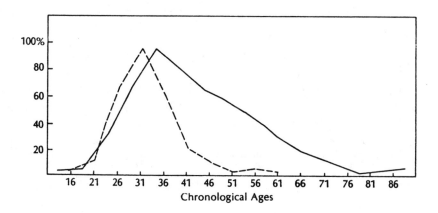

FIGURE 11.9. *Age versus output in science and proficiency in certain vigorous skills. Solid line: scientific output. Broken line: 1,175 championships in 17 classes listed in table 11.3. (From Harvey C. Lehman,* Age and achievement. *Published for the American Philosophical Society by Princeton University Press, Princeton, 1953. By permission of the American Philosophical Society.)*

age of maximal proficiency coincides with that of the maximal number of superior contributions in the scientific fields, although the rate of decline in maintenance of such performance remains much steeper (figure 11.10). A further comparison of proficiency in billiards, a fine neuromuscular skill, with output in chemistry indicates an identical age of maximal proficiency and very similar curves for performance at other age levels (figure 11.11). The surprising similarity of curves of proficiency in billiards and outstanding contributions in chemistry is not the only instance of such a relationship between activities which are primarily of a physical nature and those that are considered to be in the realm of the intellectual. Similar curves are also found for football professionalism and lyric writing and for proficiency in billiards and golf and oil painting (Lehman, 1953).

One may also consider geographical discoveries and explorations to require both a high degree of intellectual capacity and physical proficiency. Graphing such achievements with output in science reveals remarkably similar curves. Figure 11.12 indicates that peak performances in geographical exploration and output in science coincide, and the slope of the declining performance in both areas is very similar.

It would appear, therefore, that optimal performance in very vigorous physical activities is the domain of the young adult. However, high levels of performance may be maintained over a longer period of time in those activities requiring a lesser degree of vigorous functioning but with a high degree of fine neuromuscular coordination and precision of

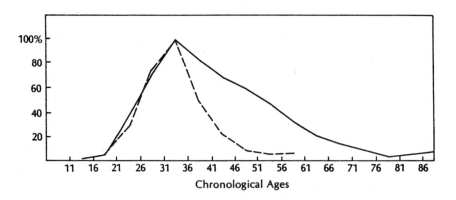

FIGURE 11.10. *Age versus output in science and proficiency in certain skills. Solid line: scientific output. Broken line: 577 championships at golf, billiards, rifle and pistol shooting, bowling, and duckpin bowling—skills of the nicest neuromuscular coordination. (From Harvey C. Lehman,* Age and achievement. *Published for the American Philosophical Society by Princeton University Press, Princeton, 1953. By permission of the American Philosophical Society.)*

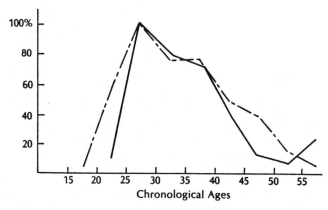

FIGURE 11.11. *Age versus output in chemistry and proficiency in billiards. Solid line: 52 greatest chemical contributions of all time (selected by three university chemistry teachers). Broken line: 136 professional championships at billiards. (From Harvey C. Lehman, Age and achievement. Published for the American Philosophical Society by Princeton University Press, Princeton, 1953. By permission of the American Philosophical Society.)*

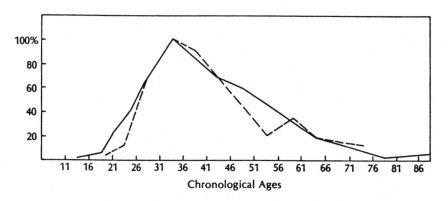

FIGURE 11.12. *Age versus output in science and geographical exploration. Solid line: scientific output. Broken line: 202 geographical explorations and discoveries (including polar expeditions) by 152 persons, now deceased, averaging 1.33 achievements per individual. (From Harvey C. Lehman, Age and achievement. Published for the American Philosophical Society by Princeton University Press, Princeton, 1953. By permission of the American Philosophical Society.)*

movement. Moreover, there is a marked similarity in performance curves for areas which require a superior physical capacity, but not necessarily championship performance, and contributions in various scientific, literary, and artistic fields.

The decline in scientists' productivity with increasing age as indicated by Lehman (1953) has been questioned by researchers who propose the thesis that a scientist's productivity does not vary with age. A more recent study by Diamond (1986) examined longitudinal data for scientists (physics and chemistry) and mathematicians (mathematics and economics) at the University of California at Berkeley and the University of Illinois at Urbana. These individuals were in departments that ranked in the top 15 in their respective fields over the period 1925 to 1977 and the salaries of these individuals, who eventually became full professors, was publically available. Diamond's analysis of the data indicated that salaries peak from the early to mid-60s whereas the number of annual citations of an individual's work appears to peak from age 39 to 89 for different departments with a mean age of 59 for the examined groups. However, the quantity and the quality of the current research output for these academics appeared to decline continuously with age. Therefore, it appears that the curves for mental and physical productivity tend to be similar in actual output but that academic productivity may be delayed in recognition due to lags in publication time, etc. whereas the achievement of world records or Olympic performance receives instant recognition through the news media.

ROLE OF EXERCISE

The growth during the period of adolescence is the final surge of genetic endowment toward the goal of a biologically mature individual, and any increments in performance subsequent to the cessation of growth are confined to the limits established at the termination of growth. With some individuals the range of limits is much greater than with others, but this, too, is a feature of the numerous differences that make each individual unique. A good example of an extreme range of limits within one individual is that of Wilma Rudolph, who overcame a crippling condition in her legs during childhood to attain her optimal physical performance by becoming the fastest woman runner in the world during the 1960 Olympics.

Young adulthood, between 20 and 30 years, marks the period of optimal physical achievement for the average individual, although championship performance is not uncommon at a later age in those activities involving a high degree of experience. The individual then faces the slow, but inevitable, decline in physical and physiological functioning termed *aging* which, barring previous decease due to illness or accident, eventually results in the death of the individual. The rate at which this decline occurs appears to be greatly influenced by the amount of physical activity of the individual.

Numerous studies indicate the beneficial effect of physical activity upon motor ability (Landis, 1955); physical fitness (Larson, 1946; Landis, 1955); circulatory changes (Michael & Gallon, 1959; Golding, 1961; Rochelle, 1961); oxidative capacity of muscles (Gollnick et al., 1972); and strength changes (Clarke, Shay, & Mathews, 1955; Berger, 1962, 1963). Studies such as those by Larson (1946) and Sloan (1963) show a higher level of physical fitness for individuals who are professionally engaged in physical education. Army Air Force physical training instructors were found to have consistently higher physical fitness ratings from ages 21 to 35 in comparison with other Air Force personnel (Larson, 1946). Similarly, physical education majors, both men and women, had significantly higher physical fitness indices than sophomore college men and women (Sloan, 1963). Moreover, the longitudinal data on Dill (1942, 1958) and the cross-sectional studies by Jokl (1954) indicate that above-normal performance levels are maintained over the years by individuals who partake regularly in vigorous physical activity.

Exercise is only one facet of an individual's life style but is one of the health practices listed as being positively related to mortality of men and women (Belloc & Breslow, 1972). The seven identified health practices are:

- Usually sleep 7 to 8 hours
- Regularly eat breakfast
- Rarely or never eat between meals
- Roughly, weight is between 10 percent under and 20 percent over desirable amounts
- Regular exercise
- No or moderate drinking
- Never smoke cigarettes

Epidemiological data were obtained from 6928 adults in Alameda County, California, in terms of the relationship between these health practices and the life expectancy of individuals at various ages. Figure 11.13 depicts these results and clearly indicates that the average life expectation increases for both sexes at all age levels with increases in the observance of these health practices. Data for observance of four to five of the health practices is also provided and these are not included in the figure for clarity of presentation, but they do indicate life expectancies falling slightly above midway between those depicted for each sex at all age levels (Belloc, 1973).

Although the data in the Alameda study were not analyzed to determine the primary cause of mortality during the 5½ follow-up period, it may be assumed that cardiovascular disease was the primary cause of mortality for the males under 60 years of age in the zero to three health practices group as this is the major cause of death for males in this age

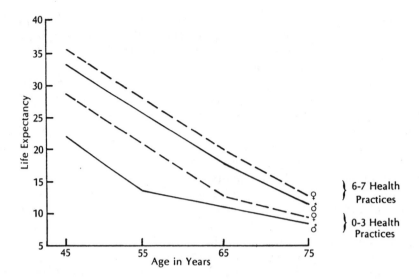

FIGURE 11.13. *Life expectancy at specific ages in relation to number of health practices. (Based on data by Belloc, N. B. Relationship of Health Practices and Mortality. Preventive Medicine, 1973, 2, 67–81.)*

group. At least three of the health habits, namely, smoking, obesity, and exercise, have been associated with coronary heart disease (Friedewald, 1985). As failure to observe these health habits results in lower life expectancy in males before 60 years of age in comparison with the rate of decline in other groupings, it is logical to assume that this lower life expectancy is the result of the higher incidence of cardiovascular mortality. A study was made of the incidence and severity of coronary heart disease in postal and transportation workers in England. The postal group was subdivided into letter carriers and office workers, while the transportation group was subdivided into the more physically active conductors and the more sedentary drivers. In both general groupings, the more physically active subgroupings had relatively less coronary heart disease, with such heart disease as did occur being of less severe condition (Morris et al., 1953). A similar study of railroad clerks and railroad switchmen conducted by the Laboratory of Physiological Hygiene at the University of Minnesota, with electrocardiographic tests taken before and after treadmill work, indicated a significantly lower incidence of abnormalities in the switchmen than in the clerks (Simonson, 1957). A survey of the incidence of coronary heart disease in active versus sedentary groups by Montgomery (1976) indicated that a lower incidence was reported for active workers as opposed to sedentary workers in nine of the 10 studies surveyed. Therefore, within occupations of similar socioeconomic levels, the amount of activity appears to be an operative factor contributing to health and mortality rate.

In a study of the relationship between physical activity and cardiovascular disease, Shapiro et al. (1969) reported that persons who were more active on and off the job had fewer and less severe myocardial infarctions than did their more sedentary counterparts with the exception that the most active individuals had a somewhat higher incidence than individuals slightly less active. However, both these groups had a lower incidence than the somewhat active and a decidedly lower incidence than the least active group (figure 11.14). This pattern of incidence is very similar to the pattern for mortality and level of physical activity reported by Belloc (1973) and illustrated in figure 12.5. A survey by Haskell and Fox (1974) reported that autopsy studies indicated that physical activity may reduce myocardial damage but appears to have little, if any,

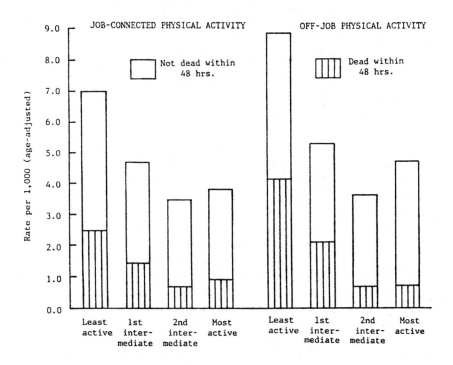

FIGURE 11.14. *Average annual incidence of first myocardial infarction among men in relation to job-connected and off-job physical activity rating (age-adjusted rates per 1000). (Based data from Shapiro, S.; Weinblatt, E.; Frank, C. W.; & Sager, R. V. Incidence of Coronary Heart Disease in a Population Insured for Medical Care (HIP).* American Journal of Public Health and the Nation's Health. *Vol. 59. No. 6. Suppl. to June, 1969.)*

effect on the atherosclerosis occurring in the major coronary arteries. Leon (1984) points out that the reduced heart rate effect of endurance exercise training is an important determinant of myocardial oxygen requirements which is especially important in the presence of advanced coronary heart disease. In addition, exercise training may significantly reduce systolic blood pressure during submaximal levels of exercise even if it does not alter resting blood pressure. The direct effects of exercise in normal individuals is a functional improvement of the heart as a pump. A partial protective effect against coronary heart disease is achieved through regular endurance activities in that they are associated with reduction in fat stores and body weight.

With our high standard of living, obesity has become a major health problem and the mortality rate for men who are 30 percent overweight is more than 40 percent greater than those of proper weight. In the Tecumseh, Michigan study of over 5000 males and females aged 10 through 69 years, fatter people at most ages tended to have higher serum cholesterol and exercise and postexercise heart rates (Montoye et al., 1976). Wilmore (1983), in his survey of appetite, body composition, and physical activity, reports that a certain minimum amount of physical activity is necessary before the body can precisely regulate food intake to balance the energy expenditure. Hard work with heavy energy expenditure requires more food but when activity is reduced below a minimal level, a corresponding decrease in appetite and food does not result and obesity develops. On the basis of his investigations, Oscai (1984) reports that exercise appears effective in correcting the increase in weight associated with short term fluctuations and the weight loss is primarily due to loss of fat. Although it is possible to correct mild obesity through exercise, severe obesity cannot be corrected by exercise alone.

Reductions in weight as well as changes in body composition can be achieved by various exercise programs. For example, Wilmore (1974) reports significant reductions in body weight and in absolute and relative body fat in men and women during a 10-week training program. Significant performance gains were also reported for both sexes in the four strength measures. Similarly, endurance types of training programs result in significant reductions in body weight and absolute and relative body fat. Pollock and associates (1975) report significant changes for males in these aspects of body composition plus a significant reduction in abdomen girth following 20-week training programs in running, walking, and bicycling. In addition, all groups had significantly lower resting heart rates and higher maximal oxygen uptake. Participation in regular endurance activities by women also results in body composition and physiological differences in comparison with sedentary females. In a comparison with age- and height-matched sedentary women, female distance runners had significantly lower resting heart rate, greater maximal oxygen uptake, less body weight and a lower percentage of fat. Although the lean body weight was slightly higher in the runners in this study by Upton et al. (1983), the difference was not significant suggesting to the investigators that most women regardless of their level of physical activity were similar in amount of bone and lean muscle mass and that lower levels of body fat in women runners is directly related to their physical activity and energy expenditure.

The emphasis upon minimization of non-productive body weight (i.e., fat) to increase the efficiency of physical actions appears to have a more profound effect upon the physiological functioning of females than on males. Frisch and McArthur (1974) have related weight with menstrual function and suggest that a minimum level of stored, easily mobilized energy (fat) is necessary for ovulation and the menstrual cycle in the human female. Loss of menstrual function (amenorrhea) is associated with below minimal weight for height indicating a low level of fatness. Ballet dancers, who have a strenuous training program and also diet to maintain the slim physique required for stage productions, have low fat levels.

In an examination of age at menarche, Frisch et al. (1980) noted that there was a relatively late mean age at menarche and delayed menarche of dancers and that their weights for height were below standard. When the ballet dancers who reported no menarche at a mean age of 14.3 years were compared with well-nourished non-dancers of the same height who attained menarche at a mean age of 12.9 years, the mean weight of the dancers was significantly less than that of the well-fed girls. It is possible that these dancers were late maturers but the hard training and low food intake typical of ballet dancers may also be factors. In a survey of eating problems, amenorrhea and eating problems were significantly related in ballet dancers with 50 percent of amenorrheics reporting anorexia nervosa as compared with 13 percent of those with normal cycles. Of the 55 adult dancers surveyed, 56 percent had delayed menarche and 19 percent were amenorrheic at the time of the study (Brooks-Gunn et al., 1987). Another survey of 75 adult ballet dancers indicated that the incidence of scoliosis was greater in individuals who had had a delayed menarche and the incidence of fractures rose with increasing age at menarche. In addition, the incidence of secondary amenorrhea was twice as high among dancers with stress fractures and its duration was longer (Warren et al., 1986).

The results of these surveys indicate that the diet of ballet dancers is an important contributing factor to amenorrhea but, as training is rigorous at all levels, it is not possible to determine the effects of differentials in training levels. Moreover, as most of the girls who aspire to careers in ballet begin training at a young age, it is not possible to determine what effect such training has on menarcheal delay. In a survey of college swimmers and runners, Frisch and associates (1981) reported that premenarche-trained athletes had a mean menarcheal age of 15.1 years whereas the postmenarcheal-trained athletes had a mean menarcheal age of 12.8 years. Moreover, 61 percent of the premenarcheal-trained athletes had irregular cycles and 22 percent were amenorrheic whereas 60 percent of the postmenarcheal-trained athletes had regular menstrual cycles and none were amenorrheic. Both these groups recorded data during an intensive training and competitive season lasting for six months and both groups reported increasing incidence of irregularity and amenorrhea during training. In a strenuous program for untrained women in which half the subjects were in a weight-loss group and half in a weight-maintenance group, the strenuous exercise disrupted cyclicity in both groups with the incidence of disruption being greater in the weight-loss group over the two-menstrual-cycle period of the study (Bullen et al., 1985). However, all subjects were again experiencing normal menstrual cycles within six months of the termination of the study and the investigators concluded that vigorous exercise, particularly if compounded by weight loss, can reversibly disturb reproductive function in women.

Decreased spinal mineral content has been noted in amenorrheic women in comparison with women menstruating normally (Cann et al., 1984). When groups of amenorrheic and normal-cycle athletes are matched for age, height, weight, sport, and training regimens, Drinkwater et al. (1984) found that the vertebral mineral density of the amenorrheic group was significantly lower than in the normal-cycle group. Two radial sites were also measured but there was no significant difference between the groups for these measures. The three-day dietary intake for the two groups was not significantly different and the groups were similar in percentage of body fat, age at menarche, years of participation, and frequency and duration of exercise. There was, however, a difference in the number of miles run per week with the amenorrheic athletes averaging 41.8 miles per week in comparison with the 24.9 miles of the normal-cycle group. Similar results have been obtained by Marcus et al. (1985) who evaluated elite women distance runners and found that mineral density of the lumbar spine was lower in amenorrheic runners than in cyclic women and age-matched controls but higher than in runners with secondary amenorrhea who were less physically active. These investigators concluded that intense exercise may reduce the impact of amenorrhea on bone mass but amenorrheic runners remain at high risk for exercise-related fractures. A survey by Lloyd and associates (1986) of the relationship between menstrual status and bone injuries of athletes indicated that premenopausal women who have absent or irregular menses while engaged in vigorous exercise programs are at increased risk for musculoskeletal injury.

In assessing the implications of the research dealing with amenorrhea and bone mass and injuries in athletes, it should be recalled that the
diet of the individuals is also related to amenorrhea. Borgen and Corbin
(1987) analyzed Eating Disorder Inventory (EDI) and questionnaire responses of college nonathletes; athletes whose sports emphasized leanness (ballet, gymnasts, bodybuilder/weightlifters, and cheerleaders);
and athletes in activities that did not emphasize leanness (swimming,
track and field, and volleyball). The results for these subjects indicated
that there were no significant differences when athletes were compared
with nonathletes in total number of EDI subscale scores above the means
of known anorexics; in preoccupation with weight; and in exceptional
preoccupation with weight or tendencies toward eating disorders.
Within the athletic groups, the athletes in activities emphasizing leanness
had more high scores (21 percent) of the total number of EDI subscale
scores than did those not emphasizing leanness (11 percent). Although
not significantly different, 23 percent of the athletic group emphasizing
leanness were preoccupied with weight whereas only 16 percent of the
nonlean emphasis group were preoccupied with weight. All of the athletes having exceptional preoccupation with weight or tendencies towards eating disorders were in the group classified as emphasizing leanness. The authors suggest that the athletes in activities not emphasizing
leanness may have a relatively low risk of anorexia because they realize
that exceptionally low body weight is not conducive to good performance in their sport. On the other hand, athletes in activities emphasizing leanness may be especially at risk of anorexia.

Amenorrhea, which may be caused by malnutrition and/or low
body weight, very vigorous training programs, and/or hormonal problems (low estrogen levels), is associated with bone loss. For women who
have regular menses, increased amounts of activity appears to have a
positive effect on bone mineral content. For example, Stillman et al.
(1986) examined the bone mineral content of women aged 30 to 85 years
who were categorized on the basis of low, moderate, and high level of
activity and found that the most active group of women had significantly
higher bone mineral content than the two less active groups. In addition,
the high activity group were significantly leaner on the basis of percent
fat estimates and skinfold thicknesses. The report of a Consensus Conference (1984) on osteoporosis states that estrogen and calcium are the
mainstays of prevention and management of osteoporosis with exercise
and nutrition being important adjuncts.

The level of estrogen is also associated with high-density lipoprotein
cholesterol (HDL-C) with a low HDL-C level being an especially good
predictor of coronary heart disease in women. Harting and associates
(1984) report that long-distance runners and joggers had higher levels of

HDL-C than inactive women and that there was a significant exercise-menopausal interaction indicating a beneficial exercise effect. These results led the investigators to conclude that endurance exercise by post-menopausal women may help prevent adverse lipid and lipoprotein changes which might predispose them to coronary heart disease. In an article (Monahan, 1986) dealing with the question of exercise for women, Barbara Drinkwater is quoted as saying, "The positive effects on the cardiovascular and musculoskeletal systems are so great, there's no doubt but that women should exercise."

In assessing the effects of varying levels of exercise on the maintenance of bone mineral content in women, it would appear that risk of bone loss is greatest for inactive women and that risk is greater for highly active women as compared with regularly active women. This trend is similar to that shown for the association between physical activity level and myocardial infarctions for males (Haskell & Fox, 1974) and for exercise levels and mortality rates for males as shown in figure 12.5. In all instances, therefore, observance of the health habit of regular exercise appears to be most beneficial at the active rather than the highly active level for both males and females. Barbara Drinkwater is cited as saying that it is important when discussing the risks of physical activity to differentiate between exercising for health and training for competition (Monahan, 1986). At high competitive levels risks grow for both men and women but, for individuals concerned with health maintenance, there is no question that regular endurance exercise has beneficial effects on general physical and mental well-being.

Health-related physical fitness goals for adults aged 25 to 65 years which have been identified by Haskell, Montoye, and Orenstein (1985) are:

a) Prevention and treatment of coronary heart disease
b) Prevention and treatment of Type II diabetes
c) Maintenance of optimal body composition
d) Enhancement of psychological status
e) Retention of musculoskeletal integrity

The recommended physical activity plan includes:

- Type of exercise: Emphasis on large muscle dynamic exercise; some heavy resistive and flexibility exercises.
- Intensity: Moderate intensity (more than 50 percent maximal oxygen uptake).
- Duration: Total of more than 30 minutes per session (more than 4 kilocalories per kilogram of body weight).

- Frequency: At least every other day. Lower level activities, such as walking are recommended on a daily basis.

In a study of the effectiveness of fast walking as an adequate aerobic stimulus for 30- to 69-year-old men and women, Porcari and associates (1987) found that, for each sex and age category, subjects who attained training heart rates walked 0.1 to 0.5 mph faster than those who did not. At all age levels, the minimum pace required to attain training heart rate was faster for males (range 4.0 to 3.5 mph) than for females (range 3.5 to 3.0 mph) with the speed decreasing progressively with increasing age.

In summary, adulthood marks the period of highest performance levels and also the greatest variability in human physical performance. Levels of achievement are influenced by interest, socioeconomic environment, and cultural patterns as well as inherent ability. The life style of the individual together with genetic endowment are important determinants of the health and life span of the individual. Participation in physical activities is a major contributor to a balanced life with a healthy mind in a healthy body.

SUMMARY

1. The peak in maximal work output ranges from 22 to 25 years for women and 25 to 28 years for men.

2. Physical activities requiring a high degree of strength, speed, and endurance components peak earlier and decrease earlier than less vigorous activities requiring more experience.

3. Because of the different biomechanical and physiological demands of the various sports, the physique of the individual is a major determinant of success in a particular sport.

4. Although body build is primarily determined by the genetic endowment of the individual, the degree to which the individual attains maximal potential is determined by interest, opportunities for and degree of training.

5. In general, a mesomorphic body build is most favorable for most activities with a higher degree of endomorphy associated with distance swimming and weight events and a higher degree of ectomorphy associated with distance running events.

6. The secular trends toward increased height and weight, together with improved equipment and training methods, have resulted in increases in Olympic and world performance records. However, average performance data does not show such a consistent secular improvement

in performance levels in association with the secular trend of increased height and weight.

7. The life style of the individual and observance of health habits, which include regular exercise, are important determinants of the health maintenance of the individual and of the potential life span.

8. Although genetic factors are an important aspect of risk of cardiovascular disease, other factors such as obesity, lack of exercise, and smoking, are major contributors to such risk. As participation in physical activity can reduce fat levels, such participation impacts two of these contributors to cardiovascular disease.

9. In terms of activity level only, inactive individuals have the highest risk of cardiovascular disease whereas regularly active individuals have the least risk. Highly active individuals have a slightly higher risk than regularly active individuals.

10. Weight levels have been associated with regularity of menstrual cycle in females with women who have low levels of body fat for height having a higher incidence of amenorrhea. Fat levels can be lowered by diet or training, or by a combination of both. As amenorrhea is associated with low estrogen levels and low estrogen levels are associated with bone mass loss, the risk of bone mass loss is higher in women who participate at high activity levels in leanness-desirable activities. For women who do not have menstrual irregularities, regular activity enhances bone mineral content whereas inactivity results in reduced bone mass.

11. Although exceptionally high levels of training may have somewhat higher risk factors for both men and women than regular active physical participation, the risk factors are not nearly as great as they are for an inactive life style.

ACTIVITY SUGGESTIONS

1. Any individual who has cardiovascular or other health problems should undergo a medical examination before undertaking an exercise program.

2. Young adults who have no cardiovascular or other health problems but have low levels of fitness should begin their cardiovascular (aerobic) training program at lower levels of intensity and gradually increase the intensity level.

3. Intensity level is based upon the degree to which exercise heart rate is elevated above the resting heart rate. Starting from an assumed maximum heart rate of 220 beats per minute, the potential exerciser should substract the exerciser's age in years to determine the potential maximal heart rate. After calculating the resting heart rate in minutes, this value is subtracted from the exerciser's maximal heart rate to determine

the heart rate reserve (range). The heart rate reserve is multiplied by the desired training percentage (e.g., 60 percent) to determine the amount the heart rate must be raised above the resting heart rate to produce the desired training effect (e.g., training increase + resting heart rate = training heart rate).

4. The duration of the aerobic exercise is also important in achieving a training effect and is inversely related to the intensity of the exercise. For example, a low intensity activity requires participation for a longer period of time in any one session to achieve similar training effects as that of high intensity participation over a shorter period of duration. Walking is an example of low intensity exercise whereas running at high speed is a high intensity exercise.

5. Individuals who are beginning their excercise programs at low levels should begin aerobic exercise programs at minimal, or even lower, levels to reduce potential muscle soreness and then gradually increase the duration and, if possible, the intensity of the exercise.

6. Exercise programs may be designed to be completed within one training session or they may be distributed over at least two periods in any one day. The distributed practice program is better suited to individuals who do not have large blocks of time available for exercise and/or prefer to be active at more than one period in the day. In the distributed practice design, at least one of the sessions should be devoted to aerobic exercises and the others to general conditioning activities. In the one session design, both aerobic and general conditioning exercises should be included.

7. Aerobic exercises include any large muscle, rhythmic activities such as running, jogging, walking, hiking, swimming, skating, bicycling, rope skipping, jazzercise or aerobic dancing, rowing, cross-country skiing, and various endurance game activities.

8. General conditioning exercises are specific exercises or activities undertaken to condition body segments and functions not optimally utilized in aerobic activities. For example, running contributes little to arm strength and endurance. In addition to strength and strength endurance, other general conditioning components include flexibility, balance, and coordination. Exercises and/or activities should be selected which will enhance maintenance of these physical activity components in all parts of the body. Some specific suggestions for activities are included in Appendix A and an effective general fitness program is included in Appendix B.

9. In selecting the time of day in which to exercise, the beginning exerciser should give consideration to the variations in the exerciser's personal daily activity levels. For example, some individuals are what is called "morning persons" who are most active in the mornings whereas others are "evening persons." The beginning exerciser will probably en-

joy the aerobic activities more if undertaken during the more active part of the day whereas the general conditioning activities can provide breaks at other times during the day.

10. The personal involvement of the exerciser in the development of a personalized exercise program can result not only in greater enjoyment and satisfaction but also can provide intellectual stimulation and a better understanding of each individual's own personal limitations and competencies.

12

Older Adulthood

The technological and scientific advances that have been made in most aspects of human endeavours have resulted not only in environmental conditions that have enabled individuals to optimize their inherited motoric performance potential. They have also resulted in reductions in the mortality rate so that more individuals are living longer. This means that more individuals have the potential of attaining the optimal species life span. However, the multiplicity and the complexity of the factors that ultimately determine longevity are such that Wright and Blass (1984) believe there is no certainty that the life span will exceed the 85 to 100 years that is rapidly becoming the norm in many developed societies.

LONGEVITY AND DEMOGRAPHIC TRENDS

The longevity of an individual is influenced by the same factors that bear a relationship to growth, namely: heredity, sex, socioeconomic status, race, geographic area, and temporal era. The records of 3,000,000 men insured with 34 American and Canadian companies were categorized into those individuals whose parents both lived to age 75 and those whose parents both died under the age of 60 (Dublin et al., 1949). Figure 12.1 indicates that the mortality of the men with long-lived parents was distinctly lower than that of the group whose parents had died before the age of 60 years, with the difference averaging 20 percent. At 27 years of age, the individuals with long-lived parents had a life expectancy of 2⅓ years more than those with short-lived parents. Lansing (1959), in a comprehensive discussion of the biology of **senescence**, contends there is an extensive collection of data supporting an heritable component to longevity.

The previously mentioned greater propensity of females for survival at all ages is reflected in longer life spans in comparison with males. In 1952, a white man of 64 years could look forward to 13 years of life, whereas a white woman of the same age had a life expectancy of 15¾ years (Wilson, 1957). By 1975, the sex discrepancy in white survival rates increased so that, although males could look forward to an increased life

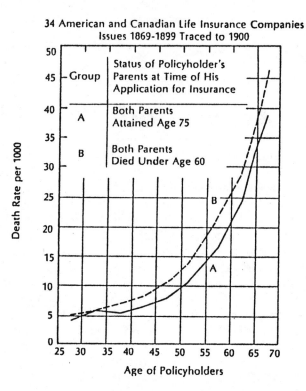

34 American and Canadian Life Insurance Companies
Issues 1869-1899 Traced to 1900

Group	Status of Policyholder's Parents at Time of His Application for Insurance
A	Both Parents Attained Age 75
B	Both Parents Died Under Age 60

Death Rate per 1000

Age of Policyholders

FIGURE 12.1. *Death rates at successive ages among white male policyholders classified according to longevity of parents. From Louis I. Dublin; Alfred J. Lotka; and Mortimer Spiegelman, Length of life. New York: The Ronald Press Company, 1949. Reprinted by permission of John Wiley & Sons, Inc.*

expectancy of 13.7 years, females could anticipate an additional 18.1 years of life at age 65. The greatest sex difference in life expectancy occurs during the first year of life when white males, in 1975, had an expectancy of 69.4 years, whereas females had an expectancy of 77.2 years with a 7.8 year differential. This differential in life expectancy gradually declines until 60 years of age, when the sex difference in life expectancy is 5.1 years, and becomes less marked thereafter so that the differential is only 1.9 years at 80 years of age. The life expectancy tables for blacks and other racial classifications also show a greater life expectancy for females at all age levels but reveal a different trend in the differential values. In this instance, the higher sex differential of 8.7 for males and females under one year of age is reflected in a higher differential of 2.5 at 80 years of age, but the most marked decline in the sex differential for life expectancy occurs between ages 30 and 50 years when the differential is reduced from 7.3 to 5.5 years (U.S. Bureau of the Census, 1977).

The different racial patterns for the sex differential between males is to some degree associated with racial differences in the incidence of cardiovascular mortality. Although the male/female coronary risk is greater than 1.0 at all ages, it is largest for whites between ages 30 to 50 years when it is approximately 7:1 (Hazzard, 1986). Associated with the higher incidence of cardiovascular mortality at younger ages for males is the sex differential in sex hormone levels which gives rise to the sex differential in lipoprotein metabolism (i.e., cholesterol level) which in time (based on lifestyle) leads to the sex differential in atherosclerosis and this in turn to the sex differential in longevity (Hazzard, 1985). The effects of life style are illustrated by the data of Belloc (1973) for the life expectancy of individuals based upon their observance of the seven health habits (figure 11.13). As with the coronary risk ratio, the pattern for the life expectancy for males who follow 0 to 3 of the health habits indicates appreciably less years of life expectancy than for females of the same age and same life style but the sex differential becomes less with increasing age.

A comparison of the life expectancy data for whites in 1975 with that of blacks and other racial classifications indicate that socioeconomic factors may, in part, be influencing these data. Whereas white males have a higher life expectation of 69.4 years in comparison with 63.6 years under one year of age, blacks and other racial classification males have the same expectation of 13.7 years at age 65 but a higher expectation of 8.5 years at 80 years in comparison with the 6.7 years for white males. Similarly, white females have higher expectation rates from under one year of age until 70 years of age at which time the expectation of 14.4 years is the same for all racial groups, but nonwhite classifications have a greater expectation of 11.0 years in comparison with white female life expectancy of 8.6 years at 80 years of age (U.S. Bureau of the Census, 1977). Whether the greater life expectancy of nonwhites after 65 years of age for males and after 70 years of age for females is attributable to a real racial difference in longevity and/or physical activity patterns which may be related to socioeconomic status is purely conjectural on the basis of the limited information available.

Socioeconomic factors do, apparently, have some relationship to the life span. As table 12.1 indicates there is a rise in mortality rate with decreasing socioeconomic levels. The occupational groupings which have a high percentage of college graduates, namely, professional, technical, administrative, and managerial workers, have the lower ratio of death rates from ages 20 to 64 years. It may be argued that the occupations having the higher mortality rate, such as semiskilled workers and laborers, also have specific hazards which outweigh socioeconomic levels. However, the same pattern was observed in a British study in which wives were classified on the basis of the occupation of their husbands and, from this, it may be inferred that mortality is influenced more by socioeco-

TABLE 12.1. Mortality ratios (in percentages) by occupation*

Occupation Class	White Males United States Ages 20-64 1950	Males England & Wales Ages 15-64 1959-1963	Married Women England & Wales Ages 15-64 1959-1963	Single Women England & Wales Ages 15-64 1959-1963
I. Professional	82	76	77	83
II. Technical, administrative, managerial	83	81	83	88
III. Proprietors, clerical, sales, skilled workers	96	100	102	90
IV. Semiskilled workers	97	103	105	108
V. Laborers	121	143	141	121

* Adapted from data by Metropolitan Life Insurance Co. Socioeconomic mortality differentials by leading cause of death. *Statistical Bulletin*, January, 1977, *58*, 5–8.

nomic environment than by occupational hazards (Spiegelman, 1960). In the data listed in table 12.1, the married women were also classified according to their husbands' occupations and it is noted that their mortality closely parallels that of their husbands. This similarity in pattern is considered as indicating that the life style and living environment account to some degree for mortality differentials (Metropolitan Life Insurance Co., 1977).

Similarly, a survey of the death rates in a large number of countries shows the death rate to be much lower, or conversely the survival rate to be much higher, in countries with better socioeconomic conditions. It also indicates that the decline in death rate since 1920 has not been as great in countries where the standard of living has been consistently high, whereas the reduction in death rate is quite marked in areas which had a low standard of living in 1920 but have made efforts to raise their nutritional standards since then (Spiegelman, 1960). Life expectancies at birth for the period of 1975 to 1980 are reported by Siegel and Hoover (1984) as ranging from a low of 48.6 years to a high of 73 years in a survey of international population trends. Although there is a range of 24.4 years at birth in this projection, the range of life expectancy at age 60 for the same period of time is only 4.7 years (i.e., from 14.1 to 18.8 years). Thus increases in life expectancy are achieved mainly by reduction of mortality rates at the lower age levels rather than with older populations.

The reduced death rates in various countries from 1920–1924 to 1959 indicate a secular trend toward greater life expectancy. Such is indeed the case and there has been a decided increase in life expectancy over the centuries since ancient Grecian times (figure 12.2). The rapid improvement in life span following the middle of the nineteenth century coincides with the rapid increases in medical knowledge and improvements in socioeconomic conditions brought about by the industrial revolution. Therefore, increased life span over the centuries is based upon reduced death rates rather than any noted change in inheritable longevity. Wilson, in 1957, indicated that, over the past four decades, the death rate for all ages decreased for both white males and white females in the United States. This decline in death rate was also consistently greater for females than for males in that life expectancy for males was increased 18 $\frac{1}{3}$ years from 1900 to 1951, whereas it was raised by 21$\frac{1}{2}$ years for females over the same time span.

The increases in life span of the population have resulted in shifts in the proportion of individuals within selected age groupings. The popula-

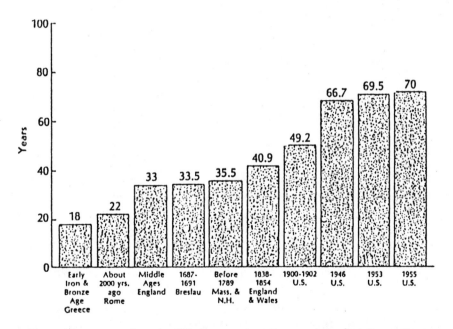

FIGURE 12.2. *Average length of life from ancient Greece to modern times. (From Otto von Mering and Frederick L. Weniger, Social-cultural background of the aging individual. In J. E. Birren (Ed.),* Handbook of aging and the individual. *Chicago: The University of Chicago Press, 1959. By permission of the publisher.)*

tion structure of the United States at various times from 1860 to the estimated percentage grouping in 2000 is depicted in figure 12.3. The most dominant trend is the increasing proportion of the population within the 45 years and older age groups and the corresponding reduction in the percentage of younger individuals so that the median age is projected to increase from 30.2 in 1950 to 37.3 years by 2000 (U.S. Bureau of the Census, 1977). The increased proportion of the under-5-years age grouping in the 1960s is indicative of the postwar "baby boom" and the increased proportion of the population in the 5 to 21 category in 1970 and 1975 distributions reflects the age increases of these children. The projection for 1990 reflects the further aging of this group and the projection for 2000 indicates subsequent inclusion in the 45 to 64 category. This "moving bubble," which passed through the educational system in the 1960s and early 1970s, will have further impact as the percentage of 19.7 for individuals age 55 and older in 1976 becomes the projected percentage of 27.1 in 2030 (Shepard & Martz, 1977).

A survey of world demographic trends indicates that, in 1980, those

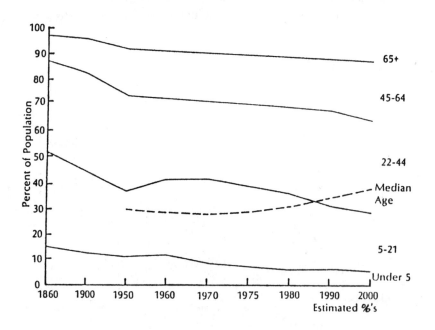

FIGURE 12.3. *Percentage distribution for the population of the United States in selected age groupings. (Data for 1860 and 1900 adapted from O. von Mering and F. L. Weniger, Social-cultural background of the aging individual. In J. E. Birren (Ed.), Handbook of aging and the individual. Chicago: The University of Chicago Press, 1959. Other data adapted from U.S. Bureau of the Census, Statistical abstract of the United States: 1977 (98th ed.), Washington, D.C., 1977.)*

over 60 years of age constituted 6.2 percent of the population in the less developed regions whereas the percentage in the more developed regions was almost 2½ times higher at 15.0 percent of the population. The proportions of older persons in all regions are expected to increase from 1980 to at least the year 2020 and it is predicted that, by the year 2000, nearly 20 percent of the population in Europe will be 60 years or older (figure 12.4). Although the more developed regions have higher proportions of the population over 60 years, the less developed regions actually have more individuals in this age grouping with the number being 205 million, or approximately 55 percent, of the approximately 376 million people aged 60 years or older in the world. The number of persons 60 years or over in the world will increase greatly by the year 2000 and it is projected that there will be approximately 590 million at that time with approximately 230 million in the more developed regions and 360 million, or 61 percent, in the less developed regions (Siegel & Hoover, 1984).

PHYSICAL ACTIVITY AND LONGEVITY

It would appear that interest and liking, conditioned by socioeconomic factors and opportunity, play important roles in the determination of an individual's participation in physical activities during adulthood. Such a complexity of factors make any assessment of the contribution of participation in physical activities upon longevity exceedingly difficult and decidedly conjectural. However, attempts have been made to examine the levels of physical activity in relation to mortality rates and, if one makes the assumption that those who have not died during the time period sampled have continued to live in part, as a result of their activity levels, then one may make the additional assumption that the level of physical activity influences longevity. In interpreting such results, one must bear in mind the fact that this "survival" longevity is a statistical measure that differs from the optimal longevity or life span of the human species.

The Framingham Study (Kannel, 1967) of 5127 men and women is frequently cited for the inverse relationship noted between coronary heart disease and habitual level of physical activity. In this study, a 24-hour history of usual physical activity for the 30- to 62-year-old men and women at entry was assessed on a rating of basal to heavy activity levels and compared to coronary heart disease death over the next 12 years. Men who had a low physical activity index had a significantly higher than normal incidence of coronary heart disease than would be expected for that particular age grouping. In addition, objective indicators of physical activity status for both men and women (i.e., weight gain, vital capacity, and resting pulse rate) indicated that those individuals who were most

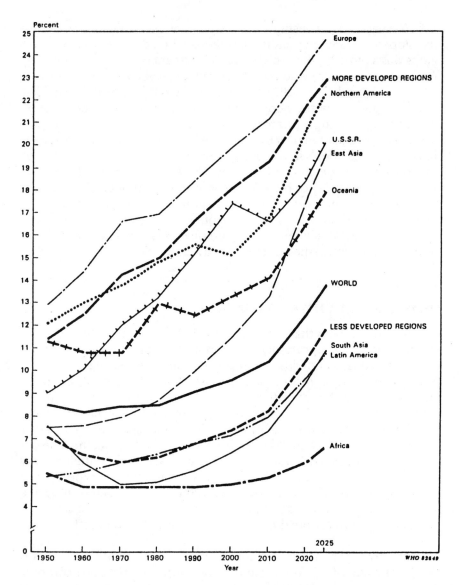

FIGURE 12.4. *Percentage of the total population 60 years and over, for regions: 1950 to 2025. (From Siegel, J. S., & Hoover, S. L.* International Trends and Perspectives: Aging. *International Research Document No. 12. Bureau of the Census, U.S. Department of Commerce, September, 1984.)*

sedentary (with adverse values for two or more of these traits) had a five-fold greater mortality from coronary heart disease than did those who had no adverse traits and were presumably more active.

In a survey-type study of health habits, Belloc and Breslow (1972) identified seven favorable health habits and Belloc (1973) reported on the mortality rates associated with these health habits during the 5½ years between the original questionnaire and the termination of the study. One of the identified health habits was regular exercise and the surveyed individuals had been asked to report on their physical activity participation. In examining the relationship between mortality rates and the amount of physical activity, an inverse relationship was shown with men and women at all age levels who never undertook regular exercise having a much higher mortality rate than those individuals who were more active on a regular basis in various types of physical activity. This inverse relationship becomes most marked after 55 years of age and figure 12.5 depicts the data reported by Belloc (1973) for both sexes in the 65 to 74

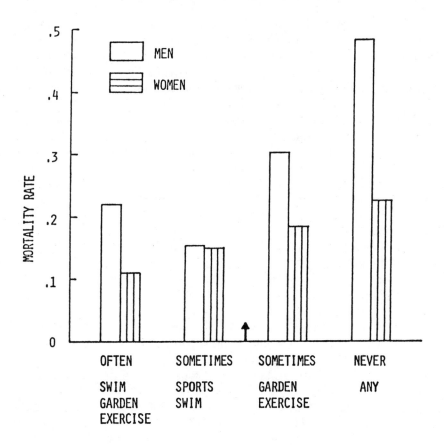

FIGURE 12.5. *Mortality rates (proportion dying in 5 1/2 years) in 65–74 year age grouping arranged by physical activity participation. (Based on data by Belloc, N. B. Relationship of Health Practices and Mortality. Preventive Medicine, 1973, 2, 67–81.)*

age grouping. In this age grouping, as in prior groupings, the differential in mortality rate with amount and level of physical activity was greater for men than for women but, in the subsequent age grouping of 75+ years, the mortality rate for women at all physical activity levels closely approximated those of men. In general, as with the 65 to 74 year age grouping, the two lowest physical participation categories are considered as associated with an unfavorable mortality risk for both men and women.

Data on physical activity and other lifestyle characteristics of 16,936 Harvard alumni, aged 35 to 74 years, were collected during 12 to 16 years of follow-up by Paffenbarger and associates (1986). A physical activity index was computed as an estimate of energy expended in walking, climbing stairs, playing sports, yard work, etc. and this index was used in the analysis of data. The results indicated that activity level was inversely related to total mortality, primarily to death due to cardiovascular or respiratory causes. The pattern of relationship between death rates and energy expenditure indicated that death rates declined steadily as energy expended on physical activity increased from less than 500 to 3500 kilocalories per week, beyond which the rates increased slightly. Mortality rates were one-quarter to one-third lower among alumni expending 2000 or more kilocalories during exercise per week than among less active men. This pattern of relationship of death rates with physical activity level is very similar to that for men in figure 12.5. Paffenbarger et al. (1986) further observed that, with or without consideration of cigarette smoking, hypertension, extremes or gains in body weight, or early parental death, the alumni mortality rates were significantly lower among the physically active. They estimated that, by the age of 80, the amount of additional life attributable to adequate exercise was one to more than two years as compared with sedentariness.

Participation in athletics requires a very high level of physical activity and associations made between the necessity for physical activity participation and the preservation of health and/or life date back to antiquity. Therefore, it is not surprising that the longevity of athletes is a matter of some concern in investigations of the validity of such claims. The results of one such study of the records of 38,269 college men, of whom 6492 were honor men, were tabulated in terms of life expectancy and mortality rates (table 12.2). Similar statistics are also recorded for the white male population in the United States over the same time period. According to the data by Dublin et al. (1949), athletes differ little from the general college population with respect to life expectancy and mortality rates, while honor college graduates have a slight advantage in these areas over the average college student and athlete. College graduates as a whole have a decided advantage in life expectancy and mortality rate in comparison with the entire white male population of the same age grouping. College graduates in general, and honor men in particular, achieve a

TABLE 12.2. Expectancy of life and mortality rates per 1,000 of college graduates compared with white males in the United States in 1900–1902*

Age	College Graduates	College Athletes	College Honor men	United States White Males 1900-1902
		Life Expectancy		
22	45.71	45.56	47.73	40.71
42	29.44	28.92	31.07	26.33
62	14.48	14.09	15.56	13.17
82	4.56	4.24	4.98	4.54
		Mortality Rate per 1,000		
22	4.38	4.04	3.68	6.68
42	6.26	6.12	5.11	11.24
62	26.14	26.39	22.10	32.76
82	138.30	151.16	123.08	155.42

* From Louis I. Dublin; Alfred J. Lotka; and Mortimer Spiegelman. *Length of life.* New York: The Ronald Press Company, 1949. Reprinted by permission of John Wiley & Sons, Inc.

higher socioeconomic status than the population as a whole and a very definite relationship has been found between socioeconomic status and death rate.

It is possible that the variations in life expectancy rates and mortality rates between athletes and graduates in general may be a function of the life style of the athlete. Although athletes have lower life expectancies at all age levels, they also have lower mortality rates until age 62 when the general graduates have lower mortality rates. This means that the lowered expectancy rates at all age levels are conditioned by the increased mortality of the athlete after 62 years of age and may be a function of the athlete's reluctance to modify behaviour with changing physical performance parameters. For example, the athlete may take more risks to prove that he is still capable of outstanding performance or may undertake such arduous tasks as snow shoveling when out of condition but push himself to the same performance level he anticipates under conditioned circumstances and hence increase the risk of heart failure.

In a very comprehensive survey of longevity of former athletes, Stephens and associates (1984) surveyed 17 athlete-population studies and found that 16 favored a lower athlete mortality, whether expressed as a mortality ratio or in additional years of life, while the remaining study had nonspecified findings. These investigators stated that it was clear from the consistent findings that athletes live longer than other individuals. However, results of these studies suggested that the caliber of athlete or level of competition may influence longevity. For example, studies of the general population have shown that the endomesomorphic types which are well adapted to line play in football have a shorter life span than do the more ectomorphic track men.

In a study of Michigan State athletes and non-athletes, Montoye et al. (1957) reported little difference in the longevity of the two groups, nor was there any difference in the longevity of the parents of the two groups. The subsequent report by Stephens et al. (1984) based upon the activity patterns of Michigan State athletes and nonathletes who had died also showed no significant differences between athletes and nonathletes on the basis of vocational and avocational activity levels. However, when the data were pooled and analyzed by activity level only, there was an avocational activity trend indicating that a higher percentage of those who were sedentary in 1960 were deceased. Analysis of the data in terms of vocational activity level indicated that, in the older age groupings, those most active in 1960 appeared to have a smaller percentage deceased between 1960 and 1976.

In general, it appears that regular physical activity of a moderate to high level is closely associated with survival rate of the individual. This factor may be more closely associated with the survival of older adults on the basis of the results reported by Stephens et al. (1984) and Belloc (1973). In addition, a longitudinal study by Milne and Maule (1984) reports that mean hand grip was significantly less at the first examination in older people who subsequently died as compared with five-year survivors. With the increased emphasis upon lifespan physical performance, more data is constantly becoming available which will help to resolve the question of the effect of physical activity on longevity. In the meantime, the data strongly suggest that only very vigorous activity, especially at older ages, may be detrimental. However, even very vigorous activity is not nearly as detrimental as a sedentary life style.

STRUCTURAL AND PHYSIOLOGICAL CHANGES

With an increasing proportion of the population in the age groupings of 45 years or older and the general increase in life expectancy, the study of aging, or **gerontology**, has become one of the major areas of research dealing with human development. Because of the recency of concentration on the problems of aging and the difficulties associated with longitudinal studies of human beings, the majority of research studies in this area are based upon cross-sectional data.

The primary mechanism in aging is considered by Bjorksten (1963) to be the phenomenon of cross-linking between the giant molecules of the body, in particular the proteins and nucleic acids, with somatic mutations, loss of elasticity, and accumulation of immobilized material being of secondary importance. Cross-linkage is favored as the primary mechanism because it is the only known process by which a single small molecule can drastically change the behavior of two giant molecules; and because the known number of cross-linking agents normally present in the body is so great the occurrence of cross-linkages, including the irreversible type, is inescapable.

Morphological examinations indicate that, with increasing age, the percentage of cells displaying intracellular accumulation of lipofuscin increases. The correlation between **lipofuscin** and age has led to its being frequently described as a "wear and tear" pigment; it accumulates at varying rates in the various body tissues. Lipofuscin pigment granules contain lipid, carbohydrate, and protein and the granule is frequently membrane bound. There is increasing research evidence that **lysosomal** enzyme activity can account for the apparent formation of lipofuscin from all other cell organelles (Feldman & Peters).

Other morphological changes that occur with aging are the increasing incidence of plaques and tangles in neural tissue with these structures appearing in the brains of 99 percent of all individuals after 80 years of age. Plaque is an extracellular focal accumulation of material which may include granular, fibrillar, and amorphous components. Senile plaques are composed primarily of glial and portions of nerve cell, amyloid fibrils, silicone, and, in later stages, macrophagic elements. In the brain, plaque is most frequently seen in the frontal, occipital, insular, and hippocampal cortices. The neurofibrillary tangle is believed to be an agglutination of the normal neurofibrillary apparatus of nerve cells, with the tangled loops and bundles of fibers sometimes remaining as inert structures after the disappearance of the cell of origin. Tangles tend to be particularly prominent in the hippocompus but are also seen with high frequency in the cerebral cortex as a whole, and in the thalamus, basal ganglia, and spinal cord. The cerebellum, however, is not involved (Feldman & Peters). In addition, a defect in protein synthesis involving ribosomal and mRNA occurs in neurons of brain tissue in Alzheimer's patients which may contribute to the decline in certain neurotransmitter enzymes and the loss of neurons in the brain with Alzheimer's disease (Tollefsbol & Cohen, 1986).

Some investigators have expressed the opinion that no single mechanism seems to cause aging, although there appears to be a progression in which genetically controlled metabolism may be involved (Sullivan et al., 1963). Aging is considered by Edington and Edgerton (1976) to bring about a gradual loss of the ability of the nucleic acids to replace functional proteins and the eventual accumulation of nonfunctional materials in the cell. In keeping with this approach, Tollefsbol and Cohen (1986) point out that protein turnover and its metabolic regulation is important in the response of specific proteins such as enzymes to a variety of stimuli but the capability of the organism to initiate adaptive fluctuations in the activity of numerous enzymes in response to a broad spectrum of stimuli is impaired with age.

Such impairment of enzyme adaptability is related to physiological decrements such as decreased immune response, impaired adaptation, and lowered hormonal response which are known to occur with age. For example, Faucheux and associates (1983) report that mean heart rate and epinephrine levels return to pre-stress values more slowly in older age men (70s) in comparison with men in their 50s. Reduced androgen production in males is related to loss of muscle mass and strength. In females, loss of estrogen is associated with loss of bone mineral content (osteoporosis) and the reduction of immune response. Tollefsbol and Cohen (1986) point out that proteins are essential to all forms of life and that it is now clear that there are specific molecular abberations in protein metabolism that are apparent both in the normal aging process and in age associated diseases.

According to Shock (1962), youth is marked by tremendous reserves in all organs of the body, whereas the aging process involves the progressive loss of body tissue from the muscles, nervous system, and many vital organs which result in increasing loss of reserve. There are great variations in the rate of loss of different functions among individuals and within each individual with respect to various aspects of function. However, there are structural changes with increasing age and a general decline in physiological functioning accompanying increases in age after 30 years which are common to most individuals.

Structural changes are reflected to some degree in body composition changes. The age related decrease in muscle mass coupled with the noted trends in weight with increased age (figure 11.5) results in changing proportions of bone, muscle, and fat with increasing age. Using computed tomography, Borkan and associates (1983) compared the body composition of middle-aged men (mean age = 46.3 years) with older men (mean age = 69.4 years) and found that the older men weighed 8.2 kilograms less than the middle-aged men with this difference being primarily the result of their having less lean tissue. The muscle area of the leg and arm were significantly less in the older men as were all lean tissues of the abdomen and chest. Analysis of the fat accumulation between muscles of the abdomen and the leg indicated fat infiltration into lean tissue in the older men. Fat mass was only slightly less in older men but there were clear distributional differences between the groups. Although the total abdomen fat area was similar in both groups, the older men had less subcutaneous fat and correspondingly greater intra-abdominal fat than the middle-aged men.

The body composition of healthy young men and women (mean age

= 20.5) and healthy older men and women (mean age = 77.8) were compared using the multiisotope method (Fulop et al., 1985). In this study, all the body components of the older men were found to be practically the same as those of young males with the exception of the red blood cell mass which was significantly lower in the older men. On the other hand, the age related changes in the body components were much greater in the women. The total body fat was significantly higher in older women but the total body water was decreased as a consequence of diminished lean body mass in the older women in comparison with the young group. Although there was no significant difference between the groups in extracellular fluid volume, the plasma volume was significantly greater in the older women. Thus, in comparison with young women, the liquid component of lean body mass was redistributed between the intracellular and extracellular spaces in the older women.

As the relative proportions of bone, muscle, and fat are known to change with different body types, age related comparison studies are dependent upon the care in selecting subjects of similar body types. Therefore, the results should not be considered as predictive of longitudinal trends for the various body types. However, such studies do point out potential degrees of and areas where muscle and fat distribution may be altered with increasing age.

The reduction in weight (figure 11.5) and in height (figure 11.6) noted in cross-sectional studies after 55 years of age is not only a reflection of the secular trend towards increased height and weight for the younger age groupings but also indicates an age related decline in height and weight after the mid-50s (Whitbourne, 1985). The decline in height with increased age may be attributed to vertebral compression due to loss of bone strength and cartilage wear. In addition, there may be postural changes involving more curvature of the spine, increased inclination of the head in a forward direction, and loss of extension (i.e., greater flexion) in the hip and knee joints in standing and walking. Decreased weight with increasing age may be associated with decreased efficiency of the digestive system, decreased muscle mass with increased age, and may also be influenced by changes in eating habits resulting from loss of taste and olfactory sensitivity and by dental problems.

The general decline in physiological functioning is reflected in changes in work rate of an individual with increased age. Figure 12.6 indicates that maximum work rate over a sustained period of time, based on a two-step climbing test, reaches its optimal level in females around the age of 25 years, while peak work performance in males occurs around 28 years of age. Following the achievement of optimal performance, there is a continuous gradual decline in work rate which is slightly greater in males than in females, so that the work differential between the sexes becomes less with increasing age.

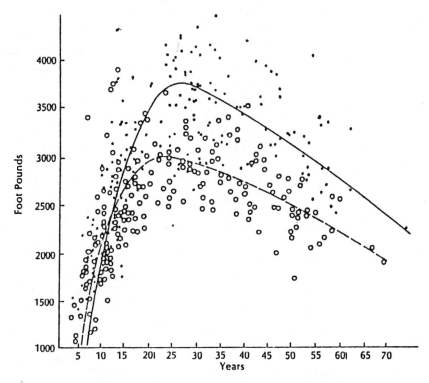

FIGURE 12.6. *Relation of age to exercise tolerance as expressed in foot pounds of work per minute. Straight line (through dots) for male and broken line (through circles) for female individuals. (From A. M. Master, The two-step test of myocardial function. Amer. Heart J., 1935, 10, 495–510. By permission of the publisher, The C. V. Mosby Company, St. Louis.)*

Although the maximum sustained work rate drops approximately 30 percent from 500 kilogram-meters per minute at 30 years to 350 kilogram-meters per minute in a 70-year-old man, there is an even greater decline during short periods of rapid work. The maximum work rate for short bursts of work on the hand ergometer falls from 1850 kilogram-meters per minute in 35-year-old men to 750 kilogram-meters for 80-year-olds— a decline of almost 60 percent (Shock, 1962). Increasing age, therefore, results in a reduced tolerance range toward physical activity as well as reduced capacity for such activity. This reduction in both range and capacity may readily be explained in terms of reduced physiological functioning in general.

Cardiac output is, of course, a significant factor in the speed of transmission of food and oxygen to areas of muscular activity and in the removal of products of such activity. Cross-sectional studies indicate a consistent decline in the highest heart rate that can be attained during maximal work with increasing age (Robinson, 1938). Longitudinal studies also show such decline in varying amounts (Dawson & Hellebrandt, 1945; Dill, 1942, 1958). The heart rate is linearly correlated with the intensity of exercise in terms of net oxygen consumption for both young and old men (Aghemo et al., 1964), but old subjects have a greater heart response during submaximal work (Norris et al., 1953) and show a delayed circulatory recuperation following exercise (Norris & Shock, 1960). Similarly, although heart rate and epinephrine levels increase in younger and older adults by the same percentages during stress, both of these variables return to pre-stress values more slowly in the older age group (Faucheux et al., 1983).

Blood circulation time is significantly prolonged in men over 70 years in comparison with the norm for young men (Diettert, 1963). However, a comparison of red blood cells and blood volumes of men over 70 years with norms of young males indicates little difference (Hurdle & Rosin, 1962). Moreover, body size, heart volume, and blood volume are not significantly correlated with maximum heart rate or maximal work in old men (Strandell, 1964), indicating that physical working capacity in old men may be limited by either vascular or muscular-metabolic peripheral factors.

Collagenous changes in the structure of various organs is undoubtedly also a factor in their reduced functioning with increasing age. The heart muscle of the rat has been found to have an almost three-fold increase in the **collagen** concentration with age (Schaub, 1964-1965). These results, coupled with the findings of Kohn and Rollerson (1959) of reduction in the swelling ability of the human heart with age, suggest that the addition of collagen to the muscle tissue reduces the structural flexibility and imposes an additional load on the contracting heart muscle.

The respiratory system shows a reduction in vital capacity, maximum ventilation volume during exercise, maximum voluntary breathing capacity, and maximum oxygen uptake during exercise with increasing age. The decline in vital capacity from 30 to 80 years is 40 percent, while the reduction in maximum breathing capacity is almost 60 percent (figure 12.7). Ventilation responses of young males are also larger during early adjustment to exercise than they are for older subjects (Norris & Shock, 1960).

The reduced blood flow undoubtedly accounts for part of the reduced oxygen uptake (Shock, 1962). However, the reduction in blood flow alone does not seem to account for the great difference in oxygen uptake between the young and the old. The arterial oxygen and percentage saturation in elderly individuals are also low, indicating either unequal ventilation of the lungs or reduced diffusing capacity or both (Dill et al., 1963). On the basis of the great changes that occur in total lung

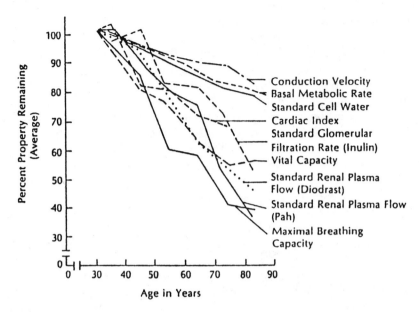

FIGURE 12.7. *Decline of various human functional capacities and physiological measurements with age. (From Bernard L. Strehler (Ed.).* The biology of aging. *Washington, D.C.: American Institute of Biological Sciences, 1960. By permission of the editor and publisher.)*

capacity and in expiration reserve volume with aging, Norman et al. (1964) concluded that a state of mild chronic obstructive emphysema occurs in old age, whereas Edge et al. (1964) contend that aged lungs show only a mild degree of emphysema. Study of the chest x-rays of 100 subjects of 75 years or older led the latter investigators to the conclusion that there is no senile lung pattern, although decalcification of the ribs is generally present and there is some shrinkage of the thoracic cage. Although vital capacity and forced expiratory volume are directly correlated with height, the percentage changes in these functions are not related to height but rather there is a longitudinal decrement which becomes more marked with advanced age. In addition, body weight gains and smoking intensify the age-dependent loss of vital capacity and forced expiratory volume (Dontas et al., 1984). Changes in ability of the individual to quantitate changes in inspiration resistive loads have also been noted with the perception of airflow resistance being blunted in older adults in comparison with that of younger adults. Such blunting of perception of airflow may be the result of impairment in the central nervous system processing of separate signals of pressure and flow (Altose et al., 1985). It is highly likely that no one factor is entirely accountable for reduction in pulmonary function and that various factors may account for varying degrees of function loss in different individuals.

Exercise tolerance is also affected by the ability of the body to remove waste products other than the carbon dioxide removed by the lungs. This is the function of the kidneys and figure 12.7 indicates that the renal plasma flow and glomerular filtration rate are reduced approximately 50 percent. The maximum excretory capacity and glucose reabsorption capacity are also reduced to a similar extent. With increasing age, there is an impairment in glucose metabolizing enzyme induction which may be related to increased glucose intolerance in elderly individuals. The slowing down of waste product removal is quite considerable between 30 and 80 years since there is a loss of 83 percent in the speed of return to equilibrium of blood acidity following exercise (Shock, 1962).

Maximal aerobic capacity is a well recognized indicator of cardiovascular/respiratory function and surveys of research in the area report age related decreases in maximal aerobic capacity following peak performances at age 20 to 30 years (Norris & Shock, 1974; Whitbourne, 1985). However, the rate of decline and the precise nature of the interrelationships and the relative contributions of the various aspects of the cardiovascular and respiratory systems to such declines has not been fully defined (Whitbourne, 1985). The activity pattern of the individual appears to be very closely associated with the level of maximal aerobic capacity as Drinkwater, Horvath and Wells (1975) report that habitual levels of activity determine the levels of maximal oxygen uptake for women in the 20 to 49 year age range with aging effects on cardiovascular and respiratory variables being minimal until age 50. Similarly, studies and surveys show that older trained athletes, while they have lower maximal aerobic power than young trained athletes, are capable of maintaining their maximal aerobic capacity above that of healthy untrained young individuals (Heath et al., 1981; Whitbourne, 1985).

The spread of scores within any one age grouping for exercise tolerance depicted in figure 12.6 clearly indicates the great variability in this performance parameter which would seem to be largely attributable to physical activity levels rather than age related variables. Longitudinal data on Dill (1942, 1958) shows that he maintained a high level of physiological functioning with regular physical activity. Moreover, cross-sectional studies by Jokl (1954) indicate above-normal performance levels are maintained over the years by individuals who partake regularly in vigorous physical activity. These earlier observations of the effects of regular physical activity on physiological performance are supported by more recent surveys (Whitbourne, 1985) and are exemplified by the performances of masters athletes which are discussed in the section on the role of exercise.

NEUROMUSCULAR AND STRENGTH CHANGES

The musculature of the body, as the only volitional means by which the body is capable of movement, is a vital factor mediating performance and the amount of work the body can accomplish. Figure 12.8 indicates a consistent loss in dominant hand grip strength in males after the age of 22 years so that the 80-year-old man is, on the average, not as strong as the 13-year-old boy. The decline is most marked after the age of 35 years, when there is a drop from 44 kilograms to 23 kilograms at 90 years of age in dominant hand grip (Shock, 1962).

Patterns of decline in strength of the dominant and subordinate hand are similar for the sexes, with the dominant hand being stronger at all ages than the subordinate hand but losing a greater amount of strength with increased age in comparison with the subordinate hand (Miles, 1950). A survey of a number of research studies by Welford (1959) indicates that other areas of the body show similar patterns of decline in strength with increased age. However, the loss of grip endurance, namely the amount that can be held for one minute, is not nearly as great as that of grip strength with the 75-year-old man having, on the average, a higher grip-strength endurance than the 13-year-old boy (figure 12.8). From a grip strength of 28 kilograms at age 20 the decline is only 8 kilograms over the intervening years to age 75 (Shock, 1962).

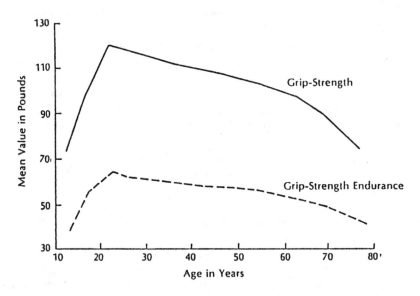

FIGURE 12.8. Changes with age in dominant hand grip and grip-strength endurance in males. (From W. E. Burke; W. W. Tuttle; C. W. Thompson; C. D. Janney; and R. J. Weber, The relation of grip strength and grip-strength endurance to age. J. Appl. Physiol., 1953, 5, 628–630. By permission of the authors and publisher.)

The degree of decline of muscle strength with age is undoubtedly conditioned by the amount and consistency of usage of muscle groups. In a study of young active (M = 22.2 yrs.), young inactive (M = 21.1 yrs.), old active (M = 68.7 yrs.) and old inactive women (M = 68.9) by Rikli and Busch (1986), the inactive groupings had never participated in vigorous physical activity on a regular basis whereas the active groupings had participated in vigorous acivity at least three times per week for the past three years for the young group or the past 10 years for the old group. Figure 12.9 clearly shows that the activity level affects preferred hand grip strength at any one age level with the more active individuals having the higher strength values. However, although activity may slow down the effects of age related decline in muscular strength, such decline appears to be an inescapable feature of the aging process.

The age related aspects of muscular strength and muscular endurance were examined by Dummer et al. (1985) who tested female masters swimmers during the 24- to 71-year age span. The women in this study were of competitive caliber and trained an average of 4.13 days per week for 64.01 minutes per session. The investigators measured the swimmers for peak isokinetic torque of shoulder and knee flexion and extension, endurance of shoulder and knee movements, and grip strength. As with previously reported studies, the grip strength for the dominant hand was greater than that for the nondominant hand. Moreover, the loss in strength over the age span was greater for the dominant hand (5.7 kilo-

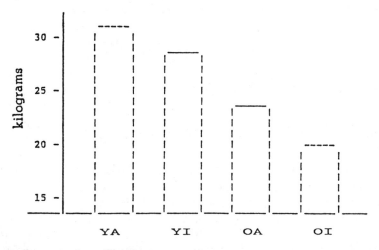

FIGURE 12.9. *Preferred hand grip strength scores. YA = young active; YI = young inactive; OA = old active; and OI = old inactive. (From data in Rikli, R., & Busch, S. Motor Performance of Women as a Function of Age and Physical Activity Level. Journal of Gerontology, 1986, 41, 645–649. Drawn by and by permission of the authors.)*

grams) than for the nondominant hand (3.0 kilograms). However, the grip strength of the swimmers was highest for both hands in the 30 to 39 age group whereas previous studies tend to show higher values in the 20 to 29 year age span. In addition, the 34.7 kilogram grip strength for the dominant hand of the 20 to 29 age group is higher than the preferred hand grip reported by Rikli and Busch (1986) for similar age groups. The comparisons made by Dummer et al. (1985) with previously published studies of hand grip strength of less active women indicated that the strength of the swimmers was approximately 4 to 10 kilograms higher for similar age levels. There was a decline of approximately 16 percent in grip strength for the swimmers from age 30 to 39 through the 60 and over age groups.

The Dummer et al. (1985) study also highlights another aspect of strength decrement with age in the examination of both flexion and extension actions around the same joint. For example, with a Cybex speed of 30 degrees per second, knee extension strength was reduced from 156.6 joules at 20 to 29 years to 103.99 joules at 60+ years. Similarly, knee flexion was reduced from 82.1 joules to 56.1 joules for the same age span. In addition, similar results were found for knee flexion and extension at a faster speed in the Dummer et al. (1985) study and for healthy women, aged 20 to 86 years, who did not participate in any regular exercise program (Murray et al., 1985). In the latter study, various knee joint angles for the isokinetic contractions as well as isometric contractions were measured to determine flexor and extensor strength. Although the isometric contractions produced the highest strength values, the relationship of flexor strength as approximately half of the extensor strength remained consistent as did the degree of decline for the strength of muscle groups in these joint actions. This aspect of differential muscle strength becomes very important when muscle strength is approaching minimal functional levels. For example, leg extensor strength is necessary to overcome the effects of gravity while standing and walking, running, etc., and flexor strength is required to lift the lower leg above the ground during locomotor activities. Because flexor strength is lower at all age levels, the associated age related decline brings this type of strength closer to the minimal level sooner so that older individuals begin to have problems associated with walking on uneven ground, etc., because they do not lift their feet high enough and their likelihood of falling increases.

In addition to its effects on muscular strength, activity level is also related to muscular endurance and Dummer et al. (1985) report that the muscular endurance data for the female swimmers do not reveal an age related pattern of decline. Although the highest mean values found were for the 50 to 59 year age groups for both knee and shoulder muscular endurance, these values were also accompanied by high variability and the investigators indicate that the higher values may, in part, be a reflection of aggression and competitiveness on the part of a few swimmers who were highly motivated. Because participation in swimming appears to have differential effects on muscle strength and muscular endurance with increasing age and because of the low correlations found between the measures of strength and endurance, Dummer et al. (1985) believe their results reinforce the notion that strength and endurance represent essentially separate influences on performance. In assessing the training of the swimmers the investigators had observed that all the subjects spent approximately the same amount of time per session in training but that the younger swimmers were moving at a faster speed and were thus averaging greater distances. If one associates greater muscular strength with potentially faster movement and endurance with time duration, then the age related loss of strength is associated with an age related loss of speed whereas the duration of the training session and the muscular endurance appear to remain relatively consistent regardless of age.

Muscular endurance is dependent upon the energy systems available to the muscle to maintain the activity over a period of time. Because sampling of the metabolic changes associated with muscle activity could only be undertaken using invasive techniques in the past, such information was based mainly on data collected using animals with measuring procedures and results being variable. With the development of nuclear magnetic resonance (NMR), a noninvasive technique became available to investigate muscle metabolism. This investigative technique was used by Taylor and associates (1984) to make a continuous and simultaneous assessment of muscle pH, phosphocreatine (PCr), adenosine triphosphate (ATP), and inorganic phosphate (Pi) for young (20 to 45 years) and old (70 to 80 years) men and women under conditions of rest and exercise. Although none of the subjects were athletes, they were all healthy and led active lives. The exercise procedures involved squeezing a rubber bulb at a rate of 22 per minute to a pressure of 100 mm Hg for five minutes followed by 300 mm Hg for 2.5 minutes. All of the subjects were able to complete the exercise and, although the subjects felt tired, they were not exhausted. NMR spectra were collected from the flexor digitorum superficialis muscle at rest before exercise, during exercise, and during the recovery period.

In normal adult subjects, the PCr concentration falls during exercise as the PCr is used to maintain ATP at its resting level and a concomitant rise in Pi occurs. At the same time, the muscle becomes more acid due to lactate production from increased glycolitic activity. When the exercise ceases, the PCr is rapidly replenished and the pH returns slowly to its resting level. The spectra taken by Taylor et al. (1984) indicated that the metabolic sequence of events for elderly subjects was qualitatively similar to those for younger individuals and no unusual compounds were noted. They concluded that the energetics of human skeletal muscle are not altered by the aging process. There is, however, a decline in oxidative capacity of muscles with aging and a study by Farrar and associates (1981) of the effects of endurance training in rats indicated that age decreased the amount of intermyofibrillar mitochondrial protein, while training increased mitochondrial protein. Their results suggested that the decrease in oxidative capacity in skeletal muscle resulted from a decrease in mitochondrial protein rather than a decrease in mitochondrial function.

Although metabolic processes during exercise may be qualitatively similar regardless of age (Taylor et al., 1984), and Dummer et al. (1985) report no significant age related differences in muscular endurance for swimmers, it is well established that work capacity (figure 12.6) and muscular endurance (figure 12.7) do decline with increasing age. The possibility exists that the lack of significant difference noted by Dummer et al. is a factor of the subjects sampled in their cross-sectional study especially as the 50 to 59 year age grouping had the highest endurance values. With the exception of this age grouping, all of the other age groupings show a consistent decline with age from 30 to 39 years for knee endurance and from 20 to 29 years for shoulder endurance. Therefore, there is definitely an age related trend for reduction of strength endurance components even under training conditions which enhance endurance maintenance. However, the reduction in muscle strength endurance is not nearly as great as that for maximal isometric strength.

Loss of strength may be explained partly by the reduction of androgen production in males, but such an explanation would not account for a similar reduction on the part of females. Perhaps an explanation may lie in the increase in collagen, which fills up the spaces between muscle fibers as the individual grows older. Such "dead" material added to the muscle structure would tend to reduce effective strength. Furthermore, the molecular changes that collagen undergoes as it ages produce stiff joints and leathery skin in the aged (Verzar, 1983). The less resilient skin of the aged (Shock, 1952) and the hampering effects of less movable and flexible joints would tend to further reduce effective strength. When the grip strength of 158 men and 112 women, aged 65 years and over, was compared with fat free mass (FFM) based on four skinfold measures, a striking decline in grip strength was noted for both men and women with increasing age, whereas the marginal decline in FFM was not statistically significant. Multiple regression analysis suggested to MacLennan and associates (1980) that age had an effect on grip strength that was independent of FFM and they offered the explanation that with aging an increasing proportion of skeletal muscle is replaced by fibrous tissue which results in the striking reduction in muscle power with only a marginal reduction in FFM.

Studies of muscle fiber changes with aging in humans have been limited as they are dependent upon muscle biopsies and are more equivocal as sampling factors have more effect on the results than occurs with animals of similar genetic stock. As type I (slow twitch) fibers are generally held to be more fatigue resistant than type II (fast twitch) fibers, various investigators have examined the proportional distribution of these types of fibers to determine if there are age associated relationships between fiber type and isometric strength and muscular endurance. One of the reasons the quadriceps muscle was chosen by Larsson and Karlsson (1978) for their muscle biopsies was because the aging processes, such as decline in maximum strength and muscle atrophy, occur relatively early in this muscle. The 50 healthy male subjects, aged 22 to 65 years, who volunteered for the study were without locomotory defects and, in general were minimally physically active. Maximum isometric and dynamic strength of knee extension decreased in the older age groups but no significant change was seen in isometric or dynamic endurance. The analysis of fiber types indicated a decrease in the proportion of type II (FT) fibers and the declines in the maximum strength measures correlated significantly with the atrophy of the type II fibers. Fiber area determinations showed that the area of type I (ST) fibers remained the same but the area decrease for the type II fibers resulted in a decrease in the Type II/I fiber area ratio from 1.30 at 20 to 29 years to 0.99 in the 60 to 65 year old group. In addition, enzyme activity analysis indicated that "anaerobic" activity decreased during aging while no change was seen in "aerobic" activity.

In a similar type of study using 12 men and 12 women, aged 78 to 81 years, Grimby et al. (1982) examined the relationship between the fiber content of the vastus lateralis and biceps brachii and strength measures for knee-extension and elbow-flexion, respectively. The men and women had the same mean fiber composition with respect to ST and FT fibers but the relative number of FTb fibers was higher in women than in men. In a comparison of sex differences for the biopsy sites, all of the fiber areas were smaller for the women in both the vastus lateralis and biceps brachii and for the mean fiber area in the vastus lateralis. For both sexes there were lower areas of FT, especially FTb, fibers in the vastus lateralis than in the biceps brachii. Atrophic fibers of both major fiber types were found in both sexes but more commonly in women with FTb atrophy in the vastus lateralis being most frequent. Isokinetic strength for knee extension correlated with mean fiber area and relative FTb fiber area in women at different torque speeds than it did for men who also had some significant correlations between these measures. The isometric strength for elbow flexion correlated with the relative areas of FT and FTb fibers in women but not in men. These investigators suggested that quantitive rather than qualitative changes may explain the reduction in work performance with age and that reduction with age in the number of muscle fibers of both fiber types must be assumed.

Muscle action depends not only on one type of muscle fiber contraction but rather on the exact timing and interplay of fast and slow motor units acting in a phasic manner. With aging, such coordination may be disrupted due to a "dedifferentiation" of the muscle fibers as a result of fast muscles showing prolonged contraction times and slow muscles a shortening of contraction time, so that there is a shift from the original mixed pattern to a more uniform group of muscles within a motor unit. Gutmann and Hanzlikova (1976) indicate such changes could result in decreases in strength, speed, and resistance to fatigue. The analyses of fiber type previously reviewed indicate a trend towards fewer fast twitch fibers with aging, suggesting that speed of muscular response may also be diminished and Davies and White (1982) have found that twitch, tetanic, and maximum voluntary strength were significantly reduced in the muscles of elderly subjects as compared with a control group of young adults. In a subsequent study (McDonagh, White & Davies, 1984), voluntary and electrically evoked muscle force of the elbow flexor group and triceps surae group of the leg were investigated in a group of old (mean age of 71.3 years) and young men (mean age of 25.8 years). When compared with the young men's responses, the leg muscle responses of the elderly subjects indicated increased time to peak twitch tension, maximal twitch tension, tetanic force, and maximum voluntary force. Although resistance to fatigue was reduced by 19 percent in the leg muscles of the older men, the amount of reduction was not significant. For the elbow flexors only tetanic force and maximum voluntary force were reduced significantly in the elderly but the loss of force was much less than that found in the calf muscles. The fact that both tetanic and maximum voluntary force reductions were greater in the leg than in the arm muscles was considered by the investigators as evidence that the different responses of arm and leg muscle to aging resides in the muscle and not solely in the control of the muscles by the central nervous system.

McDonagh et al. (1984) believe that it is likely that loss of muscle force with aging is due to a decrease in fiber number and fiber size with the increase in contraction time suggesting a preferential loss and/or atrophy of type II muscle fibers. They indicate that there is also the alternative explanation that all fiber types become slower with aging. Grimby et al. (1982) noted atrophy of both types of fibers for older men and women with greater amounts of atrophy in FT (type II) fibers in the vastus lateralis for women. The women also had larger coefficients of variance in the leg muscle than in the biceps brachii. These investigators also noted that the muscle biopsies for older subjects contained "enclosed" ST fibers with the incidence of these types of fibers being greater in the vastus lateralis than in the biceps brachii. There was also a "type grouping" of ST fibers with the incidence greater in the leg muscle. The fact that type grouping and enclosed fibers appeared almost exclusively in ST fibers could, according to the investigators, be interpreted as evidence of denervation/reinnervation on the basis of neurogenic atrophy of FT fibers. The fact that this phenomenon is more common in the vastus lateralis than in the biceps brachii may be due to an age related differential in fiber changes in the various muscle groups as there is a great deal of variability in the rate of decline in muscular strength for different muscle groups, and the flexor muscles of the lower extremities are especially affected (Gutmann & Hanzlikova, 1976).

The use of x-ray computed tomography (CT) makes possible the determination of the size and density of most of the human muscles and this procedure was used by Imamura and associates (1983) to examine 44 males and 52 females between the ages of 9 and 86 years to determine age related changes in the muscles at the level of the third lumbar vertebra. An increase in size of the major psoas and the sacrospinalis muscles occurred in males from 9 to 29 years with a gradual decrease beyond the age of 30. In women the differences in the cross-sectional size of both these muscles were relatively small with age. A two-way ANOVA analysis of the data indicated that sex had a substantial effect on the size of both muscle groups with the males showing the higher values. Age also had a significant effect on the size of both muscles (i.e., decreased size with increased age) and there was a significant interaction effect for the size of the major psoas muscle which reflected the different aging trends for the sexes. The density of the major psoas muscle was similar for the sexes and decreased with increasing age in both men and women at similar rates. On the other hand, the density of the sacrospinalis decreased markedly in women in the 40 to 49 year age bracket whereas it changed only moderately in men. ANOVA analysis showed a significant age effect for density of both muscle groups but no significant sex effect for the density of these muscle groups.

Although the Imamura et al. (1983) study does not relate the changes in muscle size and density with changes in strength such an association would seem to be logical on the basis of similar sex differences and age related changes in strength. For example, Young, Stokes and Crowe (1982) report a correlation of 0.63 between mid-thigh cross-sectional areas of the quadriceps and isometric strength of young women aged 20 to 28 years. Similarly, a correlation of 0.81 was obtained for these same measures for 10 healthy older women aged 71 to 81 years. Moreover, the ratio of the quadriceps isometric strength to its cross-section was the same for both groups, i.e., 6.7 (young) and 6.6 (old). Although the two groups had similar mean body weights, the quadriceps cross-section was 35 percent smaller in the older women and the quadriceps isometric strength was 37 percent lower with both of the differences between the old and young groups being significant. On the basis of their results, the investigators concluded that the quadriceps "weakness" of the normal elderly women in their study could be explained entirely by their smaller muscle size.

Computed tomography was used to examine the cross-sectional area of the thigh muscle in men aged 24 to 41 years who varied in their degree of participation in physical activities (Haggmark, Jansson, & Svane, 1978). The two heavyweight lifters in this study had the largest thigh muscle area whereas, the subjects with the endurance type of training background (i.e., the cross-country runner and cyclist) had muscle areas of the same size as the untrained individuals. The mean fiber area had a high correlation of 0.91 with the cross-cut area of the vastus lateralis muscle and the total number of fibers in the vastus lateralis muscle seemed to be fairly equal among the subjects. However, the heavyweight lifters had very large type II (FT) fibers and these investigators concluded that the larger cross-sectional area of the vastus lateralis muscle in well trained subjects could be explained by a larger cross-sectional area of the fiber. It is well established that weight lifting results in hypertrophy of muscles in young adults based upon external measurements of muscle size and this study by Haggmark et al., seems to indicate that most of this increased size is due to hypertrophy of the fast twitch fibers which are also the fibers in which the greatest amount of atrophy occurs with increasing age.

It is also well established that strength can be increased through resistive exercises although the degree of change is age related. A study of twelve 70-year-old men who were trained for 45 minutes three times a week for 12 weeks with dynamic and static exercises using only body weight showed that aerobic capacity and muscle strength were improved at this age level (Aniansson et al., 1980). After training, significant increases occurred in aerobic capacity and in static and dynamic strength at all measured angular velocities. In addition, fiber composition showed a significantly higher proportion of type II fibers after training. Although the fiber composition (type I and type II fibers) and mean fiber area did not differ from results previously obtained from younger age groups, the fiber area of type I fibers was somewhat larger and the area of type IIb fibers somewhat smaller for these older men. However, in comparison with 54-year-old men, the body cell mass of the 70-year-old men in this study was lower indicating a reduction in total muscle tissue with age.

The noted reduction in total muscle tissue with age and, in particular, the reduction in the type II (fast twitch) fibers is undoubtedly the major factor in the reduction of maximal muscle strength with increasing age. The rate of decline is not nearly as great for the type I (slow twitch) fibers which provide the motive power for endurance types of activities. These age related changes can be modified and/or delayed to some extent by physical activity but do eventually result in changes in activity patterns with increasing age.

As the dynamic strength pattern of decreased maximal torque with increased angular velocity is maintained even in 78- to 81-year-old men and women (Grimby et al., 1982), this means that the reduced strength is best applied at slower angular velocities as the age of the individual increases. Hence, activities such as walking, swimming, and cycling where speed can be controlled more than it can in running became more appealing for endurance types of activities. In addition, the activities requiring a high component of maximal force at maximal angular speeds such as a smash in tennis are replaced by the "softer" hit with greater control (hopefully) for the individual who continues to participate in tennis during older adulthood.

BONE CHANGE AND OSTEOPOROSIS

Because growth in height stops when the epiphyseal areas of the bones have become fused and since bones have such a solid appearance we tend to forget that bone, just as other tissues in the body, is constantly undergoing changes. Anyone who has had a broken bone is aware that replacement processes are operational in the repair of the break and is also aware of the fact that the healing process is much slower than it is with some other tissues such as the skin. Just as with other types of tissues, the building of bone tissue (apposition) and the removal of bone tissue (resorption) are lifelong processes. Obviously, the process of apposition exceeds that of resorption during the growth years and during the healing of breaks in bones but may also do so as a result of stress, usually due to physical activity, placed upon a bone. For example, an increase in shaft width occurs by apposition on the external surface of the bone due to the activity of osteoblasts in the deep layer of the periosteum. At the same time, bone is resorbed from the internal surface of the periosteum by osteoclasts and, as a result, the external diameter of the shaft and the diameter of the marrow cavity enlarge. When the speed of these processes is approximately the same, the cortex of the bone will not increase in thickness even though the width of the bone increases. However, in instances of stress when bone apposition is greater than resorption the cortex will increase in thickness at the same time the bone width increases. Conversely, when the resorption process exceeds the apposition of bone there will be loss in cortex thickness which is not readily detected without the use of x-ray as the loss results in a larger marrow area with the same external shaft width and the bone may also become more porous with less bone mineral content.

Age related changes in the width of cortical bone in the second metacarpal are illustrated in figure 12.10. Males, in part due to larger body size, have wider cortical bone after the puberal growth spurt than do females. In addition to having a lesser cortical bone width, females also have a greater loss in bone width with increasing age. Although cortical bone is apparently laid down at the periosteal surface throughout life, after about age 30-40 years, it is lost from the endosteal surface at a faster rate than it is laid down in the outer surface of the bone with females universally showing a much greater loss with age than males (Montoye, 1984).

The sex differential in age related bone loss is particularly important in that females are also more prone to osteoporosis than are males. Literally, the term osteoporosis means more porous bones and the condition is marked by thinner cortical areas and reduced bone mineral content so that the compact bone areas become more porous. As these conditions result in weak, brittle bones that break easily, it is highly desirable that each individual maintain optimal bone cortical thickness and density. We do not know all of the causes of osteoporosis but we do know that reduced calcium content is one aspect of the bone mineral loss and nutritional groups have stressed the need for sufficient calcium in the diets of women. However, a survey of activity level and bone mineral loss reports that inactivity, such as prolonged periods of recumbency, periods of immobilization in casts, and prolonged space flights leads to decalcification

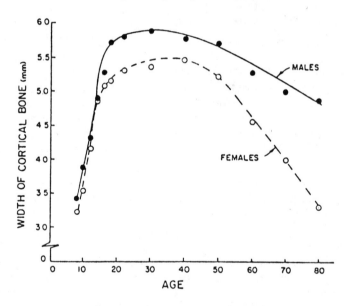

FIGURE 12.10. *Age changes in width of cortical bone in the second metacarpal. Drawn from data of Garn (1970, p. 45). (Reprinted from Montoye, H. J. Exercise and Osteoporosis. In H. M. Eckert & H. J. Montoye (Eds.), Exercise and Health. The Academy Papers. Champaign, IL: Human Kinetics Publishers, 1984. Reprinted by permission of the publishers.)*

of bones (Bailey, Malina, & Rasmussen, 1978b). As the diets of astronauts are nutritionally sound, it would appear that the additional factor of loss of physical activity and gravitational stress on the bones in space contributes to bone mineral loss.

Although estrogen deficiency is considered one of the main causes for bone loss in post-menopausal women (Heaney, 1965), the reported findings of bone mineral loss during periods of inactivity indicate that increased levels of activity may have the effect of either delaying such loss or even reversing it. This was the focus of a study of Aloia and his colleagues (1978b) who measured the total body calcium using total-body neutron activation and the bone mineral content of the distal radius using photon absorptiometry for post-menopausal women. In this investigation, nine of the 18 women exercised for one hour three times per week while the other nine maintained their sedentary routines. Both groups of women were measured before the initiation of the one-year exercise program and at the end of this period with the results indicating no significant change in bone mineral content or total body potassium for either group. However, there was an increase in the average total body calcium (TBC) for the exercise group (two of the nine had a slight decline) whereas TBC decreased in each subject in the sedentary group so that the before-after differences were significantly different in the two groups. The higher TBC values shown in figure 12.11 for the nonexercise group are due to the greater range of scores for these women (before: 1,047 to 633; after: 1,013 to 618) compared to the exercise group (before: 948 to 658; after: 968 to 631). On the basis of their results, the investigators concluded that exercise can modify involutional bone loss in post-menopausal women.

An insufficient dietary intake of calcium has also been associated with bone loss because the loss of estrogen at menopause results in an immediate deterioration in calcium balance performance in that the elderly woman absorbs calcium less efficiently from her diet and excretes it more readily through her kidneys than does a young woman (Gallagher et al., 1979). The effectiveness of supplemental calcium and/or physical activity to slow and/or increase bone mineral content for women aged 69 to 95 years, was investigated over a three-year period by Smith, Reddan and Smith (1981). In this study, control and physical activity groups were matched on the basis of age, weight, and degree of ambulation with each of these groups further assigned to a drug and placebo group using the double-blind technique. This resulted in four groups: 1) control group taking placebo tablets; 2) calcium tablet group; 3) physical activity group taking placebos; and 4) physical activity plus calcium group. There were similar dietary menus for the groups and the control group and calcium-only group made no changes in their daily activities. The physical activity group regularly participated in an exercise program three days a week for

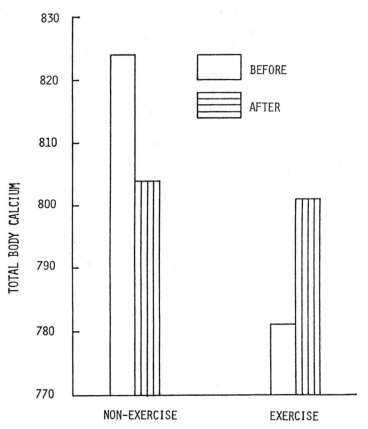

FIGURE 12.11. *Mean total body calcium values for non-exercising and exercising women taken before and after exercise period. (Based on data by Aloia, J. F.; Cohn, S. H.; Ostuni, J. A.; Cane, R.; & Ellis, K. Prevention of Involutional Bone Loss by Exercise. Annals of Internal Medicine, 1978, 89, 356–358.)*

30 minutes per day. The severity of the exercise was determined by the results from a modified Balke treadmill test and the low values plus the limited movement capabilities of the subjects resulted in an exercise program designed around a chair. When the four groups were compared using regression analysis, Smith et al. (1981) found that the bone mineral content change over the period of three years was a decline of 3.29 percent for the control and of 0.32 percent for the physical activity plus calcium groups whereas the physical activity group and the calcium groups demonstrated increases in BMC of 2.29 and 1.58 percent, respectively. The slopes of the physical activity and the calcium groups were significantly different from the control group whereas the physical activity plus calcium group demonstrated only borderline significance. Although both the activity and calcium groups improved bone mineral content of

the radius, the combined treatment group of physical activity plus calcium did not improve BMC although they maintained it better than the control group. The investigators indicate that one reason for the lack of improvement by the physical activity plus calcium group might be the older age (2.6 years) for this group with a higher overall rate of decline in comparison with other groups. Although the physical activity plus calcium group declined over the three-year period, (mean age of 87.3 years at final measurement) they demonstrated a positive slope in BMC during the first 12 months of the program.

The higher overall rate of decline in physical function noted by Smith et al. (1981) for the physical activity plus calcium group may be indicative of decreased osteoblast function as well as the increasingly decremental cumulative effect of the decrease in estrogen production and the associated inefficiency in calcium absorption. In addition, it may reflect age related differences in bone mineralization patterns. For example, a study which used rats to determine the effect of treadmill running reports that young rats increased mineralization in those cortical bones directly involved in the exercise whereas older animals undergo a total skeletal mineralization in response to exercise (McDonald, Hegenauer, & Saltman, 1986). If this same age related trend occurs in humans, then the same amount of calcium would be distributed over more bones with the amount available to one bone, such as the radius, being reduced. Moreover, other trace elements may be equally as important as calcium as a news release reports that Paul Saltman, at the University of California, San Diego, has shown that there was a significant decrease in the serum manganese in those women who had osteoporosis when they are compared with women who had normal bone (Pollock, 1987).

The differential effects of an exercise program on bone mineral loss have been reported by Krolner et al. (1986) for healthy women, aged 50 to 73 years, who had previously suffered a fractured forearm. Of the 27 women who completed this study, 14 served as controls while 13 participated in an exercise program for one hour twice weekly for a duration of eight months. These groups were comparable with regard to age, duration of menopause, time elapsing from forearm injury, physical performance capacity, and mineral metabolism before the beginning of the experimental period and all maintained their usual diet. Both distal forearms and the lumbar spine were measured using dual-photon absorptiometry at the beginning of the program and eight months later. The BMC of the lumbar spine for the exercise group increased by 3.5 percent whereas that of the control group decreased by 2.7 percent, a rate which equalled that of age-matched normal women. On the other hand, there was no significant difference between the two groups for the forearm measures as the BMC remained practically unchanged for the exercise group and dropped slightly for the control group. Surprisingly, the amount of loss in the uninjured forearm was somewhat greater than in the fractured forearm but, in both forearms, the exercise group recovered some BMC during the exercise period although none of these differences were significant. On the basis of their results, the investigators concluded that exercise can inhibit or reverse the involutional bone loss from the lumbar vertebrae in normal women and may prevent spinal osteoporosis.

In a related study, Krolner and Toft (1986) examined the effects of bed-rest on the rate of decrease and subsequent recovery of BMC in the lumbar spine. A mean decrease of 0.9 percent per week was observed in the BMC of the lumbar spine and, for a mean duration of 27 days bed-rest, the restoration of the BMC of the lumbar spine was nearly complete after four months. Thus, the rate of bone restoration was much lower than the rate of bone loss leading the investigators to suggest that recurrent bed-rest periods may predispose to spinal osteoporosis. On the other hand, the post-ambulation gain of 1 percent per month suggested the spinal osteoporosis may be prevented to some extent by increasing the functional loading on the vertebrae by either physical training or by weight bearing.

The effects of weight bearing on the bone mineral content (BMC) in the heel bone of the right foot was determined with dual photon absorptiometry in a cross-sectional study of 70- and 75-year-old men and women (Rundgren, Eklund, & Jonson, 1984). In this study, the males exceeded the females at both age levels in thickness of the right heel bone mineral content per unit length. In addition, there was a significant decline in all three variables with increasing age in men but only in the bone mineral content variables was there a decrease with age for females but these decreases were not significant. The females were similar at both ages for both body weight and heel thickness whereas the 75-year-old men had significantly lower body weight compared to the 70-year-olds. Thus, when the body weight was kept constant, there were significantly lower BMC values at age 75 for the women but not for the men. The correlation between body weight and BMC for females at 70 years was 0.41 and for males at the same age was 0.22. When percentiles for the BMC values were developed for men and women at 70 years of age and the mean body weight calculated for each percentile, there were pronounced differences in body weight between the higher and lower percentile groups for both sexes. These results indicated that the more weight the heel bone has to carry, whether it is muscle or fat tissue, the more mineral is found in the bone and the investigators concluded that, for the lower extremities, body weight must be taken into account in studies of bone mineral content changes. Based on their own findings and cited research indicating relatively low weight for female patients with hip fractures, the investigators suggest that it might be possible to point out risk groups for hip fractures among elderly females just from body weight.

Hip fractures increase with age for both males and females and, as with reduced bone mineral content with increasing age, the incidence of hip fractures is higher for females than for males. For example, one study reports the annual incidence of hip fracture per 1000 of similar age as being 8.4 for males and 19.8 for females at 80+ years (Kreutzfeldt, Haim, & Bach, 1984). In a follow-up study one year after a hip fracture, the survival curve was found to depend upon: sex (men had a higher excess mortality rate than women); age (excess mortality rate increased with age); and additional disabling disease. If the functional level of the patients was limited by disease before the fracture, the mortality rate was 33 percent whereas it was only 7 percent for those without disabling diseases. Of the 117 fractures that were examined, 86 were caused by falls indoors and 13 by falls outdoors, with nine of the patients (eight women and one man) suspected of having spontaneous fractures. Whereas falls may be the result of loss of balance and/or reduced strength (e.g., not lifting a foot high enough to clear a stair riser), spontaneous fractures are associated with loss of bone strength (i.e. low BMC and/or osteoporosis). As all of these factors are to some degree associated with physical activity level, it is interesting to note that Kreutzfeldt et al. (1984) reported that 72 percent of the surviving patients had unchanged activity levels one year after the fracture and approximately half had almost unchanged mobility with the remainder exhibiting only slight decreases in both variables.

The need for physical activity to recover the loss of bone mineral occasioned by the bed-rest associated with hip fracture was emphasized by the results of Krolner and Toft (1986) with respect to BMC changes of the lumbar spine. In addition, Krolner et al. (1986) found that fracture repair also affects the BMC of limbs differentially. It has been well established that physical activity is an important factor not only in maintaining and/or reducing the amount of age related bone mineral decrement but also plays a crucial role in increasing bone mass especially during the developmental years when the action of osteoblasts in building new bone most readily exceeds the absorptive action of osteoclasts. Therefore, the goal should be to achieve the highest possible peak bone mass before old age and to maintain that peak as long as possible. It is suggested that a program of physical exercise and prophylactic calcium supplement (for women) is a preventative program that might account for as much as 10 to 20 percent additional bone mass later on and that this differential may be crucial in preventing injury and fractures from falls in later years (Korcok, 1982).

Although a number of studies have examined the effects of exercise on dominant and nondominant hands and arms of young adults in various types of activities, data for older adults is not so readily available. Of particular interest is a study by Montoye and associates (1980) who examined the width and BMC of male participants in the National Senior Clay Court Tennis Championships held in Knoxville, Tennessee. The men, who averaged 64 years of age, had been playing tennis for a mean of 40 years and averaged about eight hours of playing time per week. The results of the measurements of bone width and BMC using photon absorptiometry, are shown in figure 12.12 for the comparisons between the playing and nonplaying arms. Clearly, there is a greater width and BMC of the bones on the dominant side for the tennis players. Montoye (1984) also points out that the differences between the dominant and nondominant hands are greater than those found in non-tennis players of the same age as the tennis players. For example, in the second metacarpal of the non-tennis players, the difference between the two hands was only 2.8 percent for total cross-sectional area and only 0.4 percent for cortical cross-sectional area with the dominant hand being the larger for both measures.

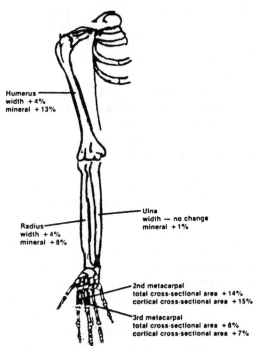

Humerus
width +4%
mineral +13%

Ulna
width — no change
mineral +1%

Radius
width +4%
mineral +8%

2nd metacarpal
total cross-sectional area +14%
cortical cross-sectional area +15%

3rd metacarpal
total cross-sectional area +8%
cortical cross-sectional area +7%

FIGURE 12.12. *Comparison of bones in the two limbs of senior tennis players. Percentages indicate the increase in bone of the dominant (playing) arm and hand compared to the non-dominant arm and hand (Montoye et al., 1980). (Reprinted from Montoye, H. J. Exercise and Osteoporosis. In H. M. Eckert & H. J. Montoye (Eds.), Exercise and Health. The Academy Papers. Champaign, IL: Human Kinetics Publishers, 1984. Reprinted by permission of the publishers.)*

Similarly, bone mineral density of 124 athletic and 1105 non-athletic Caucasian women aged 18 to 98 years has been examined by Talmage et al. (1986). The athletic group included those women who exercised regularly three times per week nine months of the year and had done so for at least five years. The minimum intensity level of the exercise program had to be equivalent to that of playing tennis for one hour per session. The non-athletic group was composed of all the other women in the study. When the results of the single and dual photon absorptiometry at the mid-radius, distal radius, and lumbar spine were analyzed an age related loss of bone mineral density (BMD) occurred at all three sites for the non-athletic women and in the two radial measures for the athletic women (too few lumbar spine measures were available for analysis). The athletes generally had higher BMD values at each of the radial sites than the non-athletes and there were higher negative correlations between age and the radial measures for the non-athletes (-0.65 and -0.53) than for the athletes (-0.25 and -0.20). The decline in BMD of the lumbar spine with increasing age for the non-athletes was reflected in the negative correlation of -0.48.

Talmage et al. (1986) also applied regression techniques for data analysis and found that a single break in the regression line (BMD versus age) best fit the data for the age range between 45 and 55 years. For the non-athletic women, the cutpoints for all three bone site decreases occurred between 47 and 52 years of age, corresponding roughly to the time of menopause, and following this cutpoint the rate of bone loss increased at all three locations. On the other hand, no cutpoint in BMD values could be demonstrated in the athletic women for this age range for the two radial sites. Although the investigators indicate that the absence of a significant change in the rate of bone loss could be due to the relatively small number of subjects (53 between 40 and 59 years), they indicated that the data could also suggest that regular sustained exercise programs may delay or minimize the increased rate of BMD loss which occurs in non-athletic women in the peri-menopausal period.

In summary, the best way to prevent the age related bone loss for both men and women is a vigorous physical activity program during the early adult years to maximize the amount of bone mass and bone density. As the age related loss of bone mineral tends to be fairly consistent at different age levels, the individual with the greater bone mass and density can theoretically lose mineral content over a longer period of time before the lower levels of bone stress tolerance (i.e., fracture point) are reached. Similarly, a regular sustained exercise program throughout the adult years has a marked potential for minimizing and even delaying the increased rate of BMD loss that occurs in the 45+ years especially for women. Moreover, regular sustained exercise programs undertaken at any age level have the potential of minimizing, and perhaps even reversing for a period of time, the age related loss of bone mineral density. Certainly, physical activity is a crucial factor in the regaining of BMD following prolonged bedrest and/or immobilization.

CHANGES IN BALANCE

The importance of the development of balance as well as strength was stressed in discussions of basic motor skill development. To the bipedal human, balance remains a vital performance parameter for the entire life span if the individual is to achieve the goal of remaining active. As with other physical performance parameters, there is improvement in balance during the growing years (figure 9.17) with decreasing performance levels following the plateauing during the young adult years.

With increasing emphasis placed upon research stressing the functional capacity of older adults, the age related changes in balance have become an area of vital concern. In a pioneering study, Hellebrandt and Braun (1939) tested postural sway of males and females aged 3 to 86 years. They reported that the magnitude of the sway about the center of the base tended to be larger in the very young and the very old with postural stability being greatest in the young adult and middle-aged subjects. A similar study was undertaken by Hasselkus and Shambes (1975) who examined postural sway in an upright stance and a forward lean stance of women in the two age groups of 20-30 year olds and 70-80 year olds. These investigators found that the postural sway area of the older adults was significantly larger than that of the young adults in both stance positions with the mean area of postural sway for the young group being .23 percent of the base of support in comparison with the .43 percent for the older women.

In order to determine the effects of disturbance of balance on postural sway, Era and Heikkinen (1985) asked 318 men, aged 31 to 75 years, to stand with both feet on a force platform under conditions of eyes open and arms hanging freely at the sides. Analysis of the sway was performed for the period before and after the disturbance of suddenly collapsing the platform. Both the anterioposterior and lateral sway increased with increasing age but only the lateral sway increases were significantly different for the three age groups of 31 to 35, 51 to 55, and 71 to 75 years. Significantly increased postural sway with increasing age was also reported for these same subjects under conditions of normal standing/eyes open; normal standing/eyes closed; and standing on one foot/eyes open with the latter condition showing a much greater degree of sway at all age levels. In the normal standing positions, the anterioposterior sway was greater than the lateral sway with the difference being most pronounced in eyes closed stand. The importance of vision in the control of postural sway was shown by a two- to three-fold greater postural sway when the eyes were closed as compared with eyes open stand.

As depicted in figure 9.17, there is some sex difference in balance performance. Females have better rail-walking performance levels prior to 8 years of age, whereas the performance of males is better thereafter. On the other hand, Hellebrandt and Braun (1939) have reported greater postural sway for males where the 1.59 cm^2 sway for an average base of support of 462.1 cm^2 indicated the area of maximal sway occupied 4.4 percent of the total base, whereas the 1.06 cm^2 sway for the females with an average base of 433.8 cm^2 occupied only 3.28 percent of the total base. The lesser amount of postural sway, over the 3- to 86-year-age range, for the 66 females in this study in comparison with the total percentage of sway in a three-minute stand for the 43 males indicates the greater stability of the female physique. An unpublished study of physical performance capabilities of 68 subjects aged 55 and older by Eckert indicates that the males in the study were slightly superior, but not significantly so, to females in the balance items of foreward and sideways rail-walking, balancing on one foot with eyes open and closed, and walking up and down stairs. The mean age of the 20 males was 71.06 and that of the 48 females was 69.04 so that the lack of a significant sex difference would not appear to be attributable to the age groupings in the sample. The lack of a significant sex difference in balance for these subjects may be a function of the sample population in that the subjects were all participants in community center programs that included varying amounts of physical activity. No sex difference in sway as measured by an ataxiameter are also reported for 151 frail elderly of 65 years and older (Brocklehurst et al., 1982).

In a study of the effects of training on 69-year-olds, Heikkinen (1975) reports pretraining balance test score means of 14.1 for the 14 males and 7.6 for the 12 females. Although pretraining sex differences are not reported, the published standard deviations indicate a significant sex difference in the balance test means. The eight-week training program consisted of five weekly sessions of one hour each in which the 69-year-old men and women participated in walking-jogging, ball games, gymnastics, and swimming. Only the females improved significantly in balance test during the eight weeks, but their mean of 9.0 was still significantly lower than the posttraining score of 15.2 for the men. On the basis of this study, which also indicated significant improvement in the cardiovascular measures for both sexes, Heikkinen concluded that the trainability of old persons seems to be better than was earlier assumed. The improvement in balance for women was commented on and considered to have some importance when possibilities in the prevention of falling accidents are evaluated.

The marked sex difference in the liability to falls in older people (figure 12.13) is of considerable concern to the medical profession in that the increased incidence for females is also associated with greater prevalence, by a ratio of four to one, of osteoporosis in females (Smith, 1971). The decrease in bone mineral mass and enlarged medullary cavity that characterizes osteoporosis results in a higher incidence of bone fracture. In females, where the angle of insertion of the head of the femur into the acetabulum of the hip creates some structural weaknesses, a fall will often result in a fracture in the hip joint area. For example, in a study of the health status of 609 patients who suffered hip fractures in one community in Sweden, 446 (73 percent) were women and only 163 (27 percent) were men with 12 percent of the women and 10.5 percent of the men having had earlier hip fractures (Johnell & Sernbo, 1986). The marked sex difference in liability to falls is not solely conditioned by the fact that females have greater longevity, although this factor undoubtedly accounts, in part, for the higher liability to falls for females aged 85 and over. The higher liability for females at all age levels clearly indicates that this is a physical performance parameter that has its genesis in other factors.

In a double-blind study undertaken by Fernie and associates (1982), they found that the average speed of sway was significantly greater for

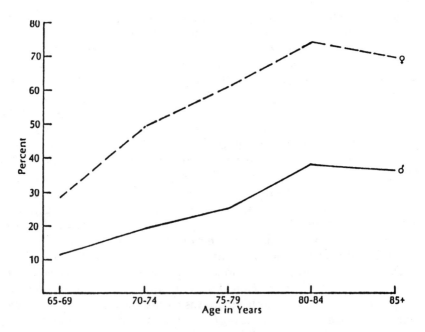

FIGURE 12.13. *Percentage of liability to falls. (Adapted from data by J. H. Sheldon, Medical-social aspects of the aging process. In M. Derber (Ed.),* The aged and society. *Champaign, Ill.: Industrial Relations Research Association, 1950.)*

those who fell one or more times in a year than for those who did not fall. The average age of the 205 subjects in the study was 81.8 years with 30 percent of the men and 46 percent of the women having had one or more falls. The investigators found no sex-related difference in the mean speed of sway in this group of institutionalized elderly but they did note that the mean speed of sway even for the non-fallers was greater than that previously measured in a sample of non-institutionalized elderly subjects. This latter observation suggests that the restricted mobility opportunities associated with institutionalization may be a factor in reducing balance.

If one examines anatomical sex differences which may be indicative of a predilection for falling, then the female with her lower center of gravity would appear to have a stability advantage or, at worse, should be no more prone to falling than males. The apparent paradox of greater stability but less balance suggests the possibility of sex differences in balance-related sensory input and/or of environmental influences which mediate against optimal balance development in the female.

The maintenance of balance is dependent upon vestibular and visual sensory input. There are indications that anatomical changes with age are minimal in the vestibular system (Weiss, 1959) and Brocklehurst et al. (1982) report only a 6 percent vestibular impairment for elderly subjects using a tilt test. However, subjects who had neck movements of 20 degrees or more towards the side of the tilt also tended to have more falls than the group as a whole. In addition, increases in vertigo have been reported (Orma & Koshenoja, 1957) and Guedry (1950) notes that an older group of 30 to 53 years showed a significantly longer subjective duration of postrotational effect than a young group of 19 to 21 years. No sex differences have been reported for vestibular function, but in an anatomically closely associated sensory function, the auditory, the prevalence of impairment for males exceeds that of females to the extent that there are approximately 20 more cases per 1000 population at 65–74 years (Weiss, 1959). A more recent follow-up study of 60- to 79-year-olds also indicated greater hearing loss for men and better hearing for women at higher frequencies (Eisdorfer & Wilkie, 1972). A very thorough review by Weiss (1959) of changes in vision of the aged does not indicate any sex differences that would account for the observed sex difference in the incidence of falling, and the marked elevation in the minimum dark-adapted light threshold after 60 years of age is the same for the sexes (Birren et al., 1948).

It appears, then, that there are few, or no, sex differences in visual or vestibular functioning; those that do exist would seem to favor females for balancing mechanisms as do the anatomical differences. The investigations of Held (1965) into the plasticity of the sensory-motor systems indicates that the activation of the kinesthetic system is crucial to the development of locomotion in kittens. When visual input is restricted as during movement in the dark, it is to be expected that greater reliance will be placed upon kinesthetic sensory modalities. Sheldon (1950) has reported sex differences in the difficulty experienced by people in the dark which are very similar to those reported for falling. Dark difficulties for 60- to 64-year-old women were similar in percentage to those of 75-to 79-year-old men. After 85 years of age, approximately 70 percent of men experienced difficulty in the dark, whereas the percentage is approximately 95 for women of the same age.

Visual acuity has been found to be significantly related to age (i.e., decreases with increasing age) by Brocklehurst et al. (1982) who also found increased postural sway with increasing age. As both of these measures are age related, a highly significant correlation was found between visual acuity and postural sway. These investigators also examined the relationship of postural sway to proprioception as measured by recording the subject's interpretation of five movements at each ankle and five movements at each great toe. These aggregate proprioception scores showed no sex differences; did not relate to age; and had a non-significant relationship with sway. On the other hand, vibration sense, based on tuning fork vibration and as measured at the lateral malleoli and each of the patella, was related to age (decrease with increasing age) and similarly related to sway in the 75- to 84-year-old grouping but not in the other age groupings. These latter reults led the investigators to conclude that there is a close relationship between increased postural sway and impaired vibration sense in the legs.

An unpublished study (Eckert) indicates some relationship between anthropometric mesures and balance in males in that positive correlations of .4 or higher were obtained between shoulder width and forward railwalking; foot width and balance on one foot with eyes open; weight and right foot, eyes closed balance; and a negative correlation between sitting height and forward railwalking. For females, no correlations above .3 occurred between the seven anthropometric measures and the eight balance items. In addition, the number of intercorrelations, of .4 or higher, among balance items was greater for males than females in that 13 such values were found in the correlation matrix for males, whereas only six were this high in the female balance matrix. The relationship between anthropometric measures and balance items for males suggests the hypothesis that males are more reliant upon kinesthetic input associated with body build during balance maintenance than are females. Moreover, the greater number of intercorrelations between balance items for males suggests that they tend to utilize similar sensory input for balance maintenance in a variety of activities to a greater degree than do females.

The hypothesis of greater reliance upon kinesthetic cues for balance by males would seem to account for Sheldon's observed sex difference in difficulty in the dark. However, the hypothesis as stated should not be interpreted as indicative of genetically mediated sex difference in kinesthetic reliance as various balance studies indicate similar rates of learning. Bachman (1961) found that, although initial trial scores were higher for males, the amount of learning on a series of 10 trials on the ladder climb was the same for the sexes at all age levels from 6 to 25 years. This same investigator also examined balance learning as measured by the stabilometer and found poorer initial performance for females at all age levels. However, after 9 years of age, the amount of learning for females over the series of 10 trials exceeded that of the males to the extent that the final trial scores were better for females from 16 through 25 years.

It would seem, then, that sex differences in balance appear to be conditioned to some extent by environmental influences in that females are not encouraged to excel in railwalking or ladder climbing. However, in culturally acceptable events such as the balance beam, females achieve exceptionally high levels of performance which excels that of males. Kinesiological considerations indicate that the superiority of females in balance beam events is mediated by the lower center of gravity and hence, greater stability of the female physique. The practice associated with developing facility on the balance beam undoubtedly involves the kinesthetic sensory system for optimal balance development which, coupled with the greater stability associated with the female physique, gives the female an advantge in balance beam events.

For the average female who does not participate in activities which encourage optimal balance development, the greater stability of the female physique can mediate against balance development in that a more stable individual does not have to activate as many sensory systems, kinesthetic or otherwise, to maintain a stable position. In support of this hypothesis, it should be noted that girls have better balance before 8 years of age (figure 9.17) at which time they have longer legs and a higher center of gravity than males (figure 9.5), whereas the inverse holds after this age. Moreover, the higher balance scores for 69-year-old men was associated with higher participation percentages in different types of physical activities, especially those which involved high levels of balance. In the 66-year-old group from which the 69-year-old training sample was drawn, the participation percentage in skiing for the men was 27.0, and that for the women was 7.5. Similarly, the percentage of men participating in bicycling was 24.8, and that for women was 9.0 (Heikkinen, 1975).

In a more recent investigation of postural sway, Era and Heikkinen (1985) found that the functioning of the postural control system was correlated with vibratory threshold on the ankles, grip strength, as well as with aerobic and anaerobic capacity within the age groups of 31 to 35, 51 to 55, and 71 to 75 years. In addition, the functioning of the postural control system was poorer in the youngest age group for those who had been subjected to noise at work. The investigators suggested that the results may indicate the partly parallel and similar effects of aging, poor physical fitness, and harmful environmental factors in the functioning of the postural control system. In addition, they suggested that it could be possible to improve the control of postural sway by physical training programs. The most difficult of the balance tests (i.e., eyes open/one-foot stand) used by Era and Heikkinen was also used by Rikli and Busch (1986) to determine the effect of age and physical activity level on balance performance. A limit of 60 seconds was placed on this balance task and figure 12.14 indicates that both active and inactive young women achieved this level. However, the old active women were significantly better at balancing than the old inactive women. Therefore, although participation in physical activity does not prevent age related declines in balancing ability, it does appear to modify the degree of decline.

The decline in balancing ability with increasing age is exemplified by reversions in basic locomotor patterns. Older individuals tend to demonstrate a wider base of support in standing than do younger subjects (Hellebrandt & Braun, 1939; Hasselkus & Shambes, 1975). The noted decrease in stance stability for women may be due in some degree to the noted preponderance of foot abnormalities (Hasselkus & Shambes, 1975) but such a widening of base of support also tends to occur for men with increasing age. A similar reversion in pattern has been noted for stair climbing where there is a trend in the elderly to abandon the young-adult practice of ascending and descending stairs with an alternate foot pattern without help for the same pattern with help followed by the

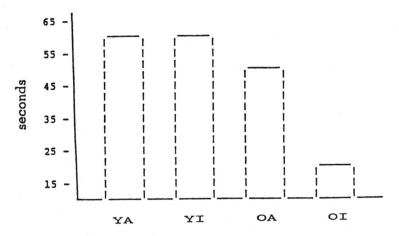

FIGURE 12.14. *Balance on the preferred foot for a maximum time of 60 seconds. YA = young active; YI = young inactive; OA = old active; and OI = old inactive. (From data in Rikli, R., & Busch, S. Motor Performance of Women as a Function of Age and Physical Activity Level. Journal of Gerontology, 1986, 41, 645–649. Drawn by and by permission of the authors.)*

mark-time foot pattern. There is also a trend towards the lesser balance demanding patterns occurring during the descending of stairs prior to the utilization of the same pattern in the ascending of stairs (Eckert, 1975).

Changes in gait pattern also occur with increasing age and may be influenced by other factors in addition to the age related decreases in strength and balance. When Visser (1983) measured the gait and balance of 11 elderly ambulant patients suffering from moderately severe senile dementia of Alzheimer type in comparison with an equal number of healthy, non-demented, age- and sex- matched controls, the demented patients had significantly shorter step length; lower gait speed; lower stepping frequency; greater step-to-step variability; greater double support ratio; and greater sway path. The surface on which individuals walk has also been noted as affecting the gait patterns of elderly hospital patients with Willmott (1986) reporting that the gait speed and step length were significantly greater on a carpeted surface than on a vinyl surface. Some of these patients expressed fear of walking on vinyl but no patient expressed difficulty in walking on carpet where they were also more confident in their walking pattern. Although vinyl floors may be preferable in a hospital and in other settings where sanitary considerations and ease of cleaning are important factors, some attempt should be made to provide areas, such as carpeted common rooms, where individuals may walk more confidently.

MOTOR BEHAVIOR CHANGES

In addition to the increase in plaques and tangles previously noted with respect to morphological changes in neural tissue, brain autopsy reveals a reduction in brain weight from 1375 grams (3.03 pounds) at 30 years to 1232 grams (2.72 pounds) at 90 years (Shock, 1962). Computed tomography (CT) was used by Takeda and Matsuzawa (1984) to determine the cranial cavity volume, cerebrospinal fluid (CSF) space volume and a brain atrophy index (BAI) for men and women ranging in age from 10 to 88 years. All the subjects were free from neurological deficits on CT examinations and the data were organized into age groups by decades. The cranial cavity volumes differed very little among the age groups studied although they were larger for the males (range 1049 to 1051 milliliters) than for females (949 to 951 milliliters). The CSF space volume decreased from the 20s to the 30s and then started to increase after the 30s in an exponential manner for both males and females. However, the rate of increase for the men from the 30s to the 40s was twice that of the females in the same age group indicating that considerable brain atrophy began to occur in the 40s in men and in the 50s in women. Similarly, the brain atrophy index began to increase in the 40s in both sexes with the increase in BAI being large for the men from the 30s to the 40s but small in the women for the same age grouping. The larger increase in BAI occurred for the women from the 40s to the 50s and, as with the CSF, the BAI increased exponentially with age after the 30s in both men and women. Although there are sex differences in the CSF space volume, the BAI adjusts these values on the basis of cranial cavity volume and there are no sex differences in the BAI other than its noted earlier increase in males.

The functioning of neural connections is based not only upon the number of neurons but also on the number and type of receptors that serve as binding sites for neurotransmitters. Neurotransmitter receptor numbers can be unaltered, increase, or decrease across the lifespan, generally in a region specific manner characteristic of each receptor. In addition to changes in neurotransmitter receptors, the concentrations and dynamics of neurotransmitters themselves can be altered and anatomic substrates of neural function, neuronal elements and eventually neurons can decline with advanced age. Severson (1984) points out that, across the lifespan, brain function may be more properly considered as a constant shift in neuronal equilibria caused by changing relationships between neuronal systems resulting from remodeling of local anatomy and biochemistry, and hence, neuronal circuitry. For example, tongue motion is a highly necessary aspect of speech production but older persons show a significant diminution of tongue thickness at rest and significant differences in direction and extent of tongue displacement during production of the "a" sound in comparison to young adults. However, the variation in tongue posture does not impair the message (Sonies et al., 1984).

Standard tests have been developed for various aspects of intellectual performance and some of these show age related trends (age-sensitive) whereas others show little or no performance change (age-irrelevant) with increasing age. Cornelius (1984) examined groups of young (mean age = 26.0), middle age (mean age = 49.2), and older (mean age = 69.9) men and women on three age-irrelevant and four age-sensitive tests. Results indicated that age-sensitive tests were rated as less familiar, more difficult, and more effortful than age-irrelevant tests by all age groups. For both types of tests, performance was associated positively with ratings of test familiarity and associated negatively with ratings of test difficulty, effortfulness, and speed. In general, the differences between the ratings for the age-sensitive and age-irrelevant tests increased with increasing age indicating that the older subjects found the age-sensitive tests more difficult than did the younger subjects.

Memory recall is another way in which intellectual functioning is assessed, but the testing procedures and test items or tasks vary widely and hence, results tend to vary. Numerous studies have investigated a variety of cognitive tasks with these generally showing that older persons normally perform more slowly than younger persons. In addition, older persons often use less optimal or different processing strategies than younger persons leading Macht and Buschke (1984) to question whether the age differential was due to strategy differences or was due to a real decline in processing rate. They used a verbal recall task which induced both the young (mean age = 31.9) and older (mean age = 65.6) men and women to carry out the same processing during learning and recall. Overall the older subjects recalled fewer items than the young; however, recall by both groups increased across successive intervals of the recall period and the cumulative item recall curves for both age groups were essentially parallel (i.e., rate of recall is the same). The noted age difference in the number of items was due to the greater number of items recalled by the young group during the first 30 seconds of recall. Following this period, the number of items recalled by both age groups during the remainder of the recall period was very similar.

In another study of rate of processing, Lorsbach and Simpson (1984) found that young and older adults were equivalent in their ability to identify recently presented identical words, homonyms and synonyms. However, age differences were observed in the speed of response latency with older subjects responding significantly slower than young adults and these differences were greatest on tasks requiring retrieval of semantic information from the secondary memory of short-term memory. A sorting task resulted in an equally high overall initial recall for both young and older adults in a study by Worden and Meggison (1984) but the effect of increasing numbers of categories on recall differed dramatically with young adults who sorted high-frequency words into six or eight categories remembering significantly more words than older adults. In addition, long-term recall showed a greater memory loss for the older adults who had forgotten an average of 11.5 words, almost double the 6.0 words forgotten by young adults, and indicating the effects of decay or interference may be more pronounced in older adults.

During the discussion on the development of perceptual-motor integration stress was placed upon the fact that the various perceptual concepts develop at different rates. Similarly, the potential exists that there may be differences in age related declines in the various types of perceptual functions and such is indeed the case as indicated by the age related declines in ability to recall shape and location. The Tactual Performance Test, which requires that participants recall the shape and location of a number of tactually experienced geometric blocks, was administered to 24 men and women ranging in age from 19 to 76 years (Moore, Richards, & Hood, 1984). Figure 12.15, based upon the results obtained by these investigators, shows that the recall for the location of the geometric

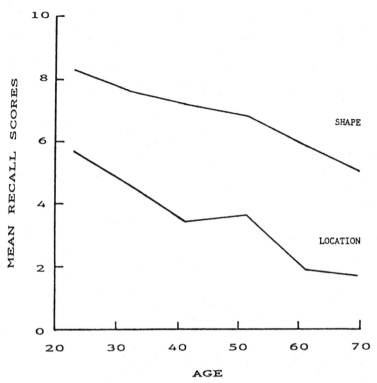

FIGURE 12.15. *Mean recall scores for shape and location on Tactual Performance Test for various age groups. (Adapted from data in Moore, T. E.; Richards, B.; & Hood, J. Aging and the Coding of Spatial Information.* Journal of Gerontology, *1984, 39, 210–212.)*

blocks was less at all age levels and the amount of decline tended to be greater with increasing age in comparison with recall of geometric block shape.

Just as the type of test affects the results obtained in studies of perceptual-motor development, so also the type of test appears to affect the results obtained from investigations of age related effects on the various perceptual abilities. For example, in a task which required the subjects to sort targeted words into one of four input spatial locations, McCormack (1982) found that awareness of the location requirement had no effect on performance and both the young and older female adults were equivalent on overall spatial accuracy. On the other hand, Perlmutter et al. (1981), using the location of buildings on a map as a spatial memory task and the priority of presentation of two pictures as a temporal memory task, found no age difference between younger and older adults on the temporal task but the older adults performed worse than the younger on the spatial task. Similarly, in a study of spatial location of picture and word stimuli, Park et al. (1983) found that young people were significantly better at recognizing items than older people but, for both groups, spatial memory was markedly superior for pictures compared with matched words. Shelton et al. (1982) used structurally similar verbal and visuospatial paired-associated learning tasks to determine if there were different age related decrements in the right hemispheric dominant (visuospatial) and left hemispheric dominant (verbal) tasks. These investigators found that older males made more errors on both the verbal and visuospatial learning tasks than did middle-aged males. In addition, similar patterns were noted in decade cohorts (i.e., both the middle-aged and older males exhibited significantly poorer performance on verbal than on visuospatial learning tasks) and these investigators concluded that they found no evidence to support the notion of a hemispheric laterality effect associated with aging.

The integrity of the nervous system is vital to the initiation and coordination of muscular responses. Figure 12.7 indicates the rate of decline in nerve conduction velocity with increasing age. The nerve conduction velocity loss is more prominent in the distal segments of the body than in proximal areas (Mayer, 1963), and is greater in inferior parts of the body than in the superior members of the trunk (Graux et al., 1962). In addition, there is a decrease, particularly in the lumbrosacral regions, in the number of neural fibers with each decade of life (Corbin & Gardener, 1937) which amounts to a reduction of 27 percent in the number of nerve trunk fibers with advanced age (Shock, 1962). Such changes in the nervous system suggest impairment of function and this is indeed the case, with greater slowing of reaction and movement time being noted with increased age (Pierson & Montoye, 1958; Dupree & Simon, 1963). The differential effects of such neural decline are exhibited in the differential loss of movement time of various segments of the body (figure 12.16). In general, greater reduction in both reaction and movement times tends to occur in the lower parts of the body and reduction tends to be least in areas of most frequent use, e.g. the fingers. Moreover, the rate of decline is also affected by the complexity of the task with increasing complexity of the performance task being associated with increased rates of decline (Birren et al., 1962). Increased synaptic delay in neural impulse transmission with increasing age (Wayner & Emmers, 1958) is undoubtedly one of the factors contributing to these increased rates of decline with increasing complexity.

Age related changes in the sensory input systems may also have profound influences on the motor behavior of individuals. For example, the previously reported investigation by Brocklehurst et al. (1982) of the age related relationships between various sense modalities and postural sway stressed the close relationship between increased postural sway and impaired vibration sense in the leg. Similarly, Kline et al. (1983) used contrast

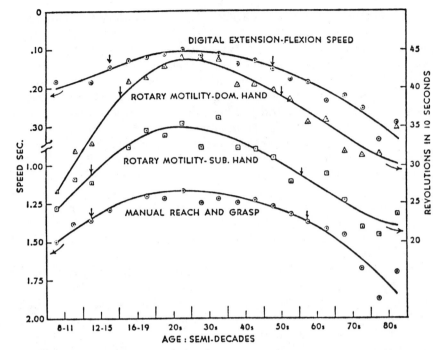

FIGURE 12.16. *Changes in manual motility with age. (Reprinted from Miles, W. R. Changes in Motor Ability during the Life Span. In R. G. Kuhlen & G. G. Thompson (Eds.),* Psychological Studies of Human Development. *New York: Appleton-Century-Crofts, 1952. Meredith Publishing Co., 1963. By permission of G. G. Thompson.)*

sensitivity functions to examine spatial vision and assessed the response speed to varied spatial frequencies for young (mean age = 18.3) and older (mean age = 64.4) adults who had normal visual acuity. They observed an age related loss in contrast sensitivity primarily for stimuli of intermediate and high spatial frequency with older adults being significantly less sensitive than their younger counterparts. Differences in sensitivity as a function of spatial frequency were more pronounced in the older adults with greatest age differences at the intermediate and high spatial frequencies. Reaction time rose significantly with increasing spatial frequency with the reaction time for the older adults being significantly slower than for those of young adults and this difference was especially marked at the higher spatial frequencies. To the investigators, these results suggested a slowing in the speed of operations of individual visual channels and/or a change in the relationship between classes of visual channels with increasing age.

In addition to the age related decrease in visual acuity and accommodation, decreased sensory input function is also exhibited in adjustments to recovery from work in heat (Brouha, 1962); pain (Sherman & Robillar, 1964); auditory sensitivity (Schaie et al., 1964) acoustic processing (West & Cohen, 1985); control of body sway (Sheldon, 1963; Brocklehurst et al., 1982); memory (Shock, 1962); sleep deprivation (Webb et al., 1982); vibration sense (Brocklehurst et al., 1982); and to sensory thresholds in general (Hinchcliffe, 1962). Although many studies tend to look at only single and/or one aspect of sensory modality functioning, changes in one sensory modality may have ramifications for functioning of other sensory modalities and/or operations. For example, Smith et al. (1983) report that the presence of proprioceptive loss in stroke patients is indicative of a more extensive lesion and a larger portion of such patients also have impairment of intellectual function, motor power of the upper and lower limb, and postural function. They stress the importance of diagnosing the loss of proprioception because it influences rehabilitation.

Physical activity is important not only for rehabilitation but also serves a vital role in preventative maintenance. In her survey of exercise as a factor in aging motor behavior plasticity, Spirduso (1984) points out that the hypothesis that exercise may prevent premature aging of the central nervous system is supported by the observation that psychomotor speed is faster in healthy, physically active individuals when compared with the speed of sedentary individuals. Age related changes in reaction time and movement time have been investigated for various groups under varying conditions and activity level is one factor that influences performance. Spirduso (1975) who investigated reaction time in young and old, active and inactive men, reports that active individuals are considerably faster in simple reaction time than inactive individuals with choice reaction time also being faster for the active group but less markedly so. Young groups, when averaged over activity level, were faster than old groups. Similar results were found for movement time and the old nonactive subjects were the group having the slowest reaction and movement times under both simple and choice conditions.

In a similar design of young and old, active and inactive women, Rikli and Busch (1986) noted significant differences between old active and old inactive participants in simple reaction and in choice reaction times. No other significant differences were reported for simple reaction time (figure 12.17). In choice reaction time the young active and young inactive women also differed significantly but the relative ordering of the groups was the same as it was for simple reaction time, i.e., the young active group was the fastest and the old inactive group the slowest.

Spirduso (1985), in her survey of age as a limiting factor in human neuromuscular performance, indicates that practice enhances the performance of older individuals on most psychomotor tests but whether it benefits the older individuals to the extent that it does younger individuals is dependent upon the motor behavior being tested. According to

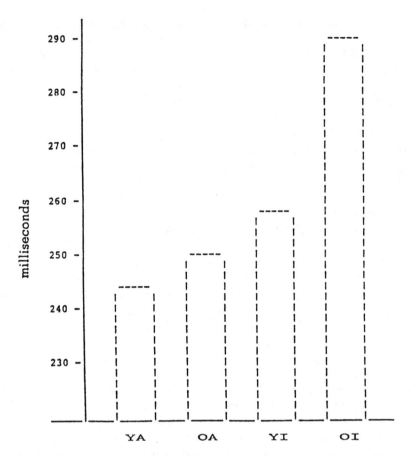

FIGURE 12.17. *Simple reaction time scores. YA = young active; YI = young inactive; OA = old active; and OI = old inactive. (From data in Rikli, R., & Busch, S. Motor Performance of Women as a Function of Age and Physical Activity Level.* Journal of Gerontology, *1986, 41, 645–649. Drawn by and by permission of the authors.)*

Spirduso, exercise effects appear to be significant for those psychomotor performances requiring quick perception and discrimination of environmental stimuli, as well as control of motor overflow requiring rapid initiation and termination of discrete movements. On the other hand, tasks that required perceptual and/or memory scanning or short- or long-term memory seem to be unassociated with physical fitness. The results of a test battery of seven psychomotor tasks in which 11 components of task performance were analyzed indicated that all subjects, both old and young, improved with practice. However, only in choice reaction time and tapping between targets was an interaction between age and days of practice detected. In all other tasks, which included simple reaction time, digit symbols, trailmaking, and movement time, the older individuals improved in the same ways as did the young.

Spirduso (1985) points out that one of the reasons that the old may need more practice to achieve their optimum performance is that they have greater memory deficits so that the task is more novel in the early stages. As a result, a single administration of some psychomotor tests may not provide a true indication of the aged individual's capabilities on such cognitive functions as visual discrimination, signal detection, reaction time, and digit symbol substitution. This pattern of response, that is, early responses being better for young subjects followed by a subsequent period in which there is little or no difference in response between young and old subjects, also occurred for cumulative number of items recalled in the previously reported study by Macht and Buschke (1984).

In general, then, age related changes are noted in most parameters of motor behavior which vary greatly in terms of the type of motor behavior and the amount of experience and/or practice of the individual in a particular task. Practice may enhance performance in most types of psychomotor tasks but the degree to which age related decrements in psychomotor behavior can be postponed and/or moderated is greatly affected by consistent practice and the maintenance of a healthy and physically fit life style.

ROLE OF EXERCISE

Cardiovascular disease is the primary health problem of our society and the incidence of death from this condition increases markedly for both sexes after 65 years of age in comparison with the next major killer, cancer (figure 12.18). It is, therefore, understandable that a great deal of research has been directed towards identification of factors associated with cardiovascular disease. In his survey, Leon (1984) points out that age, male sex, and a strong family history of coronary heart disease are biological factors that increase susceptibility and cannot be modified. Living habits are, however, among the factors that can be modified and figure 11.13 shows the effect of differences in health habits on life expectancy with one of these health habits being regular exercise. The survey of exercise and risk of coronary heart disease by Leon (1984) did not identify lack of physical activity as a major cause but it did contribute to conditions which aggravated the underlying atherosclerotic process and unfavorably disturbed the balance between myocardial oxygen supply and demand. It was suggested that the most important mechanism for partial protective effect of regular endurance activities against coronary heart disease was the reduction of fat stores and body weight.

An investigation of the physiological effects of an exercise training

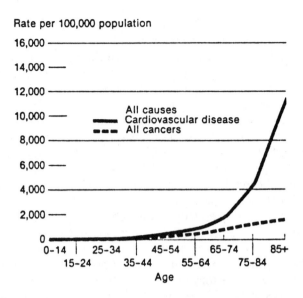

FIGURE 12.18. *Mortality rates for selected causes of death, United States, 1976, by age group. (From Brody, J. A. Facts, Projections, and Gaps Concerning Data on Aging.* Public Health Reports, *1984, 99, 468–475.)*

program upon men aged 52 to 88 by deVries (1970) indicated that the most significant improvements were related to the oxygen transport capacity. The vigorous physical conditioning program, which consisted of calisthenics, jogging, and either stretching exercises or swimming in each workout of approximately one hour three times per week, resulted in significant improvements in percent of body fat, physical work capacity, and both systolic and diastolic blood pressure after six weeks. Similar significant improvements in physiological functioning were also reported by Heikkinen (1975) for 69-year-old men and women during an eight-week physical training program but no differences occurred in weight during this period.

The lack of change of body composition in the Heikkinen study in comparison with the results of the deVries study may have been a result of differences in intensity of training. For example, Vaccaro and associates (1984) report that there were significant differences between highly trained and not highly trained female masters swimmers on measures of weight, body density, percent fat and lean body weight with the more highly trained swimmers having lower body fat at all age levels from 20 to 69 years. In comparison with data reported for normal untrained women of similar ages, both of the training groups had a considerably lower percentage of body fat. However, training does not appear to overcome all age associated increases in body fat in women as these investigators also noted that percent of body fat showed significant increases within each training group at approximately 40 years of age. Heath et al. (1981) also report a slightly higher body fat for male masters endurance athletes in comparison with young endurance athletes and again the athletes had lower percentages of fat than did untrained men.

Both the Vaccaro et al. (1984) and Heath et al. (1981) studies also measured maximal oxygen uptake and in both instances this measure was lower in the older athletes than the younger athletes. However, the highly trained female swimmers had a higher maximal oxygen uptake at all age levels than did the not highly trained swimmers. Although no significant differences are reported, the mean values for maximal oxygen uptake for the highly trained 60-69-year-old swimmers were higher than those of the 20-29-year-old not highly trained female swimmers (Vaccaro et al., 1984). Similarly, Heath et al. (1981) report that highly trained masters endurance athletes (mean age = 59 yrs) had a 60 percent higher maximal oxygen uptake than middle-aged untrained men when this value was expressed in terms of lean body mass to correct for differences in body fat content. Therefore, for individuals who partake regularly in vigorous physical activity, no improvements may occur with increasing age, or may be minimal, but performance values are maintained at higher than average levels (Dill, 1942, 1958; Jokl, 1954). Age related decrements in performance do occur, however, and these are somewhat greater for shorter, higher speed activities (anaerobic) than for longer, slower speed (aerobic) activities. For example, figure 12.19 indicates that the decline in output in terms of yards per second with increasing age in masters swimming competition is greater for the shorter distances than it is for longer distances for both men and women (Hartley & Hartley, 1984).

There are also instances of unusual endurance levels such as that of Walt Stack who has always been a physical fitness enthusiast.

> Walt usually rises at 2:30 A.M. (after sleeping about five hours). He peddles his old three-speed bicycle up and down the steep San Francisco hills to his swimming club, where he begins a leisurely 17-mile jog across the Golden Gate bridge to Sausalito and then back to San Francisco. After this run he dives into the icy cold waters of the San Francisco Bay and swims for at least an hour. By now it is 8 A.M. and time to begin his working day as a hod-carrier, which requires him to carry 100-pound bags of cement up and down ladders on various construction sites throughout the city. At 69, Walt Stack's stamina and energy are extraordinary for a man of any age (Simo-witz, 1977).

The unusual accomplishments of individuals who compete in masters tournaments and/or are physical fitness enthusiasts are undoubtedly closely associated with their previous life styles as well as their ge-

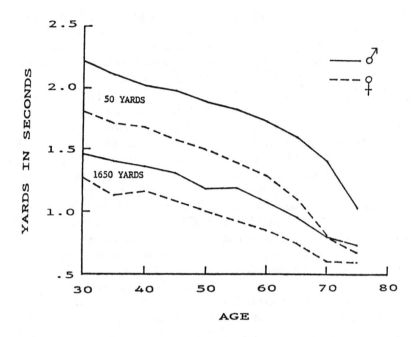

FIGURE 12.19. *Mean performance (in yards per second) for short and long distance masters freestyle swimming events at various ages. (Adapted from data by Hartley, A. A., & Hartley, J. T.* Performance Changes in Champion Swimmers Aged 30 to 84 Years. Experimental Aging Research, *1984,* 10, *35–42.)*

netic endowment. However, what hope is there for older persons for whom physical fitness was not a prominent part of previous life style? Numerous studies, of which the deVries (1970) and Heikkinen (1975) studies are examples, indicate that improvement can occur in the various health-fitness components for older adults. In some instances such improvement is remarkable.

Ben Hirsch, a retired librarian, began jogging when he was sixty-five. That first run was devastating for him. He couldn't run more than a quarter of a mile without almost fainting from exhaustion. But he persisted. And devoted more and more time to running. At age sixty-eight, Ben entered the first race of his life, a four-mile run. This was only the beginning. This past May, he completed his second full marathon at the Avenue of the Giants in Humbolt Redwoods State Park. And on August 1, 1976, Ben Hirsch ran to the summit of Pike's Peak for the second time in his life. This is a grueling fourteen and a half mile run complicated by rocky terrain, adverse weather conditions, loose gravel and high altitudes. The runners ascend from the base, which is 6000 feet, to the summit, which is 14,100 feet high. Ben made it to the top without the help of supporting oxygen and, as he said, "was only slightly fatigued." He says he was surprised how good he felt and how easy the climb was for a man of seventy-four (Simowitz, 1977).

Similar outstanding performance levels have been achieved by Ed Delano of Vacaville, California, who is one of the few expert cyclists to begin racing in his late 50's. He won the very first race he entered in 1958 and decided to make it a life-long hobby. At age 72 (in 1977), Delano cycled more than 125 miles per week and participated in races across the United States and Europe. In July of 1977, he achieved his fastest speed ever of 33.69 mph. and placed 11th in the race where the fastest speed was 49.93 mph. He has also gone on bicycle tours of 3,000 miles or more across the country having cycled to his 40th class reunion at Wurter Technical Institute in Massachusetts in 1969 and then covering the distance of 3,260 miles to satisfy his urge to see Quebec, Canada in 1975 (Lawson, 1977).

In his training study, deVries (1970) also examined changes in strength and noted significant improvements in arm strength of 11.9 percent associated with a decrease in muscle girth of 1 percent. To deVries these results seemed to indicate that the improvement in strength was due to greater activation of the central nervous system than to any hypertrophic changes in the muscle. Liemohn (1975) also found significant improvement in both upper-extremity and lower-extremity strength during a six-week strength training program for 52 men ranging in age from 42 to 83 years. However, strength trainability appeared to decrease as age increased. Differential rates of muscle decline are associated with muscle use. For example, the diaphragm muscle, where respiration requires continuous activity of the motor units, shows only a small, if any, decrease in number and diameter of muscle fibers and in transmitter synthesis. Moreover, the mixed pattern of the motor unit is maintained in old age (Gutmann & Hanzlikova, 1976).

As with physiological functioning, strength levels are maintained at higher levels for individuals who regularly participate in physical activities at high performance levels. In addition, as with physiological functioning, age related declines are greater for maximal strength than they are for muscular strength endurance (Dummer et al., 1985). An unusual example of strength maintenance in an elderly individual is that of Joseph Greenstein, of Brooklyn, N.Y., who "was reduced to breaking chains with his chest muscles, and bending 60-penny nails with his fingers," six months before his death at age 84. He was a former vaudeville strongman who had long ago earned the nickname of "Mighty Atom" by performing feats such as "biting tire chains in half and stopping airplanes (on the ground) with his body." (This World, 1977b)

Heikkinen (1975), in his eight-week training study, reported significant improvement in balance for women and improvement in this performance parameter was also registered for men but not significantly so. The training program also resulted in significantly faster reaction time for men whereas the slight improvement for women was not significant. Additional studies of the relationship between physical activity level and measures of balance and reaction time have been discussed in previous sections and support the conclusion that training can improve performance in these parameters at any age level. Moreover, although there are age related declines in these parameters, individuals who partake regularly in physical activities tend to maintain higher than average levels of performance. For example, a very high level of balance was maintained by Karl Wallenda who was participating in high wire walking when he sustained a fatal accident at 73 years of age (*This World*, 1978b).

Physical activity and physical therapy programs have been found by Smith (1971) to result in significant improvements in bone mineral content over a nine-month period for individuals aged 55 to 94 years. Similar results have been reported in the previous discussion on bone changes and osteoporosis. However, as with structural parameters in the human, age related declines in bone mineral content occur even with regular exercise programs. Lack of activity is highly associated with a rapid decline in bone mineral content and higher incidence of osteoporosis and higher incidence of fractures especially in women. On the other hand, regular physical activity, particularly during the young adult years which is maintained in later years, provides for the optimal deposition and maintenance of bone mineral content.

Changes in the articular surfaces of the bones also affects movement and Whitbourne (1985) reports that age related losses have been documented in virtually every structural component of the joints. Some of these include the connective tissue of the tendons and ligaments which become less resilient and less able to transmit tensile forces; increased scar tissue and areas of calcification within the connective tissue and joint capsule tend to reduce flexibility and elasticity; development of hypertrophied fibers in the synovial membrane also reduces flexibility; and the decrease in the viscosity of the synovial fluid reduces the ease with which joints may move. In some individuals, such age related changes are associated with arthritis and osteoarthritis disease is marked by increased rate of decline in various structural components of the joints. Balke (1984), in his review of arthropathy, concludes that regular exercise remains essential and swimming and resistance movements in warm water are recommended for any form of chronic arthritis. In addition, carefully chosen exercises stimulate the regeneration of cartilage, the production of synovial fluid required for joint lubrication, and help maintain optimal mobility and adequate muscular strength in the afflicted body parts. Moreover, physical activity helps to prevent loss of bone mass and undesirable weight gain that might contribute to quicker joint degeneration.

Arthritis is associated with pain in the joints and many individuals believe that immobility will keep the pain at minimal levels. Exercise is known to stimulate the production of endorphins which are the body's natural way of relieving pain. Therefore, although the first few movements of an exercise routine may cause more discomfort than immobility, the subsequent movements often involve less pain and certainly contribute to the individual's maintenance of functional mobility. The effects of a regular program of physical activity on maintenance of bodily flexibility is clearly illustrated by the results of the study by Rikli and Busch (1986) in which they reported that old active women had significantly greater sit and reach (trunk) flexibility than old inactive women. Figure 12.20, which records the mean performance values for old and young, active and inactive women, shows that old active women were even slightly more flexible than young inactive women. The ability of individuals to maintain enough flexibility to reach feet and toes becomes extremely important if the elderly are to maintain the functional capacity to put on their own shoes and clip their own toe nails.

As indicated by the training studies of deVries (1970) and Heikkinen (1975), exercise and training programs tend to impact many aspects of bodily functioning because of the interdependence of the various bodily systems and the unitary nature of the human being. An aerobic exercise training program conducted over a four-month period by Dustman and

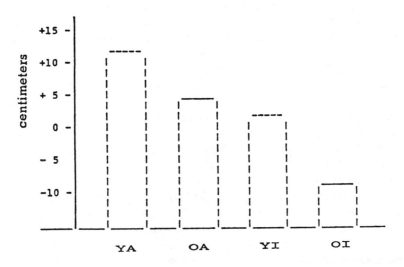

FIGURE 12.20. *Trunk flexibility as measured by a sit-reach test. YA = young active; OA = old active; YI = young inactive; and OI = old inactive. (From data in Rikli, R., & Busch, S. Motor Performance of Women as a Function of Age and Physical Activity Level. Journal of Gerontology, 1986, 41, 645–649. Drawn by and by permission of the authors.)*

associates (1984) resulted not only in the anticipated significantly greater improvement in maximal oxygen uptake but also in neuropsychological tasks purported to measure response time, visual organization, memory, and mental flexibility. The study design included an aerobic exercise group, a strength and flexibility exercise group, and a control group of 55- to 70-year-olds who had previously been sedentary. Both exercise groups improved as a result of the training programs in the maximal oxygen uptake and the neuropsychological measures but the improvement in the aerobic exercise group was greater than that in the strength and flexibility group where aerobic demands were kept low. The investigators suggested that the improved neuropsychological performance of the aerobically-trained group occurred as a result of enhanced cerebral metabolic activity. As the aerobic exercise group participated in fast walking or slow jogging which are speed and coordination activities, it is also possible that training may have resulted in increased dendritic connections (Coleman & Buell, 1983) and/or alterations in EEG patterns as active elderly individuals who are healthy tend to have EEGs that are indistinguishable from the young (Long, 1985).

Although Dustman et al. (1984) report no changes in depression scores for any of the groups during the four-month period, such a result does not appear to be unusual in mentally healthy individuals and cannot be interpreted as indicating that no change in attitude has occurred as a result of the training program. The attitude of the individual is extremely important not only with respect to the desirability of participation in physical activities but also with respect to the individual's functional capacity to undertake everyday activities. Research in this area is much more limited than in areas where performance parameters can be more precisely measured. However, a study of the effects of mastering swimming skills on the personal self-efficacy of older adults gives an indication of the potential in this area. Hogan and Santomier (1984) asked 35 volunteers who were 60 years of age or older and living in non-institutional settings to rate themselves on their ability on 11 swim-skill related items. Following this initial rating, 18 of the subjects (four men and 14 women) were given five weeks of swimming lessons which were designed and paced according to each subject's skill level. During these five weeks, the 17 control subjects were requested not to alter their lifestyles, and at the end of the period, the same rating test was readministered to both groups. The self-efficacy rating for the control group remained virtually the same whereas the change for the group which had received five weeks of swimming lessons was dramatic as well as statistically significant for their ratings of their self-efficacy.

In their comments, 14 of the subjects indicated a change in feeling regarding their ability to perform or achieve as a result of the swim experience and many of these comments suggest that there was a generalizing effect as a result of increased swim self-efficacy. These comments expressed an ability to do other things as well as swimming more easily; more confidence in physical endurance activities such as walking and climbing; and the opinion that one is never too old to learn a new skill. On the basis of their results, these investigators expressed the belief that self-efficacy intervention procedures may be effective ways to counteract the social breakdown of older adults and that involvement in physical activities may do much to counteract stereotypes depicting older adults as inefficacious, dependent individuals.

Persons who take part regularly in physical activities should have a better knowledge of their capabilities in interacting with the environment, thus alleviating to some degree the loss of confidence as well as physical weakness that have been noted as concomitants of the aging process. Measures of cognitive style, which is considered to be the way an individual perceives stimuli, are also considered to reflect the individual's characteristic way of interacting with the environment. One type of cognitive measure is field-dependence/independence and Panek (1985) reports that older adults (mean age = 73.96 years) were significantly more field-dependent than young adults (mean age = 18.65 years). Similarly, Markus (1971) noted progressively lower field-independence perception over age (i.e., more field-dependence). In addition, he reported significant differences between institutionalized and club-going older adults in field-independence perception (i.e., evidencing considerable self-esteem and confidence in the body) with the institutionalized having less field-independence perception as may be expected in a less stimulating environment. Although no sex differences were noted, the field-independence scores were generally higher for men than for women in both these studies. Such difference may reflect less self-confidence in older women that, to some degree, may account for their previously noted increased incidence of falling and difficulty in moving in the dark. However, similar sex differences do not occur for those activities which have traditionally been culturally acceptable for women and which have been part of their daily lives, namely, cleaning house, cooking, and washing clothes. Here fewer women than men reported they would have difficulties although the differences were not marked (Kleemeier, 1959).

Although participation in physical activities tends to increase field-independence and self-confidence, there are other factors that may discourage individuals from even trying to undertake physical activities. For example, Ostrow and Dzewaltowski (1986) reported that older adults viewed participation in all physical activities, with the exception of ballet, as more appropriate for males than females. Moreover, both sexes viewed participation in each of the listed physical activities as less appropriate with increasing age. For instance, basketball was given a high rating as an appropriate activity for 20-year-olds but a low rating for 80-year-olds. However, swimming retained a high rating for appropriateness at all age levels for both sexes. This factor becomes extremely important when planning facilities in the increasing number of retirement communities and in communities in general.

One of the outstanding examples of a housing development designed for the retired age grouping is that of Leisure World at Laguna Hills in Southern California. Of the 22,000 residents at this well-planned retirement community, more than 9000 take advantage of Leisure World's sports opportunities which range from shuffle board and lawn bowling to tennis and swimming with 15 sports-related clubs being responsible for organizing most of the community's athletic events. Swimming is the most popular event with about 4000 to 5000 residents regularly using the five pools while more than 2000 golfers regularly play the two golf courses in the second most popular activity. Additional sports facilities at Leisure World include three lawn bowling greens, a 40-stall stable, a gymnasium where exercise classes are conducted by two full-time instructors, a badminton court, an indoor area for table tennis and six tennis courts. Of the approximately 13,000 residents who do not participate in active sports, all except about 3000 residents use the community facilities regularly for some form of non-sport recreational activity such as chess, bridge, and handicrafts while gardening may be undertaken on a community or individual plot basis (Arp, 1985). It is obvious that in this retirement community, physical activity participation is maintained at high levels and is highly acceptable socially.

Another factor influencing an individual's attitude towards and participation in physical activities is the health of that individual. In a two-year investigation of the degree of compliance by 50- to 65-year-old women in a walking program, Kriska and associates (1986) reported that the compliers (average 7+ miles walked per week over the two years) claimed significantly less illnesses than did the non-compliers who walked less than five miles per week. The compliers also tended to be more active, lighter in weight and non-smokers at baseline; therefore, the higher degree of compliance may reflect their greater observance of health habits and better health. The compliance in the walking program undoubtedly maintained this association between activity level and health.

Elderly people are generally perceived as having more illnesses and "old age" appears to be attitudinally correlated with functional ill health. Therefore, it is not surprising that Milligan and associates (1985) reported that healthy older veterans viewed themselves as more like a younger than an older person whereas the more impaired elderly tended to view themselves more like the stereotyped "old" person. Physical health variables, therefore, are important in the determination of self-concept of the elderly. Indeed, a survey of the concerns of elderly individuals has shown that concern for health (especially lengthy disease and/or disability) and concern for loss of functional capacities rank only slightly behind the primary concern of economic survival (Stein et al., 1984).

The importance of the degree to which an older individual maintains a "younger" self-concept (i.e., more independent and functionally capable) is highlighted in a study of mortality in homes for the elderly undertaken in England by Booth and associates (1983). In the initial phase of their study of 6947 residents living in 175 homes for the elderly, the investigators administered four separate scales which were designed to provide a composite rating of personal functioning. The assessments based on the four scales (i.e., self-care, continence, social integration, and mental orientation) were conflated into a three-point summary measure of dependency.

Twelve months following the initial assessment, the characteristics of the 4763 "survivors" and the 1336 "lost cohort" individuals from the original group were examined to determine the relationship between dependency level and mortality rate. Three risk groups were identified. (1) A low risk group with mortality rates in the range of 11 to 15 percent. This group comprised independent residents under 90 years of age and moderately dependent residents under 80 years of age. (2) A medium risk group with mortality rates in the range of 22 to 26 percent. This group comprised independent residents over 90 years and moderately dependent residents between 80 and 90 years old. (3) A high risk group with mortality rates ranging from 34 to 49 percent. This group comprised moderately dependent residents over 90 years and all severely dependent residents irrespective of age. Booth et al. (1983) noted that the direct relationship between mortality and dependency was found to hold irrespective of the time spent in care.

In their study of the immune status of healthy centenarians whose immune systems appeared to be similar to that of younger elderly subjects, Thompson and associates (1984) also examined the emotional and activity independence of their 17 subjects who ranged in age from 100 to 103 years. All subjects had daily contact and very positive support from family and/or close friends, and each individual felt a sense of self-worth. Four of the centenarians were quite independent, maintained active social lives, and routinely left their residences. Another seven were quite active but required assistance from their family and friends and only one individual was dependent upon others for most daily activities and never left her residence. Thus, a very large proportion of these individuals were able to maintain a certain degree of independent functional capacity which undoubtedly contributed to their sense of self-worth and also, to some degree, to their health maintenance.

Clearly, then, the maintenance of functional independence becomes a crucial aspect of life style for the elderly themselves and for all the individuals and agencies closely associated with the elderly. The role of governmental and social agencies in encouraging functional independence for older adults is beyond the scope of this discussion. However, it is important to note that research, much of which has been sponsored by governmental agencies, has provided strong evidence pointing to regular participation in physical activities as a mitigation factor in age related health and functional independence and/or capabilities problems. Indeed, the crucial need for retention of mobility among the elderly has focused attention on performance-oriented assessments of mobility problems to provide diagnoses that cannot be obtained through the disease-oriented approach (Tinetti, 1986). These performance-oriented assessments of balance and gait include descriptions of normal, adaptive, and abnormal responses during various balancing and walking activities. Further analyses include possible etiologies, possible therapeutic or rehabilitative measures, and possible preventive or adaptive measures for abnormal maneuvers in balance and gait.

In a review of health-related physical fitness components, Haskell, Montoye and Orenstein (1985) identify the following major health-fitness goals for older adults over 65 years:

a) Maintain general functional capacity;
b) Retain musculoskeletal integrity;
c) Enhance psychological status;
d) Prevent and treat coronary heart disease and Type II diabetes.

To achieve these goals, the recommended physical activity plan includes:

Type of exercise: Emphasis on moving about, flexibility, and some resistive exercises;
Intensity: Moderate intensity (overload with slow progression);
Duration: Based upon capacity of individual; up to 60 minutes per day;
Frequency: Every day. Lower level activities (e.g., walking) every day.

Although older adulthood is the age at which declining performance parameters become increasingly evident, it is also evident that participation in physical activities is extremely necessary in enabling older people to stay active and feel good about themselves. The habits and attitudes as well as the skills developed during the growing years play a vital role in the health, both mental and physical, of the individual throughout the entire life span. Motor skills learned during childhood and/or youth provide the tools which encourage participation and provide enjoyment in vigorous activity in young adulthood and form the base upon which older adults build healthful and functionally independent "golden years." As Wright and Blass (1984) point out in an editorial on aging and longevity research, "The path of wisdom seems to be to concentrate on helping people have as healthy, productive, and meaningful a life as possible, until as close as possible to their death."

SUMMARY

1. There is a secular trend towards decreased mortality and, hence, increased longevity which is the result of technological and scientific advances rather than any change in the optimal biological life span of the human species.

2. Factors, in addition to the secular trend, associated with longevity are: the sex of the individual; the genetic endowment (e.g., age at which parents died); the socioeconomic status; and the life style of the individual (e.g., adherence to the seven health habits).

3. In general, it appears that regular physical activity of a moderate to high level is inversely related to mortality rate.

4. There are age related changes in body composition resulting in redistribution of fat, and decreases in height and weight in older adults.

5. There are age related changes in physiological functions such as the cardiovascular system, the respiratory system, and the filtration system of the kidneys which result in greater decreases in maximal exercise tolerance than in submaximal endurance.

6. Decreases in maximal strength with increased age are much greater than decreases in muscular strength endurance with age. The loss in maximal strength is associated with increased atrophy of type II (fast twitch) fibers and/or conversion of some type II fibers to type I (slow twitch) fibers with increased age. In addition, there is a reduction in muscle mass with increased age associated with the reduction in the size of muscle fibers particularly of the type II fibers.

7. Activity level affects the rate of change and decline of muscle fibers and, hence, strength. Therefore, there is a differential in the rate of decline in strength for the various muscle groups (e.g., flexors of the leg decline more quickly than extensors).

8. There is an age related decrease in bone mineral content which is associated with the decline in estrogen production in females and with activity level and calcium metabolism in both males and females.

9. The decline in bone mineral content is much greater in females after 50 years of age than it is in males and may lead to osteoporosis and, hence, greater liability to bone fractures especially during falls.

10. The increased bodily sway during standing which has been ob-

served with increased age is associated with decreases in visual acuity; increases in vibratory threshold in the ankles; the activity level of the individual; lowered strength; and low aerobic and anaerobic capacity.

11. Although there are no marked sex differences in balance with increasing age, the likelihood and incidence of falls is greater in females than in males. This sex difference is greater than can be accounted for by the high ratio of females to males during older adulthood and may be a feature of sex differences in physical activity level.

12. The reduction in brain weight after 30 years of age is associated with brain atrophy which results in a reduction in functional capacity in tests which are less familiar, more difficult, more effortful, and require speed responses.

13. In recall types of tests, differences between young and older adults are usually due to more items recalled during the early recall period by young adults whereas the rate of recall is similar during later recall. However, increasing the complexity or number of categories of recall increases the differences between the responses of young and older adults for both short- and long-term memory.

14. There are differential rates of decline with increasing age for various types of perceptual functions such as recall of shape and location (visuospatial) and verbal stimuli.

15. Reduction in sensitivity to sensory input systems with increasing age is associated with reduction in motoric responses, e.g.:

Sensory input	Motor behavior
visual acuity	reaction time
	balance
auditory threshold	reaction time
vibratory threshold	balance
tactile threshold	reaction time

16. Although the age related changes in sensitivity of the sensory input systems are not associated with levels of physical activity, the responses to these changes also include a neuromuscular component which may be modified by physical activity. For example, training can improve the neuromuscular components of reaction time and balance in older individuals but has no effect on visual acuity.

17. Exercise can reduce the risks associated with cardiovascular disease by improving cardio-respiratory functioning and reducing fat stores and body weight.

18. Similarly, exercise, at any age level, can improve strength, balance, reaction time, and, in general, slow down the age related "slowing down" that occurs in all neuromuscular activities.

19. Age related structural changes in the joints and functional aspects of joint action (i.e., flexibility) can be modified by exercise. Exer-

cises in warm water (e.g., swimming) are recommended for any form of chronic arthritis.

20. Participation in physical activities can enhance the individual's concept of self-efficacy not only in a particular activity but also in functional capacity in general.

21. Risk of mortality tends to be greater for individuals who are inefficacious and dependent ("old" persons) than it is for individuals who have good functional capacity and are independent ("young" persons).

22. In general, older adults tend to regard participation in physical activities as more appropriate for males than females and both sexes consider participation in physical activities to be less appropriate with increasing age. Swimming is an exception to these trends as is walking.

23. The main concerns of older adults are economic survival; concern for health; and concern for loss of functional capacity. Participation in physical activities can make a major impact on two of these concerns through improved physical health (better cardiorespiratory functioning, strength, balance, reaction time, etc.); mental health (better self-efficacy and more independent); and better functional capacity. A balanced life—a healthy mind in a healthy body—is the key to a vigorous old age.

HELPFUL HINTS

Those of you who have not exercised for some time should consider the following guidelines in developing or selecting an exercise program:

1. If you have not done any physical activity for a long period of time, you should have a thorough medical examination before undertaking an exercise program, especially exercises designed to improve cardiorespiratory endurance.

2. You may wish to separate your aerobic rhythmic exercise activities from your more general activity exercise session; for example, do one exercise program in the morning and the other in the afternoon. Don't forget to do some stretching and warm-up exercises before doing your rhythmic aerobic activity.

3. For the aerobic portion of your exercise program, select activities such as walking, swimming, or cycling where it is easy for you to set your own pace. These are activities where muscle and bone stress are low while the rhythmic muscle contractions required for the activity improve overall muscle tone and cardiorespiratory fitness.

4. Limit the time spent in any one exercise session to 15 minutes until muscle discomfort disappears and then gradually increase the time limit especially in aerobic exercise sessions. Remember, exercise stimulates the endorphin system which is the body's natural way to relieve pain.

5. Your general activity exercise program should include exercises

which will improve strength, strength endurance, coordination, flexibility, and balance. In addition, you should select exercises which will develop these physical performance components in all parts of the body; for example, shoulder strength, ankle flexibility, and arm-leg coordination.

6. In your general activity exercise program, begin by doing only a few repetitions of each exercise to reduce the potential for muscle stiffness. For the beginner, it is much better to do a few repetitions of each of the exercises for the various components and parts of the body as indicated above than it is to do many repetitions of only a few exercises.

7. When you first do exercises that involve flexibility and range of joint action beyond what you are accustomed to, only do the movement to the extent that it is comfortable until you are confident that you are not over-stressing the joint. You will find that you can then gradually increase the range of movement once your muscles have become stronger and the joint has become more flexible. Do not take part in exercises where someone else is pushing your limit to increase the range of joint action unless that individual is a licensed physical therapist. In some instances, for example, where there is reduced joint movement in the fingers, you may wish to push the joint to get more range, but the push should not cause excessive pain. Increase in joint action can be gained only by *gradually* increasing the range as the required changes to the muscles, tendons, and joints occur gradually.

8. In order to make sure that you are getting the maximum benefit from your exercise program, vary the exercises you use for both your rhythmic aerobic activity session and your general exercise program. For example, in your rhythmic aerobic activity sessions, you may wish to vary your activity from walking to swimming or bicycling. This provides variety, which keeps up interest, as well as contributing to different aspects of over-all fitness in addition to the goal of cardiovascular fitness. Similarly, changing the exercises you select for your general activity program will not only contribute to different aspects of overall fitness but will prove to be mentally stimulating as you select the exercises most appropriate to your needs. For those of you who are just beginning your exercise program and wish some help in this regard, please see the suggested exercise routine variations listed in the Julius Palffy-Alpar Fitness Program in Appendix B.

9. Make sure that you undertake your exercises under *warm* conditions. Cold will cause muscles to tighten up and this increases the possibility of discomfort and injury if one then tries to move too quickly or too strenuously. Rubbing a joint before moving the joint will increase surface circulation and reduce discomfort from moving the joint. In order to ensure that the muscles are warm, some individuals may prefer to begin their exercise program as soon as they get out of their warm beds in the

morning. This is the time preferred by Julius Palffy-Alpar for his exercise routine.

10. Remember, you never know if you can do something until you *try* it, and you only maintain and improve your physical fitness level by *doing* physical activity. Knowing you can do something improves your self-confidence and ability to be independent, and being fit makes you feel better and more vigorous so you can meet life's challenges more easily and with less worry and stress.

Appendix A

Exercise Program Development

Exercise may be undertaken at times other than a specially allotted time period. Included below are suggestions for exercises to accompany TV watching and during tension-relieving breaks at work as well as suggestions for a self-developed exercise program.

The following general conditions apply to all the exercises listed below:

1. Begin at a slow pace and gradually increase speed and/or intensity.
2. Begin with a few activities and/or repetitions and gradually increase the number of activities and/or repetitions.
3. It is better to do a variety of different activities using few repetitions than only a few activities with a large number of repetitions. That is, select activities that cover all aspects of movement and all sections of the body rather than concentrating on one type of movement for one body part.

WHILE WATCHING TV

1. During program:
   a) jogging or high stepping on the spot;
   b) arm swings standing facing TV;
   c) squeeze a tennis ball as hard as possible;
   d) sitting toe touches;
   e) balance on one foot facing TV;
   f) use a doubled-over bicycle tube to do resistive movements of arms and legs;
   g) combination arm and leg movements (jazzercise if the music program is right tempo).
2. During commercial break:
   a) pushups;
   b) sit-ups;
   c) standing toe touches.

AT THE OFFICE

This section is divided into upper body, trunk and leg exercises. It is recommended that you select one exercise from each of these areas for any one exercise bout and also that you change the selected series of exercises for each bout so as to provide a greater overall coverage.

1. Upper Body Exercises

Chicken wings: Bend your elbows and place your thumbs into your armpits (same side), then rotate your elbows starting in a forward and upward movement and doing five complete rotations. Repeat the rotary action five times but starting in a backward and upward direction for the completed rotation. This exercise uses the same muscles as full arm circle swings but reduces the arm length so that you can do the activity while seated behind your desk.

Neck and eye relief: Often office work requires that the head remain in the same position and that vision be concentrated in a fairly small field. Larger movements of both the head and the eyes are, therefore, a relief from the muscular tension of maintaining approximately the same position. In this exercise the movements of the eyes should be synchronized with the movements of the head as would occur normally and each cycle of action should be repeated 10 times before doing the next exercise. Keep your back straight and against the back of your chair for all the exercises.

    a. Drop the chin as low as possible and then stretch up as far as possible while looking down and then up as far as possible.

    b. While holding the head erect, turn the head to look to one side as far as possible then to the other side as far as possible.

    c. With eyes looking forward, bend the head sideways as far as possible in one direction and then in the other direction.

    d. Starting with the chin dropped as low as possible and looking downward, rotate the head and eyes to the side, upwards, and then the other side to complete a rotary action first in a clockwise direction 10 times and then in a counterclockwise direction the same number of times. The exercise can be varied by alternating the direction of rotation after the completion of each cycle.

Shoulder and arm strength: Sitting towards the front of your chair with back straight, put your hands behind your back and curl the fingers of your hands against each other. Try to pull your hands away from each other while holding with your curl fingers. Hold the pulling action for six long counts.

Shoulder abduction and adduction: In a chicken-wing position, raise the elbows upwards at the sides of the body to touch your ears if possible and then lower back to the sides. Repeat 10 times. This exercise can also be done in the fully extended arm position if there is enough room and your office mates do not object to your waving your arms around. It would undoubtedly create some discussion and may even encourage "exercise breaks" for others in the office.

2. Trunk Exercises

Trunk rotation: With back straight and sitting somewhat forward on your chair, turn your shoulders and head first to the right as far as possible and then to the left as far as possible. Make sure your feet are firmly placed on the floor and slightly apart for greater stability while you rotate your trunk. Repeat in each direction five times.

Sideward trunk flexibility: Sitting with straight back and slightly spread feet placed firmly on the floor, bend sideways to the right while reaching towards the floor with the right hand. Placing the left hand on the left side of the chair back will give you a greater feeling of security and may allow you to bend sideways a bit more. Return to the upright position and then reverse direction to bend sidewards to the left and use the right hand for support on the chair side before returning again to the upright position. Repeat the entire sequence five times.

Trunk forward flexion: With your chair placed sideways to your desk and sitting toward the front of your chair, extend one leg straight out in front of you while keeping the other foot firmly on the floor. Bend forward with your fully extended arms to try to touch the toes of your extended foot. (*Caution*: If your chair has wheels be careful while doing this exercise as only a slight pressure from your feet when you are in the forward leaning position may push the chair from under you.) After reaching as far as possible return to an upright, straight back position. The exercise may be varied by keeping both feet firmly placed on the floor in the normal sitting position and reaching towards the left foot with the extended right hand and vice versa. The reaching sequence should be repeated the desired number of times.

3. Leg Exercises

Cycling: With your chair placed sideways to your desk and gripping the back of your chair at seat level with both hands, lift both feet off the floor and perform a cycling action with your legs. You should keep the action going for six seconds or longer. Increasing the speed of the cycling action increases the amount of energy used and better fitness results.

Leg extensor strength: With a straight back and feet placed firmly on the floor, raise yourself slightly off your chair and hold this raised position for six seconds or longer. The length of time you are able to hold this position will depend upon your leg endurance strength. This exercise is an office version of the leg endurance exercise recommended for skiers.

Leg stretch: With straight back and hands gripping the back of your chair at seat level, raise both legs and hold at seat level for six seconds or longer. You can vary this exercise by spreading your legs and bringing them back together again while in the extended position.

Toe flexibility: Slip off your shoes and then, with heels resting on the floor, spread out your toes as much as you can and then curl them. Repeat the spreading and curling sequence 10 times. You may wish to see if you can do a variant of this exercise by dropping a pencil and then picking it up with your toes. Because we confine our feet in shoes, many of us greatly reduce the functional capability of the muscles controlling flexion and extension of our toes. Exercising your toes promotes circulation of blood in the feet and helps to maintain neural innervation which is vital to balance.

YOUR EXERCISE PROGRAM

The important thing about your exercise program is that it is designed by you to meet your personal needs. Do not be afraid to experiment with various arrangements of timing during the day as to when you exercise as well as with various combinations of what types of exercise components you feel most comfortable with during the various times of the day. There is no fixed exercise program that will meet the needs of everyone and trying to follow precisely a program devised by someone else often leads to frustration with the ultimate result that the program is abandoned.

It is easy to follow the few simple guidelines of 1) selection of a rhythmical activity you enjoy to provide for development of cardiovascular fitness; 2) selection of activities that develop the other components of general physical fitness such as flexibility, coordination, balance, strength and strength endurance; and 3) selection of exercises that provide for general physical fitness for all parts of the body. You are the most knowledgeable person for determining how these guidelines can best be used to meet your needs as you have the most accurate knowledge of your past experience and your present capabilities. In addition, you have the most knowledge of your daily habits, schedule, and work conditions and requirements. Such contributions are vital to a viable exercise program so use your personal knowledge to develop your own personal exercise program. In short, become intellectually involved in your exercise program as well as physically for *overall* fitness.

1. Rhythmic Activities for Cardiovascular Fitness

The most desirable types of rhythmical activities for improving the cardiovascular fitness of healthy, young adults are listed and each of these makes additional contributions to other aspects of physical fitness as indicated:

   a) Swimming: strength and strength endurance for all parts of the body; coordination.

   b) Running: strength and strength endurance of legs; some balance.

   c) Bicycling: strength and strength endurance of legs; excellent for balance.

   d) Rope Skipping: leg strength and strength endurance; excellent for coordination if skipping pattern changed during exercise, balance.

   e) Jazzercise: depending upon movements used—strength and endurance; strength of all parts of body; coordination; balance, flexibility.

   f) Skating: leg strength and strength endurance; excellent for balance.

   g) Rowing: arm, shoulder, and trunk strength and strength endurance; coordination.

   h) Cross-country Skiing: strength and strength endurance of all parts of body; coordination; balance.

2. General Component Exercises

Included here are exercises for flexibility, strength, coordination, and balance.

a. Flexibility and Stretching Exercises

The following exercises are designed to improve and maintain flexibility in various parts of the body. They are also recommended as stretching and relaxing exercises to limber up and warm up the various parts of the body prior to undertaking strenuous activities. The selected exercises should be repeated until you feel comfortable and relaxed about the movement of the concerned joint actions.

Leg stretch: With legs spread forward and backward as far as possible, shift weight to forward leg while bending the forward knee. This stretches the back leg and increased stretch can be achieved by bouncing up and down gently. Hands placed on the forward knee are a help in controlling the weight of the upper body during the bouncing action. Alternate the leg position and repeat exercise.

Arm and body stretch: Interweave the fingers of the hands, then lift hands, with palms extended upwards, as far as possible above the head and stretch the entire body upwards as much as possible raising up on the toes. Hold stretched position for a period of time.

Trunk twisting: While standing with feet in a comfortable spread sideways position, place hands on hips, rotate body as far as possible to the right slowly, then to the left. Repeat desired number of times. This exercise can also be performed with arms extended horizontally at the sides of the body but extending the arms reduces the balance aspects.

Back stretch (flexion): Sitting on the floor with the legs stretched out in front, reach forward with the extended arms as far as possible. Slight bouncing of the trunk forward should extend the distance you can reach towards and beyond your toes. Repeat as many times as desired.

Back stretch (extension): In a front lying extended body position, place the hands behind the neck, then raise the head and the extended legs simultaneously and hold for a period of time. The longer the extended position is held the greater the contribution to back extensor strength endurance. Repeat number of desired times.

Shoulder flexibility: In a comfortable standing position, starting with one arm raised above the head and the other down at the side, reach down the back with the hand that had been raised and reach up the back with the hand that had been held down to touch fingers at the upper back level. Try to overlap fingers if possible. Repeat while alternating the up and down reaching of the hands.

Knee and hip flexion: In a standing position, raise one leg with bent knee to bring leg as close as possible to the chest. Placing the hands at shin level and pulling the leg gently towards the body increases the amount of flexion. Alternate leg action and repeat desired number of times. This exercise can also be performed in a back lying position but this eliminates the balance component.

Ankle flexibility: While standing, raise one leg and move the foot up and down as far as possible using the ankle joint. Repeat for 10 counts, then rotate the foot to the right five times and then to the left five times using only the ankle joint. Repeat the up and down rotation action with the other foot and then repeat the entire sequence for alternate ankles the desired number of times. This ankle flexibility exercise can also be performed in a sitting down or lying position but doing so removes the balance contribution to general fitness.

Finger flexibility: With hands held at the sides of the body, extend the fingers of both hands as far as possible and spread them out as far as possible. Then curl the fingers as tightly as possible. Repeat the extension and flexion as many times as desired and then shake the relaxed fingers vigorously.

Wrist flexibility: With hands at sides or in front of the body, move the hands up and down using only wrist action for a count of 10, then rotate wrists in an inward direction for five counts followed by rotation in an outward direction for five counts. Repeat entire sequence as many times as desired.

b. Strength and Strength Endurance Exercises

The rhythmic activities recommended to develop and maintain cardiovascular fitness of young adults also contribute considerably to strength and especially strength endurance. However, the rhythmic activity may not contribute to strength and strength endurance for all parts of the body. Therefore, you should examine the relative contributions of these activities and be sure to select additional strength and strength endurance exercises that will complement the rhythmic activity in your program of over-all physical fitness.

Push-ups (arms strength endurance): From a front lying position with the hands flat on the floor at shoulder level (elbows are bent), extend the arms by pushing up the straight held body. In the arm extended position, the straight body is supported by the toes and the hands only. Lower the upper body again by bending at the elbow. Repeat the extending and bending of the arms as many times as desired. Restricting the bending of the straight arms to a 90 degree position at the lowest part of the push-up cycle makes the exercise somewhat easier. In addition, using the knees, rather than the toes, as the lower point of contact for the straight body also decreases the amount of arm pushing strength required.

Leg strength endurance: From a standing position with the extended arms held in a horizonal position in front of the body, assume a bent knee position with the angle at the back of the knee approximately 100 degrees. Hold this position as long as possible.

Bent knee sit-ups (abdominal strength endurance): From a back lying position with knees bent (approximately 120 degrees at back of knee) and with hands clasped behind the head, lift the upper body (hip serves as fulcrum) to touch the right elbow to the left knee. Resume the back lying position and on the next sit-up touch the left elbow to the right knee. Repeat this sequence of alternate elbow-knee touches as many times as desired.

Toe touching (back strength endurance): With feet comfortably placed in a side-by-side position, extend the arms at shoulder level to the sides of the body. Then bend forward and twist the trunk to touch the toes with the right hand while the left is extended vertically. Resume the original upright position and then bend and twist to touch the toes with the left hand while the right is vertically extended. Repeat the alternate right hand - left hand toe touch sequence as many times as desired.

Push and pull arm strength endurance: With the heels of the hands pressed together in front of the body and the arms held at chest level, push the hands together as hard as possible for 10 counts (use the thousand and one, etc., counting method). Lower the arms and shake for a while. Then curling the fingers of one hand around the curled fingers of the other hand with the hands in front of the body and at chest level, pull against the intercurled fingers as hard as possible for 10 counts. Lower the arms and shake for a while and then repeat the entire push-pull sequence as many times as desired.

Trunk endurance strength: Assume a back lying position with the arms extended out to the sides of the body and the extended legs held vertically above the body. Keeping the shoulders on the floor, turn the hips to lower the extended legs to the floor on the right side. Raise the extended legs back to the center position and then lower them to the floor on the left side. Raise the legs back to the central vertical position and repeat the alternate side leg lowering as many times as desired.

Jump and hop (leg endurance strength): In a standing position jump as high as possible off the floor with both feet three times. Then using the right foot only, hop as high as possible three times. Jump again with both feet three times and then hop as high as possible with the left foot three times. Repeat the entire sequence as many times as desired. The endurance requirements can be made harder by increasing the number of repetitions for each of the both foot, left and right foot jumps before changing over; for example, repeat each type of jump six times before changing the type of jump.

V-sit (abdominal endurance strength): Sit on the floor with legs extended in front of the body and arms folded across the chest. Lean the upper body backwards and raise the legs to form a V position and maintain this balanced position on the hips as long as possible. Balancing in the V position is somewhat easier if the arms are extended in front of the body to help maintain balance while supported on the hips only.

c. Coordination Exercises

Neuromuscular coordination is required for every movement in the body and becomes more complex with each increase in the number of body segments involved and/or the variations in the types of movement involved. Therefore, it is strongly recommended that participation occur in a wide variety of activities, especially those requiring variations in patterns, for the development of good overall coordination.

Jumping jack: Starting from a feet-together standing position with the arms down at the sides, do a straddle jump (legs apart to the sides) while at the same time bringing the extended arms up at the sides to slap the hands together over the head. Then from the straddle position jump to bring the legs back to the feet-together position again while bringing the extended arms back down to slap the hands together behind the back. Repeat the complete cycle 10 times.

Jumping jack variations:

a) Same pattern as above but slapping the hands together in the down position first behind the body then in front of the body during alternating cycles.

b) Start with extended arms in front of the body at shoulder level when feet are together; then move arms apart as legs move apart and slap hands in front when feet move together.

c) Do a forward and back straddle jump while extended arms move forward and back: 1) with right leg going forward and left arm going back (alternate arm-leg action) and reverse; 2) with right arm and right leg going forward while left arm and leg go backwards (ipslateral action) and reverse.

d) Combinations of the above in a continuous sequence. In this instance, each of the pattern cycles should be repeated several times before going on to the next pattern.

Arm patterns while cycling: In a back lying position with the legs raised and performing a bicycling action, do the following arm movement variations and repeat the cycles the desired number of times.

a) From an arms at the side position with the hands at the hips, raise the extended arms at the sides of the body to touch the backs of the hands above the head and lower again to hips.

b) Starting from an arm position with the right arm extended above the head and the left at the side of the body, alternate the position of the arms by moving the extended arms in a vertical plane above the body.

c) From a position with the arms extended out from the sides of the body at shoulder level, bring the extended arms up to pass each other at chest level, then bend arms and continue arm movement to touch the left hand to the floor on the right side of the body and vice versa before bringing arms back to original extended sidewards position.

d) Starting with both arms extended up in front of the body at shoulder level, move both extended arms up, around, down, and then back up in a rotary action. After 10 rotations, change the direction of rotation to down, around, and up, and repeat for 10 more rotations.

Patting-rubbing: With the right hand held above the stomach making a rotary rubbing movement, the left hand is placed above the top of the head doing an up and down tapping movement. After having mastered the movements for this coordination game, reverse the position and the actions of the hands.

d. Balance Exercises

Balance is required for the body to make rapid and accurate adjustments to the varying changes in the levels of the center of gravity and to the size of the base of support in all bodily positions and movements. Therefore, as with coordination, participation in a wide variety of activities, especially those involving varying levels of center of gravity and sizes of base of support, are recommended for good overall balance. Again, as with coordination, balancing skill is dependent upon the amount of practice as well as innate ability. The following exercises illustrate the balance components associated with size of base of support and the effect of rapid changes of direction. These exercises are also frequently used to measure balance.

Stork stand: While standing on the right foot, place the sole of the left foot against the calf of the right leg. This position can be maintained longest when the arms are held out to the sides to help to maintain balance. Placing the hands on the hips and keeping them there reduces the time during which balance on one foot is maintained. In addition, closing your eyes while in the stork stand position reduces the length of time balance may be maintained. Select the version that is most challenging to you and try to maintain balance as long as possible. Alternate the supporting foot to the left foot and repeat your selected version of the balancing exercise.

Rotary balance: From a feet together position, jump and turn around (rotary action) on the same spot landing with feet together and in balance. The amount you can turn and still maintain balance at the end of your rotary jump can be used as a measure of your balance ability. Repeat the exercise doing a rotary jump in the other direction. As with the previous exercise, balance becomes much more difficult if the jump-turn is made with the hands on the hips.

ENJOY THE ZESTFUL RESULTS OF YOUR SELF-DEVELOPED EXERCISE PROGRAM!

Appendix B. Julius Palffy-Alpar Fitness Program

As we grow older we become increasingly aware of the importance of good health. Regular participation in physical activity also becomes increasingly important in the maintenance, and in some instances the regaining, of good health.

Julius Palffy-Alpar, supervisor of physical education, developed his fitness program upon retirement as a method of health maintenance for older adults. Some of its features are:

1. It is a general conditioning program including exercises for flexibility, coordination, balance, strength, and endurance.
2. For endurance, it is recommended that the exercises should follow each other in continuous sequence but they should always be performed in a relaxed manner without overstretching the muscles, locking knees, or jerking the limbs.
3. The tempo of the exercises should be built gradually from a relaxed state to a more vigorous movement.
4. The number of repetitions for each exercise should begin at no more than three when first beginning the exercise routine. The repetitions should be gradually increased to as many as 20 for some of the activities that are most helpful for the individual.
5. The series of exercises begin in a reclining position, then change to a sitting position, followed by a standing position.
6. In general, the exercises alternate the use of the arms and the legs so that no one area becomes overused.
7. The beginning exerciser should not do the entire series of exercises during the first few sessions, but should select some exercises from each position and then gradually increase the number of exercises selected; until the entire sequence can be completed in one activity session.
8. While expanding the exercise program, it is better to increase the number and diversity of the exercises rather than increasing the number of repetitions of a few exercises.
9. It is recommended that the exercise program be undertaken under warm conditions and when the body is warm and relaxed (such as when first getting up in the morning).
10. It is recommended that an aerobic activity, such as walking, be undertaken during another activity session each day.

EXERCISE PROGRAM

The following exercises should be done on a mat or carpet which provides a soft but firm surface. A pillow of comfortable thickness should be placed under the head for the first series of exercises until the directions indicate it should be removed.

1. Lie on your back with legs extended and together and arms comfortably placed at your sides. Bend the left leg pulling your foot along the floor until the heel is close to your buttock, then straighten the leg again. Repeat the exercise with the right leg and then continue with alternation of legs.

2. Lying on your back with knees bent or straight, raise both arms to extended position and then lower to chest level. Close both hands to form fists at chest level and stretch fingers as arms are fully extended above chest.

3. While lying on your back with legs extended and using the hands with palms down as a cushion under the buttocks, lift the extended left leg to an upright position and then lower slowly. Repeat using the right leg and alternate leg action until desired number of repetitions are completed.

4. On the back with knees bent and straight arms at sides so that the hands are beside hips, bring straight arms up over the head and touch relaxed hands to the floor above the head. Bring straight arms back over head to touch relaxed hands to the floor at hips.

5. With the arms at sides and legs extended, bend one knee to the level of the other knee and then extend the bent knee to a straight upright position. On the return to the floor, again bend the upright extended leg to the side of the lower knee and then straighten to return it to the floor. Repeat the sequence with the other leg.

6. With knees bent, alternately raise straight arms from the level of the hips to over the head and touch floor above head. Keep hands relaxed as they touch the floor above the head and at the hips.

7. With hands under buttocks for support, lift flexed legs and do a bicycling rotation action for the desired number of times. (Bend and extend legs as much as possible during the bicycling.)

8. With legs bent, move both extended arms in a horizontal arc from the sides of the body to a position above the head and back again. Although extended, the arms should remain relaxed as they complete the desired number of "snow angel" sweeps. If desired, the legs can be extended and also moved apart and back

together again in a synchronized action with the arms to replicate the complete "snow angel" action.

9. Using the hands under the buttocks for support and as cushions if necessary, lift the extended legs and spread them apart and then together to cross over in a scissoring action alternating the leg that is uppermost during the crossing over.

10. With knees bent, scissor the arms across the body at chest level from an outspread position. Extend the fingers of the hands, when the arms are spread at the sides of the body, and then curl the fingers into a fist, when the arms are crossed over the body.

11. Extending both legs, bend one knee at a time to bring it close to chest level and keep it there for two seconds. Return leg to extended position and repeat with alternate leg. (When the knee is at chest level, the hands may be used to pull the leg closer to the chest.)

12. With knees bent and arms in an outspread relaxed position, embrace yourself with your arms at chest level as tightly as possible and hold before relaxing. Then lower them to a relaxed outspread position.

13. Extend legs, then bend one knee and reach over the other leg as far as possible. With the bent knee allow the lower back to rotate. Bring the leg back to the extended position and repeat the action with the other leg, and complete a rotation to the other side. During the action of the legs, brace the upper body with arms spread out at the sides.

14. Lying on the left side, with the left hand supporting the right shoulder in the side position, swing the extended upper leg to the front of the body and the extended right arm back from the body. Then reverse the action of the extended arm and leg. Repeat the alternate extended arm and leg swings for the desired number of times.

15. Roll over on the right side and support the left shoulder with the right hand. Then repeat the alternate extended arm and leg swings from the previous exercise for the left arm and leg.

16. Roll back to the left side, supporting the body with the left hand, and rotate the upper arm and leg in unison in a horizontal plane and starting with a forward and downward action. Extend the arm and leg fully at the lower part of the circle and bend as fully as possible at the upper part of the circle.

17. Roll over to the right side and repeat the rotational circling by using the left arm and leg as in the previous exercise.

18. Roll back onto the left side and, with the lower leg bent and the

body supported by the left arm, raise and lower the extended upper arm and leg above the side of the body.

19. Roll back onto the right side and repeat the sideways raising and lowering of the upper arm and leg.

20. On the back with legs extended together, lift bent knees and then separate legs to a side spread-extended position. Then bring the legs back to the original position. Repeat the action slowly and smoothly. (This is a frog kick action.)

21. On back with knees bent and both arms extended, move arms in full sweeping circles in an up, out, down, and in action allowing the circles to overlap above the body.

22. Keeping the feet on the floor with knees bent, and hands firmly under the buttocks, separate knees and bring them back together again. Use a controlled action and do not let knees "flop" back and forth.

23. On the back with knees bent, place the hands under the head and relax the shoulders, allowing arms to rest on the floor. Bring the bent arms up to touch the head and lower back to the floor again.

24. On the back in bent knee position, with arms spread out to the side for support, raise the hips up as far as possible, hold and then lower to floor again.

25. Using both hands, with extended fingers, massage the scalp and ears with rotary motions for a period of approximately one minute.

26. In a back reclining position, lift the legs and curl the back to bring the feet over the head. Place hands under hips and, with upper arms, support the body. Do bicycling and/or extended-leg scissoring actions with legs.

27. From the previous curled body position, embrace the back of your knees with forearms. Use a forward and upward momentum so as to uncurl upper body in order to roll into a sitting position.

Discard the cushion.

28. In sitting position with arms extended over head, bend the upper body over the knees. With the hands rub the lower leg up and down from the knees to the ankles.

29. In sitting position, do an alternate hand-to-toe touch. If you cannot reach the toe, the hand should be extended as far as possible towards the toe. Finish the desired number of repetitions in a sitting position.

30. Sit with one leg extended, and the other leg bent with the foot

placed to the outside of the extended leg. The hand on the same side as the extended leg is placed on the ankle of the bent leg. The cupped fingers of the other hand are stroked in a front-to-back arc on the carpet. This movement causes the trunk to twist, and the stroking of the nails on the carpet acts as a stimulant to circulation. After the desired number of repetitions, reverse the leg and arm position, and repeat the stroking action.

31. On the back with legs extended, wrap the arms around the body at chest level. Then roll to the left side. Return to the back and continue the rolling action to the right side. Repeat the side-to-side rolls for the desired number of repetitions. Finish the last roll to the side by continuing around to a front-lying position. Use the shoulders only to drive the rolling action.

32. Lying on stomach (front-lying position) with legs extended, place the hands at chest level, and push chest up as far as possible. Arch the back while keeping the hips on the floor. Hold position for several counts before lowering chest to floor (use controlled muscle action–do not let body drop). Repeat for desired number of times.

33. In the front lying position, with legs extended, use the arms to push up chest and hips as far as possible. Hold for several counts before using a muscle-controlled slow return to the floor.

34. In the front lying position, and keeping the entire body extended, use the arms to push up the chest, hips, and knees as far as possible. Hold. Use slow muscle action to lower body to floor. Repeat as desired. A variation of this action is to lift the extended body by using the knees as the contact point with the floor, and elevating only the chest and hips.

35. In the front lying position, pull the knees a few inches forward and keep them on the floor. Raise hip up and hold this position ("cat back") for a few seconds before lowering the hip again.

36. Support the body on the knees and extend arms (crawl position). Then bring one knee up to the chest and hold before returning to the floor. Repeat by bringing the other knee up to the chest.

37. From the hands and knees position, move your hips back until they touch your heels, sinking your chest toward the floor (not moving your hands), bounce once and return to hands and knees position.

38. From the hands and knees position, extend one leg out backwards ("mule kick position") and hold for several counts. Before returning knee to floor, repeat action using the alternate leg. Repeat sequence desired number of times.

39. From the hands and knees position, extend one arm and the alternate leg and balance for several counts. Return knee and hand to the floor and extend the opposite arm and leg in the alternate action. Repeat sequence for desired number of times.
40. In a front-lying position, lift your lower legs to a vertical position and perform the following exercises:
    a) Flex your ankles as much as possible, then do alternate leg lowering and raising—touch toes to the floor.
    b) Extend your ankles as much as possible, then do alternate leg lowering and raising—touch toes to the floor.
41. In a front-lying position with your legs in a vertical position, alternately move your ankles up and down.
42. In the same position circle your feet inward toward each other. Then circle your feet outward to each other.
43. From hands and knees support position, use arms to support the body while both feet are brought up under the body close to the arms. Use a push from the arms and an extension of the legs to stand up in a relaxed position. (Do NOT lock knees when standing.)
44. In a standing position with arms extended at chest level in front of the body, swing arms apart to sides in a horizontal plane as far as possible, and then back to the center. Repeat as desired.
45. With hands down at sides, swing extended arms to cross behind back as far as possible. Then swing them up in an arc to cross over above the head. Repeat as desired.
46. With arms extended out to the sides of the body at shoulder height, rotate arms in a clockwise direction. Start with small circles then increasing to larger circles to the full extent of shoulder rotation. Repeat sequence of rotations in a counter-clockwise direction.
47. With arms straight and starting in down position, circle arms across the body and over the head in full arm swings. After completing the desired number of repetitions, repeat swings in the opposite direction.
48. With upper arm at shoulder level at side of body, elbow bent at 90 degrees, and the hands curled in a fist, rotate the elbows in a forward direction for two cycles. Then, starting with fists at chest level, pull the elbows back to the sides of the body in a horizontal direction two times. Repeat entire sequence desired times.
49. Gradually bend the upper body forward as you swing hanging arms backward. Increase the forward body bend and backward swing of the arms until upper body is parallel to the floor.
50. With hands on shoulders and elbows out towards the sides of the

body, lift the elbows up to touch the side of the head and return to shoulder level position. Repeat desired times.

51. Bend over slowly and let arms hang relaxed in front of body. Swing arms in a scissoring motion in front of thighs and continue the return arc swinging arms sideways up to above the body. Let the momentum of the upward swing of the arms straighten the trunk to an upright position. Repeat the down and up swings and coordinate the bending and extension of the trunk with the arm action.

52. With right arm curved above head and left arm curled behind the body, bend the trunk to the left reaching with both hands as far as possible to the left and bounce. Change position of the arms and trunk in a right direction and repeat movement to that side. Repeat entire sequence desired times.

53. With arms at chest level and hands clasped together (fingers in opposite direction), swing arms from one side of the body to the other. Let the trunk rotate with the swinging action.

54. With hands on hips and elbows pointed away from the sides of the body, bend trunk first to the right and then to the left. Repeat as desired.

55. With hands on hips, rotate the trunk from left to right allowing the trunk to bend to approximately 90 degrees when in the forward position. After desired number of repetitions, repeat rotation in opposite direction.

56. Stand straight and lift one arm to stretch hand as far as possible above head. Hold for two counts while shaking your fingers and hands vigorously. Repeat stretching action with other arm and repeat entire sequence desired times.

57. In a standing position with arms at sides, swing both arms forward and up to reach above the head, then back down to the sides again. From a full sole foot support position, use the upward momentum of the arms to raise up on the toes. When the arms are extended above the head, the fingers and hands should be shaken. Coordinate the foot support with the position of the arms in further repetitions.

58. Place feet apart for stability and, from a standing position, bend forward gradually to bring hands as closely as possible to the floor (touch toes to floor if possible). A slight bounce while reaching for the toes helps give better bend. Return to standing position and repeat desired times.

59. With feet apart, bend over slowly and swing relaxed arms backward between legs. Using a bouncing action at the backward position of the swing will increase the amount of swing. Return

to front leaning relaxed arm position for upward part of swing and then repeat sequence desired times.

60. With feet apart and forward bent position with arms hanging in front of body, swing extended arms out to the sides and then up and back as far as possible. Using a bounce action on the back position increases the amount of backward flexibility. Return arms to forward hanging position and repeat sequence desired times.

61. In the bent forward position with arms stretched out towards the sides of the body, swing arms behind back to cross over as much as possible behind back. Repeat as desired.

62. From an upright position, bend forward and, using the right hand, touch the right leg as far down as possible. A bouncing action at the lowest point can increase the reach. Repeat action using the left hand to touch the left leg.

63. From an upright position, bend forward and touch one leg as far down as possible with the opposite arm. Return to upright position and repeat with alternate arm. Then repeat sequence desired times.

64. From upright position with arms raised to the sides at shoulder height, bend to touch the outside of your right knee with your right hand. Then continue the bend to touch your right ankle. Repeat the same action on your left side.

65. Raise up from bent position in previous exercise with both arms straight in front of body and continue arm swings to full stretch position when upright. Breathe in deeply on upward swing of arms. Lower extended arms in front of body and exhale with lowering of arms. Coordinate inhalation and exhalation with the raising and lowering of arms for 10 breaths.

66. With hands clasped together and extended above head, circle the entire body in a clockwise direction. Legs should be spread and knees kept slightly bent to provide balance during rotation. After desired number of rotations repeat in opposite direction.

67. Turn trunk to the right and swing both arms down and past the right side of the body in a circle action for two circles. Repeat circling action twice on left side with trunk turned to the left. Repeat sequence and use bouncing action in transition from one side to the other.

68. With the trunk bent forward and arms hanging loosely in front of body, swing arms to the right and then to the left in as full an arc as possible, so that the trunk rotates and the momentum of the swing carries the trunk towards the upright position.

69. In the upright position with arms stretched out at sides and at

shoulder height, twist the body and arms first to the right and then to the left. Repeat the sequence the desired times.

70. In upright position, swing both arms down in front of the body then up on alternate sides of the body. Allow the trunk to rotate with the swing and the momentum of the swing to raise the body on its toes at the height of the swing.

71. With hands on hips, rotate the hips in a clockwise circle (hula action) for the desired times and repeat the rotary action in a counter-clockwise direction. Keep knees bent for balance and mobility.

72. Jog on the spot or walk around the house on your toes for about three minutes, lifting the knees as high as possible and keeping the arms and hands relaxed at sides.

73. Go to a firm table or counter. Put one extended leg on the table and reach forward with the hand on the same side as the extended leg touching the toes twice (grasp edge of table with other hand for support). Change to alternate leg and arm position and repeat action.

74. With right leg extended on table (and using right hand for support) reach across right leg with left hand to touch table twice (as close to toe area as possible). Change to alternate leg and hand. Repeat reach across twice.

75. With hand holding firmly onto edge of table or counter and in a standing position, bend both knees and straighten to a standing position (moderate knee bends only). Repeat as desired.

76. Standing and holding onto the edge of the table for balance, do the following neck exercises repeating each the desired number of times:
    a) Move head up and down.
    b) Turn head from side to side in upright position.
    c) Lean head from side to side.
    d) Rotate head counterclockwise.
    e) Rotate read clockwise.
    f) Alternately rotate head clockwise, then counterclockwise.

77. While standing (hands on hips increases balance difficulty), do the following jaw exercises repeating each the desired number of times:
    a) Open mouth as far as possible then close (breathe out when mouth is open and inhale through nose when mouth is closed; use deep breaths).
    b) Move jaw slowly from side to side as far as possible.

Glossary

acetabulum   cup-shaped socket of the hip which holds the head of the femur

acoustopalpebral   blinking of the eyes in response to a sudden sound

adenine   a chemical compound found in DNA where it is associated with thymine and in RNA where it is associated with uracil

adrenergic   stimulated or activated by epinephrine

aerobic   having molecular oxygen present

agonist   a muscle that is active in a movement

Ahlfeld breathing movements   movements similar to respiration occurring prior to birth

alimentary   digestive tract

alleles   alternate forms of a gene occupying corresponding sites on homologous chromosomes

amenorrhea   absence or abnormal stoppage of menses

amniocentesis   the removal of amniotic fluid prior to birth

amniotic fluid   the fluid which is enclosed in the amnion (a protective covering for the fetus)

anabolic   the growth aspects of metabolism

androgens   male hormones

androgynic   a type of body build classification based on a masculine-feminine scale

anomaly   an irregular, or abnormal, condition

antagonist   a muscle which is located in opposition to a moving muscle

anthropometric   various body measures, e.g., calf girth

atypical   not usual

auditory   hearing

autism   developmental language disorder and social adjustment problems

aversive   to be avoided

axillary   pertaining to the armpit

axon   the long branch on a nerve

biepicondylar   widest part of the bone at joints

biochemical specificity   a change in chemical structure which results in greater differentiation or specificity

bipedal   using two legs

blastocyst   stage in development of human zygote at the end of second week of pregnancy

brachyphalangy   an inherited condition in which the middle joint of the fingers is greatly shortened

455

Caesarean section removal of fetus through the abdominal wall

castrate remove testicles

catabolic the destructive aspects of metabolism

catalytic proteins those proteins which assist a chemical process but are not changed by that chemical process

caudal pertaining to the foot region

central gyrus the central convolution of the cerebral cortex

centromere the organizing segment of a chromosome which is the last part to split during meiosis

cephalic pertaining to the head region

cephalocaudal from head to foot

cerebellum an area off the upper brain stem controlling coordination of movement

cerebral cortex the uppermost area of the brain

cervical area of the spine in the shoulder region at the base of the neck

chemoaffinity an affinity for specific chemical substances

cholinergic stimulated, activated, or transmitted by choline

chromatid reconstituted portion of the DNA chain (chromonemata) during the first phase of meiosis

chromatin material within the nucleus of the cell

chromonemata segment of the chromosome that splits during first phase of meiosis

chromosome a strand of DNA that is composed of many segments (genes) which have specific functions in reproduction and cell maintenance

chronological in sequence: usually refers to a time sequence

cinematographic photographic film

collagen a main supportive protein of skin, tendon, bone, cartilage, and connective tissue

colostrum the thin, yellow, milky fluid secreted by the mammary gland a few days before or after parturition

commissural neurons connecting neurons

concave a hollow shape

congenital a condition appearing at birth

contralateral opposite side

controls a statistical term referring to subjects who do not have the same treatment as other subjects being studied

corpuscle a type of cell body

correlation coefficient a statistical method for determining relationship

cortical pertaining to the cerebral cortex

cretinism a congenital condition resulting from a deficiency of maternal thyroxine; symptoms include arrested physical and mental development

crossing over the process whereby there is an exchange of DNA between two similar chromosomes so that the genetic structure of the resulting chromosomes is not exactly the same as the original
cutaneous of the skin
cytoplasm the nonchromosomal material in the egg cell
cytosine a chemical compound found in DNA

damping depressing the effect of
defecation bowel movement
desmosomes attachments between similar cells
diploid number the number of chromosomes in a cell before reduction division
DNA Deoxyribonucleic acid—the material in the chromosomes of all living organisms
dominant gene one of a pair of genes that has an effect in development
dorsal the area towards the back
ductus arteriosus a blood vessel connecting the pulmonary artery to the aorta during prenatal life
dynamometer an instrument for measuring the static strength of hand grip
dyslexia inability to read with understanding
dystonia disordered tonicity of muscle

ectoderm one of the early cellular differentiations during the embryonic period
efferent going away from the central nervous system
egestion casting out of material that is indigestible
elongation the process by which amino acids are joined together to form protein
embryonic period from the second to the eighth week of pregnancy; the developing organism is called an embryo at this stage
endoderm one of the early cellular differentiations during the embryonic period
endomysium the covering of a muscle fiber
enzyme a protein that acts as a messenger or catalyst
epimysium covering of an entire muscle
epiphysis layer of cells below the cartilage at the ends of a bone where longitudinal bone growth occurs
equivocal having an uncertain meaning
erythroblastosis a condition in which the red blood cells do not mature properly; i.e., retain a nucleus

estrogen   female hormone

eugenics   applied science of heredity concerned with improvement of human stock

eumenorrhea   normal menstruation

eunuch   a castrated male person

extensor   a muscle which acts to increase the angle of a joint

factor analysis   a statistical method for identifying groups of things that are related to each other

fasciculi   primary bundles of muscles

fauna   animal life

femur   the bone in the thigh

fetal period   from the second month after fertilization to birth during pregnancy; the developing organism is called a fetus at this stage

fetoscopy   the withdrawal of a small sample of blood from the fetus

fibroblasts   embryonic connective tissue cells

flexor   a muscle which acts to cause a joint to decrease its angle

flora   plant life

foramen ovale   an opening between the atria of the heart during prenatal life

gamete   general term given to mature egg and sperm

gamma globulin   a compound in blood

ganglion   a cluster of neurons

gastrocnemius   a muscle in the calf of the leg

gene   segment of a chromosome which has a specific function

genotype   the type of genes in an individual

germinal cell   immature cell in the reproductive organs which mature into sperm in the male and into an egg in the female

germinal period   the first two weeks of pregnancy after fertilization

gerontology   the study of the aging process

guanine   a chemical compound found in DNA

guanosine triphosphate   a chemical compound that releases energy

gustatory   taste

glycolytic   promotes glycolysis (breaking down of sugars into simpler compounds)

gyrus centralis   the central convolution of the cerebral cortex

haploid number   the number of chromosomes in a germ cell after reduction division

haptic system   interaction of tactile and kinesthetic senses

hemotrophic from the blood

heredity the tendency to be like one's parents

heritability contribution to population variance by genetic differences among individuals

histone a chemical compound in the nucleus of the cell

homogeneous having the same consistency

homologous cells cells having the same relationship

humerus the bone of the upper arm

hyaline membrane disease a condition resulting when the lining of the lungs is immature

induction the process whereby a chemical compound causes changes in another structure

inhibit to depress or stop

inner cell mass collection of cells in blastocyst that contain the embryonic disc

interfacial area between body cells walls

interstitial fluid fluid located between cell walls

intrinsic within an organism

in utero within the uterus

in vitro under laboratory conditions

ipsilateral same side

isometric does not involve movement; static

isotonic involves movement; dynamic

karyotype the chromosomal array for any individual

ketosteroids a steroid found in the urine of normal men and women

linearity a line shape

lipofuscin a class of fatty pigments

lumbo-sacral area of the spine in the hip region toward the base of the spine

lumbrical a muscle in the lower back

lysosomal pertaining to a lysosome, which is a minute body in many types of cells

medulla a specific segment of the brain stem

meiosis the process of cell division during which the number of chromosomes in each of the two resulting cells is reduced to one-half that of the original cell

menarche the first menstrual period

mesoderm one of the early cellular differentiations during the embryonic period

methyl testosterone an androgenic compound used like testosterone, which is a male hormone

micturition excretion of urine

mitochondria a structure in the cell which is associated with energy production

mitosis the process whereby cells divide

monovular coming from one egg

Moro response reaching out and then pulling in the limbs in response to strong stimulus

morphogenic the form, or shape, of a species

morphological the biological form or shape

mortality rate the rate at which people die; usually based upon the proportion per 1,000 individuals

morula spherical cluster of cells during the germinal period

multiple regression analysis a statistical technique for assessing relationships between a dependent and a number of independent variables

mutation a change in a gene which causes the gene to have a different effect thereafter

myoblasts embryonic muscle cells

neuroblasts immature nerve cells

neurotransmitter biochemical substance that transmits a neural impulse across a synaptic junction

nonhistone a chemical compound in the nucleus of the cell

notochord an early embryonic developmental organizer

nystagmus involuntary rapid movement of the eyeball

olfactory smell

ontogenetic the developmental characteristics of the individual

oögenesis the process whereby an egg is formed in the ovary of the female

operator gene controls the functioning of other genes

organella small structures, usually within the cell

osmosis (osmotic) the process whereby fluids pass through a cell wall

osteoblasts cells associated with the production of bone

osteoclasts cells associated with absorption and removal of bone

osteoporosis demineralization of bone

ovary   female reproductive organ
ovum   a human egg cell

palpebral response   blinking of eyelids
parabiotic   derived from the same fertilized egg
perception   the action by which the mind recognizes sensory inputs
perimysium   the covering of a small bundle of muscles
peripheral   outer parts or away from the center
phenotype   refers to appearance, physical or chemical properties, and/or behavior of an organism
phosphorylation   a chemical process
phylogenetic   the developmental characteristics of the species
plantar   the sole of the foot
plantigrade   on both hands and both feet
platysma   a muscle in the neck
polar bodies   female germ cells which do not have a nutrient protoplasm as does the egg
polarity of cell   the point in the cell to which chromosomes are drawn during the division process
ponderal   length or height of individual
pons   an area of the upper brain stem
primitive streak   believed to organize early embryonic development
primordial   primitive form or time period
prophase   the first stem or division, during meiosis
proprioceptors   internal sensory end organs which provide movement and position sensations
proteolipid   a combination of protein with a lipid
protoplasm   that portion of the cell which does not contain the nucleus
proximal-distal   from the center to the outside or extremities
punctiform   sharp point; prick
pupillary response   change in the size of the pupil of the eye in response to light changes
pursuit rotor   a piece of equipment used to test eye-hand coordination

recessive gene   one that does not have an effect in the presence of a dominant gene of the same type
reciprocal innervation   neural connections which result in inhibition of antagonist muscles during movement
regression   a statistical method for determining relationships
replication   the process whereby DNA reproduces itself
repressor   inhibits the other genes, especially the operator genes

Rh factor a blood component which appears in some individuals and not in others

rhogam gamma globulin from blood of Rh negative individuals sensitized to Rh factor

ribosome a structure in the cell which is associated with energy production

RNA Ribonucleic acid is a derivative of DNA and is operational in the production of proteins

roentgenograph X-ray

Rolandic zone area of the cerebral cortex of the brain

sartorius a muscle in the thigh

senescence the process or condition of growing old

skeletal age age calculation based upon maturation rate of the skeleton

socioeconomic status status based upon the social level and income of the individual and often closely associated with the occupation of the individual

somatic of the body

somatosensory sensory input from the body

somatotype classification based on body build

somites structures that appear along the back during the embryonic period

sonography the use of ultra sound to develop images of internal structures

spermatogenesis the process whereby sperms are formed in the male

stapedius a muscle in the ear which dampens the action of the stapes

striated having stripes

structural genes produce messenger RNA

subcutaneous below the skin surface

subscapular below the scapula (shoulder blade)

suprailiac above the upper front tip of the ilium (hip bone)

surfactant the coating of the lining of the lungs

symptomatology study of symptoms

synapse the connection point of two neurons

tactile the sense of touch

tensiometer an instrument for measuring static strength of muscle groups in the body

testes male reproductive organs

thalidomide a tranquilizer that caused birth defects

thymine a chemical compound found in DNA

thymus-lymphatic system an immunity system of the body

thyroxine   a hormone involved in metabolism and secreted by the thyroid gland

tibialis anterior   a muscle in the front of the lower leg

titre   a quantity of a substance required to produce a reaction of a given quantity of another substance

tonic neck response   extension of arm on side to which head is turned and flexion of other arm

transcription   the process whereby DNA produces RNA

transection   cutting of

translation   the process whereby RNA produces protein

traumatization   injury

triceps   an extensor muscle of the upper arm

trophoblast   outer cell covering of the blastocyst

ulnar   on the little finger side of the forearm

ulnar-radial   from the little finger to the thumb side

ulno-carpal   on the little finger side and associated with the fingers

uracil   a chemical compound derived by the addition of oxygen to thymine and found in RNA

vastocrureus   a muscle in the leg of a cat

vestibular   associated with balance; inner ear organ

viability   capable of sustaining life functions

visuopalpebral   blinking of the eyes in response to a sudden flash of light

zygote   a fertilized human egg cell

Bibliography

AAHPER youth fitness test manual. Washington, D.C.: American Association for Health, Physical Education and Recreation, 1961.

Abbs, J. H.; Gracco, V. L.; & Cole, K. J. Control of multimovement coordination: Sensorimotor mechanisms in speed motor programming. *J. Motor Behav.*, 1984, *16*, 195-232.

Acheson, R. M. A method of assessing skeletal maturity from radio-graphs. A report from the Oxford Child Health Survey. *J. Anat.*, 1954, *88*, 498-508.

———, Dupertuis, C. W., The relationship between physique and rate of skeletal maturation in boys. *Hum. Biol.*, 1957, *29*, 167-193.

Acredolo, C.; Adams, A.; & Schmid, J. On the understanding of the relationships between speed, duration, and distance. *Child Develpm.*, 1984, *55*, 2151-2159.

Aghemo, P.; Gesell, D.; & Mangili, F. The relation of work performance to heart rate in aged man. *Gerontologia*, 1964, *9*, (2), 91-97.

Aloia, J. F.; Cohn, S. H.; Babu, T.; Abesamis, C.; Kalici, N.; & Ellis, K. Skeletal mass and body composition in marathon runners. *Metabolism*, 1978a, *27*, 1793-1796.

Aloia, J. F.; Cohn, S. H.; Ostuni, J. A.; Cane, R.; & Ellis, K. Prevention of involutional bone loss by exercise. *Annals of Intern. Med.*, 1978b, *89*, 356-358.

Altose, M. D.; Leitner, J.; & Cherniack, N. S. Effects of age and respiratory efforts on the perception of resistive ventilatory loads. *J. Geron.*, 1985, *40*, 147-153.

Ames, L. B. The sequential patterning of prone progression in the human infant. *Genet. Psych. Monogr.*, 1937, *19*, 409-460.

———. Development of interpersonal smiling responses in the preschool years. *J. Genet. Psych.*, 1949, *74*, 273-291.

Aniansson, A.; Grimby, G.; Rundgren, A.; Svanborg, A.; & Orlander, J. Physical training in old men. *Age and Ageing*, 1980, *9*, 186-187.

Apgar, V. A. A proposal for a new method of evaluation of the newborn infant. *Current Researches in Anaesth. and Analg.*, 1960, *32*, 260.

Arp, D. Swimming called No. 1 sport at LW. *The Register* (Leisure World), 1985, April 9, 1, 4.

Ashley Montagu, M. F. *Adolescent sterility. A study in the comparative physiology of the infecundity of the adult organism in mammals and man*. Springfield: Charles C. Thomas, 1946.

———. *Prenatal influences*. Springfield: Charles C. Thomas, 1962.

Aslin, R. N.; Pisoni, D. B.; & Jusczyk, P. W. Auditory development and speech perception in infancy. In M. M. Haith & J. J. Campos (Eds.), *Infancy and developmental psychobiology*. Volume II of P. H. Mussen (Ed.), *Handbook of child psychology*. New York: John Wiley & Sons, 1983.

Atkinson, R. K. A study of athletic ability of high school girls, *Amer. Phys. Educ. Rev.*, 1925, *30*, 389-399.

Austin, C. R. Sperm fertility, viability and persistence in the female tract. *J. Reprod. Fert.*, 1975, Suppl. *22*, 75-89.

Bachman, J. C. Motor learning and performance as related to age and sex in two measures of balance coordination. *Res. Quart*, 1961, *32*, 123-137.

Bailey, D. A.; Malina, R. M.; & Rasmussen, R. L. The influence of exercise, physical activity, and athletic performance on the dynamics of human growth. In F. Falkner & J. M. Tanner (Eds.), *Human growth (Vol. 2). Postnatal growth*. New York: Plenum Press, 1978.

Bailey, S. W. An experimental study of the origin of lateral-line structures in embryonic and adult teleosts. *J. Exp. Zool.*, 1937, *76*, 187-234.

Baird, D. The influence of social and economic factors on stillbirths and neonatal deaths. *J. Obstet. Gynaec. (Brit).*, 1945, *527*, 217-234.

Bakwin, H. & Bakwin, R. M. Body build in infants: II. The proportions of the external dimensions of the healthy infant during the first year of life. *J. Clin. Invest.*, 1931, *10*, 377-394.

———, & ———. Growth of thirty-two external dimensions during the first year of life. *J. Pediat.*, 1936, *8*, 177-183.

———, & Patrick, T. W. The weight of Negro infants. *J. Pediat.*, 1944, *24*, 405-407.

Baldwin, B. T. Anthropometric measurements. In L. M. Terman (Ed.), *Genetic studies of genius. Mental and physical traits of a thousand gifted children* (Vol. 1). Palo Alto: Stanford University Press, 319.

Balke, B. Exercise and arthropathy. In H. M. Eckert & H. J. Montoye (Eds.), *Exercise and Health. The Academy Papers*. Champaign, IL: Human Kinetics, 1984.

Ballantyne, J. W. & Browne, F. J. The problems of foetal postmaturity and prolongation of pregnancy. *J. Obstet. Gynaec. Brit. Emp.*, 1922, 29, 177-238.

Banks, M. S., & Salapatek, P. Infant visual perception. In M. M. Haith & J. J. Campos (Eds.), *Infancy and developmental psychobiology*, Vol. II of P. H. Mussen (Ed.), *Handbook of child psychology*. New York: John Wiley & Sons, 1983.

Barcroft, J.; Barton, D. H.; Cowie, A. T.; & Forsham, P. H. The oxygen supply of the foetal brain of the sheep and the effect of asphyxia on foetal respiratory movement. *J. Physiol.*, 1940, 97, 338-346.

_____, & Karvonen, M. J. Action of carbon dioxide and cyanide on fetal respiratory movements: Development of chemo-reflex in sheep. *J. Physiol. (London)*, 1948, 107, 153-161.

Barker, R. G., & Stone, C. P. Physical development in relation to menarcheal age in university women. *Hum. Biol.*, 1936, 8, 198-222.

Barnes, L. L.; Sperling, G.; & McCay, C. M. Bone growth in normal and retarded growth rats. *J. Geron.*, 1947, 2, 240-243.

Barry, A. J., & Cureton, T. K. Factorial analysis of physique and performance in prepubescent boys. *Res. Quart.* 1961, 32, 283-300.

Barsanti, R. A. The relationship between leg strength and performance of elementary school girls in the dash and standing broad jump. Unpublished master's thesis, University of Wisconsin, Madison, 1954.

Bass, R. An analysis of the components of tests of semi-circular canal function and of static and dynamic balance. *Res. Quart.*, 1939, 10, 33-52.

Bayer, M., & Bayley, N. *Growth diagnosis*. Chicago: University of Chicago Press, 1959.

Bayley, N. A scale of motor development. Unpublished paper, Institute of Child Welfare, University of California, Berkeley (n.d.).

_____. The development of motor abilities during the first three years. *Monogr. Soc. Res. Child Develpm.*, 1935, 1 (1), 1-26.

_____. *The California Infant Scale of Motor Development*. Berkeley: University of California Press, 1936.

_____. Size and body build of adolescents in relation to rate of skeletal maturing. *Child Developm.*, 1943, 14, 47-90.

_____. Some psychological correlates of somatic androgeny. *Child Develpm.*, 1951, 22 (1), 45-60.

_____, & Bayer, L. M. The assessment of somatic androgyny. *Amer. J. Phys. Anthrop.*, 1946, 4 N.S., 433-461.

_____, & Davis, F. C. Growth changes in bodily size and proportions during the first three years: A developmental study of sixty-one children by repeated measurements. *Biometrika*, 1935, 27, 26-87.

Beasley, W. C. Visual pursuit in 109 white and 142 Negro newborn infants. *Child Develpm.*, 1933, 4, 106-120.

Beckwith, L., & Parmelee, A. H. EEG patterns of preterm infants, home environment, and later IQ. *Child Develpm.*, 1986, 57, 777-789.

Behnke, A. R., & Wilmore, J. H. *Evaluation and regulation of body build and composition*. Englewood Cliffs, N.J.: Prentice-Hall, Inc., 1974.

Belloc, N. B. Relationship of health practices and mortality. *Prevent. Med.*, 1973, 2, 67-81.

Belloc, N. B., & Breslow, L. Relationship of physical health status and health practices. *Preventive Medicine*, 1972, 1, 409-421.

Berger, R. Effect of varied weight training programs on strength. *Res. Quart.*, 1962, 33, (2), 168-181.

_____. Comparison between static training and various dynamic training programs. *Res. Quart.*, 1963, 34 (2), 131-135.

Berry, W. T. C.; Cowin, P. J.; & Magee, H. E. Haemoglobin levels in adults and children. *Brit. Med. J.*, 1952, 1, 410-412.

Birch, H. G., & Lefford, A. Visual differentiation, intersensory integration, and voluntary motor control. *Monograms of the Society for Res. in Child Develpm.*, 1967, 32 (2), Serial No. 110.

Birren, J. E.; Bick, M. W.; & Fox, C. Age changes in the light threshold of the dark adapted eye. *J. Geront.*, 1948, 3, 267-271.

_____; Riegel, K. F.; & Morrison, D. F. Age differences in response speed as a function of controlled variations of stimulus conditions: Evidence of a general speed factor. *Gerontologia*, 1962, 6 (1), 1-18.

Bjorksten, J. Aging, primary mechanism. *Gerontologia*, 1963, 8, (2/3), 179-192.

Blanton, M. G. The behavior of the human infant during the first thirty days of life. *Psychol. Rev.*, 1917, 24, 456-483.

Boas, E. P., & Goldschmidt, E. F. *The Heart Rate*. Springfield: Charles C Thomas, 1932.

Bojlen, K., & Bentzon, W. Seasonal variation in the occurrence of menarche. *Danish Med. Bull.*, 1974, *21*, 161-168.

Bolaffio, M., & Artom, F. Richerche sulla fisiologia del sistema nervosa del feto umano. *Arch. Sci. Biol.*, 1924, *5*, 457-487.

Bolk, L. Untersuchungen über die Menarche bei der niederlandischen Bevolkerung. *Z. Geburtsh. Gynak.*, 1926, *89*, 364-380.

Booth, T.; Phillips, D.; Barritt, A.; Berry, S.; Martin, D. N.; & Melotte, C. Patterns of mortality in homes for the elderly. *Age and Ageing*, 1983, *12*, 240-244.

Borgen, J. S., & Corbin, C. B. Eating disorders among female athletes. *The Physician and Sportsmed.*, 1987, *15*, 88-95.

Borkan, G. C.; Hults, D. E.; Gerzof, S. G.; Robbins, A. H.; & Silbert, C. K. Age related changes in body composition revealed by computed tomography. *J. Geront.*, 1983, *38*, 673-677.

Bouchard, C.; Lesage, R.; Lortie, G.; Simoneau, J.; Hamel, P.; Boulay, M. R.; Perusse, L.; Theriault, G.; & Leblanc, C. Aerobic performance in brothers, dizygotic and monozygotic twins. *Med. and Sci. in Sports and Exer.*, 1986, *18*, 639-646.

Bower, T. G. R. Repetitive processes in child development. *Sci. Amer.*, 1976, *235* (5), 38-47.

————. *Human development*. San Francisco: W. H. Freeman and Company, 1979.

Boynton, B. The physical growth of girls: A study of the rhythm of physical growth from anthropometric measurements on girls between birth and eighteen years. *Univ. Iowa Stud. Child Welfare*, 1936, *12* (4), 1-105.

Braun, P. Contribution to the study of postnatal changes in skeletal muscle in man. *Folia Morphologica*, 1967, *15*, 11-17.

Brazelton, T. B. *Neonatal Behavioral Assessment Scale*. Philadelphia: J. B. Lippincott Co., 1973.

Breckenridge, M. E., & Vincent, E. L. *Child development*. Philadelphia: Saunders, 1949.

Breitinger, E. Body form and athletic achievement of youths. (Trans. and cond. by Ernst Thomas.) *Res. Quart.*, 1935, *6*, 83-91.

Bridgman, C. S., & Carmichael, L. An experimental study of the onset of behavior in the fetal guinea-pig. *J. Genet. Psychol.*, 1935, *47*, 247-267.

Broadhead, G. D., & Church, G. E. Movement characteristics of preschool children. *Res. Quart. for Exer. and Sport*, 1985, *56*, 208-214.

Brocklehurst, J. C.; Robertson, D.; & James-Groom, P. Clinical correlates of sway in old age—sensory modalities. *Age and Ageing*, 1982, *11*, 1-10.

Broman, B.; Dahlberg, G.; & Lichtenstein, A. Height and weight during growth. *Acta. Paediat. (Upsala)*, 1942, *30*, 1-66.

Brooks-Gunn, J.; Warren, M. P.; & Hamilton, L. H. The relation of eating problems and amenorrhea in ballet dancers. *Med. and Sci. in Sports*, 1987, *19*, 41-44.

Brouha, L. Heat and the older worker. *J. Amer. Geriat. Soc.*, 1962, *10* (1), 35-39.

Brundtland, G. H., & Walloe, L. Menarcheal age in Norway: Halt in the trend towards earlier maturation. *Nature*, 1973, *241*, 478-479.

Bruner, J. S. Organization of early skilled action. *Child Developm.*, 1973, *44*, 1-11.

Bullen, B. A.; Skrinar, G. B.; Beitins, I. Z.; von Mering, G.; Turnbull, B. A.; & McArthur, J. W. Induction of menstrual disorders by strenuous exercise in untrained women. *New England J. Med.* 1985, *312*, 1349-1353.

Bullock, M.; Gelman, R.; & Baillargeon, R. The development of causal reasoning. In W. Friedman (Ed.), *The developmental psychology of time*. New York: Academic Press, 1982.

Burke, B. S.; Harding, V. V.; & Stuart, H. C. Nutrition studies during pregnancy, relation of protein content of mother's diet during pregnancy to birth weight, length and condition of infant at birth. *J. Pediat.*, 1943, *23*, 506-515.

Burke, W. E.; Tuttle, W. W.; Thompson, C. W.; Janney, C. D.; & Weber, R. J. The relation of grip-strength and grip-strength endurance to age. *J. Appl. Physiol.*, 1953, *5*, 628-630.

Buskirk, E. R. Observations of extraordinary performances in an extreme environment and in a training environment. In D. H. Clarke & H. M. Eckert (Eds.), *Limits of human performance. The Academy Papers*. Champaign, IL: Human Kinetics, 1985.

Cann, C. E.; Martin, M. C.; Genant, H. K.; & Jaffe, R. B. Decreased spinal mineral content in amenorrheic women. *J. Amer. Med. Assoc.*, 1984, *251*, 626-629.

Carlson, A. J., & Ginsburg, H. Contributions to the physiology of the stomach. XXIV. The tonus and hunger contraction of the stomach of the newborn. *Amer. J. Physiol.*, 1915, *38*, 29-32.

Carmichael, L. Ontogenetic development. In Stevens, S. S. (Ed.), *Handbook of experimental psychology*. New York: John Wiley & Sons, Inc., 1951.

_____. The onset and early development of behavior. In L. Carmichael (Ed.), *Manual of child psychology* (2d ed.), New York: John Wiley & Sons, Inc., 1954.

Carpenter, A. The measurement of general motor capacity and general motor ability in the first three grades. *Res. Quart.*, 1942a, *13* (4), 444-465.

_____. Strength in testing in the first three grades. *Res. Quart.*, 1942b, *13*, 328-332.

Carter, J. E. L. Morphological factors limiting human performance. In D. H. Clarke & H. M. Eckert (Eds.), *Limits of human performance. The Academy Papers*. Champaign, IL: Human Kinetics, 1985.

Cavanagh, P. R., & Williams, K. R. The effect of stride length variation on oxygen uptake during distance running. *Med. and Sci. in Sports and Exer.*, 1982, *14*, 30-35.

Cearley, J. E. Linearity of contributions of ages, heights, and weights to prediction of track and field performances. *Res. Quart.*, 1957, *28*, 218-222.

Chugani, H. T. & Phelps, M. E. Maturational changes in cerebral function in infants determined by [18]FDG positron emission tomography. *Science*, 1986, *231*, 840-843.

Clark, J. E., & Phillips, S. J. A developmental sequence of the standing long jump. In J. E. Clark & J. H. Humphrey (Eds.), *Motor development. Current selected research*. Princeton, NJ: Princeton Book, 1985.

Clarke, D. H. Sex differences in strength and fatigability. *Res. Quart. for Exer. and Sport*, 1986, *57*, 144-149.

Clarke, H. H. Strength development and motor-sports improvement. *Physical Fitness Res. D.*, (Series 4, No. 4). Washington, D.C.: President's Council on Physical Fitness and Sports, 1974.

_____. Exercise and aging. *Physical Fitness Res. D.*, (Series 7, No. 2). Washington, D.C.: President's Council on Physical Fitness and Sports, 1977.

_____, & Carter, G. H. Oregon simplification of the strength and physical fitness indices. *Res. Quart.*, 1959, *30*, 3-10.

_____, & Degutis, E. W. Comparison of skeletal ages and various physical and motor factors with the pubescent development of 10, 13, and 16 year old boys. *Res. Quart.*, 1962, *33*, 356-368.

_____, & Harrison, J. C. E. Differences in physical and motor traits between boys of advanced, normal, and retarded maturity. *Res. Quart.*, 1962, *33*, 13-25.

_____; Irving, R. N.; & Heath, B. H. Relation of maturity, structural, and strength measures to the somatotypes of boys 9 through 15 years of age. *Res. Quart.*, 1961, *32*, 449-460.

_____, & Petersen, K. H. Contrast of maturational, structural, and strength characteristics of athletes and nonathletes 10 to 15 years of age. *Res. Quart.*, 1961, *32*, 163-176.

_____; Shay, C. T.; & Mathews, D. K. Strength decrements from carrying various army packs on military marches. *Res. Quart.*, 1955, *26*, 253-265.

Clarke, M. F., & Smith, A. H. Recovery following suppression of growth in the rat. *J. Nutr.*, 1938, *15*, 245-256.

Clayton, I. A. A study of the evidence of motor age based on technique of standing broad jump. Unpublished master's thesis, University of Wisconsin, Madison, 1936.

Coghill, G.E. *Anatomy and the problem of behaviour*. New York: Macmillan, 1929.

_____, & Legner, W. K. Embryonic motility and sensitivity. (Trans. of W. Preyer, *Specielle physiologie des embryo*.) *Monog. Soc. Res. Child Develpm.*, 1937, *2*, 1-115.

Coleman, P. D., & Buell, S. J. Dendritic growth in aging brain? In W. H. Gispen & J. Traber (Eds.), *Aging of the brain*. Amsterdam: Elsevier Science Publishers, 1983.

Comfort, Alex. *Ageing, the biology of senescence*. New York: Holt, Rinehart and Winston, Inc., 1964.

Consensus Conference. Osteoporosis. *J. of the Amer. Med. Assoc.*, 1984, *252*, 799-802.

Conel, J. L. *The postnatal development of the human cerebral cortex. Vol. I, The cortex of the newborn*. Cambridge: Harvard University Press, 1939.

_____. *The postnatal development of the human cerebral cortex. Vol. II. The cortex of the one-month infant*. Cambridge: Harvard University Press, 1941.

Cooley, D. G. Medicines of tomorrow. *Today's Health*, November 1963, 38-42.

Cooper, J. M., & Glassow, R. B. *Kinesiology*. St. Louis: C. V. Mosby Co., 1963.

Cooper, L. Z. German measles. *Sci. Amer.*, 1966, *215* (1), 30-37.

Corbin, K. B., & Gardner, E. D. Decrease in number of myelinated fibers in human spinal roots with age. *Anat. Rec.*, 1937, *68*, 63-74.

Corey, E. L. Causative factors of the initial inspiration of the mammalian fetus. *Anat. Rec.*, 1931, *48* (Suppl.), 41.

Cornelius, S. W. Classic pattern of intellectual aging: Test familiarity, difficulty, and performance. *J. of Geront.*, 1984, *39*, 201-206.

Coronios, J. D. Development of behavior in the fetal cat. *Genet. Psychol. Monogr.*, 1933, *14*, 283-386.

Cowan, E., & Pratt, B. The hurdle jump as a developmental and diagnostic test. *Child Develpm.*, 1934, *5*, 107-121.

Cowan, N.; Suomi, K.; & Morse, P. A. Echoic storage in infant perception. *Child Develpm.*, 1982, *53*, 984-990.

Cratty, B. J. A comparison of fathers and sons in physical ability. *Res. Quart.*, 1960, *31*, 12-15.

Cron, G. W., & Pronko, N. H. Development of the sense of balance in school children. *J. Educ. Research*, 1957, *51*, 33-37.

Croucher, J. S. An analysis of world weightlifting records. *Research Quart. for Exer. and Sport*, 1984, *55*, 285-288.

Crum, J. F., & Eckert, H. M. Play patterns in primary school children. In J. E. Clark & J. H. Humphrey (Eds.), *Motor development. Current selected research*. Princeton, NJ: Princeton Book, 1985.

Cullumbine, H. Oral, rectal and axillary temperatures of adult Ceylonese. *Ceylon J. Med. Sci. D.*, 1949, *6*, 88-90.

Cumbee, F. Z. A factorial analysis of motor co-ordination. *Res. Quart.*, 1954, *25* (4), 412-428.

———; Meyer, M.; & Peterson, G. Factorial analysis of motor coordination variables for third and fourth grade girls. *Res. Quart.*, 1957, *28*, 100-108.

Cureton, K. J.; Hensley, L. D.; & Tiburzi, A. Body fatness and performance differences between men and women. *Res. Quart.*, 1979, *50*, 333-340.

Cureton, T. K., Jr. *Physical fitness of champion athletes*. Urbana: The University of Illinois Press, 1951.

Cutting, J. E.; Proffitt, D. R.; & Kozlowski, L. T. A biomechanical invariant for gait perception. *J. Exper. Psychol.: Human Perception and Performance*, 1978, *4*, 357-372.

Danzinger, L., & Frankl, L. Zum Problem der Funktionsreifung. *Z. Kinderforsch.*, 1934, *43*, 219-254.

Dargassies, S. S. Neurological maturation of the premature infant of 28 to 41 weeks' gestational age. In F. Falkner (Ed.), *Human development*. Philadelphia: W. B. Saunders Company, 1966.

Davies, C. T. M.; Mbelwa, D.; & Dore, C. Physical growth and development of urban and rural East African children, aged 7-16 years. *Annals of Hum. Biol.*, 1974, *1*, 257-268.

Davies, C. T. M., & White, M. J. The contractile properties of elderly human triceps surae. *Gerontology*, 1983, *29*, 19-25.

Davies, P. A., & Stewart, A. L. Low-birthweight infants: Neurological sequelae and later intelligence. *Br. Med. Bull.*, 1975, *31*, 85-91.

———, & Tizard, J. P. M. Low birth weight and subsequent neurological defect. *Dev. Med. Child Neurol.*, 1975, *17*, 3-17.

Dawson, G. Lateralized brain dysfunction in autism; Evidence from the Halstead Reitan Neuropsychological Battery. *J. Autism and Develpm. Disorders*, 1983, *13*, 269-286.

Dawson, G.; Finley, C.; Phillips, S.; & Galpert, L. Hemispheric specialization and language abilities of autistic children. *Child Develpm.*, 1986, *57*, 1440-1453.

Dawson, G.; Warrenburg, S.; & Fuller, P. Cerebral lateralization of individuals diagnosed as autistic in early childhood. *Brain and Language*, 1982, *15*, 353-368.

Dawson, P. M., Hellebrandt, F. A., The influence of aging in man upon his capacity for physical work and upon his cardio-vascular response to exercise. *Amer. J. Physiol.*, 1945, *143*, 420-427.

Deach, D. F. Genetic development of motor skills in children two through six years of age. *Microfilm Abstracts*, 1951, *11*, 287.

Deford, F. Nadia awed ya. *Sports Illus.*, 1976, *45* (5), 28-31.

de Garay, A. L.; Levine, L.; & Carter, J. E. L. *Genetic and anthropological studies of Olympic athletes*. New York: Academic Press, 1974.

Deglin, V. L. Our split brain. *UNESCO Courier*, January 1976, pp. 4-16; 31-32.

Dennis, W. A description and classification of the responses of the newborn infant. *Psychol. Bull.*, 1934, *31*, 5-22.

———. The effect of restricted practice upon the reaching, sitting and standing of two infants. *J. Genet. Psych.*, 1935, *47*, 17-32.

———. Infant development under conditions of restricted practice and of minimum social stimulation: A preliminary report. *J. Genet. Psych.*, 1938, *53*, 149-158.

———. Does culture appreciably affect patterns of infant behavior? *J. Soc. Psychol.*, 1940, *12*, 305-317.

———. Spalding's experiment of the flight of birds repeated with another species. *J. Comp. Psych.*, 1941, *31*, 337-348.

———, & Dennis, M. G. The effect of cradling practices on the age of walking in Hopi children. *J. Genet. Psych.*, 1940, *56*, 77-86.

Desroches, H. F., & Kaiman, B. D. Stability of activity participation in an aged population. *J. Geront.*, 1964, *19* (2), 211-214.

Deupree, R. H., & Simon, J. R. Reaction time and movement time as a function of age, stimulus duration, and task difficulty. *Ergonomics*, 1963, *6* (4), 403-411.

deVries, H. A. Physiological effects of an exercise training regimen upon men aged 52 to 88. *J. Geront.*, 1970, *25*, 325-336.

Diamond, A. M. The life-cycle research productivity of mathematicians and scientists. *J. Geront.*, 1986, *41*, 520-525.

Diettert, G. A. Circulation time in the aged. *J. Amer. Med. Assoc.*, 1963, *183* (12), 1037-1038.

Dill, D. B. Effects of physical strain and high altitudes on the heart and circulation. *Amer. Heart J.*, 1942, *23*, 441-454.

_____; Graybiel, A.; Hurtado, A.; Taquini, A. C. Gaseous exchange in the lungs in old age. *J. Amer. Geriat. Soc.*, 1963, *11* (11), 1063-1076.

_____; Horvath, S. M.; & Craig, F. N. Responses to exercise as related to age. *J. Appl. Physiol.*, 1958, *12*, 195-196.

Dimock, H. S. A research in adolescence. I. Pubescence and physical growth. *Child Develpm.*, 1935, *6*, 177-195.

Dobbing, J. Undernutrition and the developing brain: The use of animal models to elucidate the human problem. In R. Paoletti and A. N. Davison (Eds.), *Chemistry and brain development*. New York: Plenum Press, 1971.

_____, & Smart, J. L. Vulnerability of developing brain and behavior. *Br. Med. Bull.*, 1974, *30*, 164-168.

Dockeray, F. C., & Rice, C. Responses of newborn infants to pain stimulation. *Ohio State Univ. Stud., Contrib. Psychol.*, 1934, *12*, 82-93.

Dodge, P. R.; Prensky, A. L.; & Feigin, R. D. *Nutrition and the developing nervous system*. St. Louis: C. V. Mosby, 1975.

Dontas, A. S.; Jacobs, D. R.; Corondilas, A.; Keys, A.; & Hannan, P. Longitudinal versus cross-sectional vital capacity changes and affecting factors. *J. Geront.*, 1984, *39*, 430-438.

Douday, D., & Tremolières, J. Persistances d'importants deficits de croissance chez les enfants d'age scolaire en 1945-46. *Pr. Evnt. Med.*, 1947, *55*, 599-600.

Downing, M. E. Blood pressure of normal girls from 3 to 16 years of age. *Amer. J. Dis. Child.*, 1947, *73*, 293-316.

Drillien, C. M. Abnormal neurological signs in the first year of life in low-birthweight infants: Possible prognostic significance. *Dev. Med. Child Neurol.*, 1972, *14*, 575-584.

Drinkwater, B. L.; Horvath, S. M.; & Wells, C. L. Aerobic power in females, ages 10 to 68. *J. Geront.*, 1975, *30*, 385-394.

Drinkwater, B. L.; Nilson, K.; Chesnut, C. H.; Bremner, W. J.; Shainholtz, S.; & Southworth, M. B. Bone mineral content of amenorrheic and eumenorrheic athletes. *New England J. Med.*, 1984, *311*, 277-281.

Dublin, L. I.; Lotka, A. J.; & Spiegelman, M. *Length of life*. New York: The Ronald Press Company, 1949.

Dummer, G. M.; Clarke, D. H.; Vaccaro, P.; Vander Velden, L.; Goldfarb, A. H.; & Sockler, J. M. Age-related differences in muscular strength and muscular endurance among female masters swimmers. *Res. Quart. for Exer. and Sport*, 1985, *56*, 97-110.

Dupertuis, C. W.; & Hadden, J. A. On the reconstruction of stature from long bones. *Amer. J. Phys. Anthrop.*, 1951, *9*, 15-54.

_____, & Michael, N. B. Comparison of growth in height and weight between ectomorphic and mesomorphic boys. *Child Develpm.*, 1953, *24*, 203-214.

Du Randt, R. Ball-catching proficiency among 4-, 6-, and 8-year-old girls. In J. E. Clark & J. H. Humphrey (Eds.), *Motor development. Current selected research*. Princeton, NJ: Princeton Book, 1985.

Dusenberry, L. A study of the effects of training in ball throwing by children ages three to seven. *Res. Quart.*, 1952, *23*, 9-14.

Dustman, R. E.; Ruhling, R. O.; Russell, E. M.; Shearer, D. E.; Bonekat, H. W.; Shigeoka, J. W.; Wood, J. S.; & Bradford, D. C. Aerobic exercise training and improved neuropsychological function of older individuals. *Neurobio. of Aging*, 1984, *5*, 35-42.

East, W. B., & Hensley, L. D. The effects of selected sociocultural factors upon the overhand-throwing performance of prepubescent children. In J. E. Clark & J. H. Humphrey (Eds.), *Motor development. Current selected research*. Princeton, NJ: Princeton Book, 1985.

Easter, S. S.; Purves, S.; Rakic, P.; & Spitzer, N. C. The changing view of neural specificity. *Science*, 1985, *230*, 507-511.

Eccles, J. The synapse. *Sci. Amer.*, 1965, *212* (1), 56-66.

Eckert, H. M. Linear relationships of isometric strength to propulsive force, angular velocity, and angular acceleration in the standing broad jump. *Res. Quart.*, 1964, *35*, 298-306.

_____. A concept of force-energy in human movement. *J. Amer. Phys. Therapy Assoc.*, 1965, *45*, 213-218.

_____. The effect of added weights on joint actions in the vertical jump. *Res. Quart.*, 1968, *39*, 943-947.

_____. A developmental theory. In H. M. Eckert (Ed.), *Motor development symposium*. Berkeley: University of California, 1971.

_____. Variability in skill acquisition. *Child Develpm.*, 1974, *45*, 487-489.

_____. Physical activity and developmental aspects of aging. In U. Simri (Ed.), *Physical exercise and activity for the aging: Proceedings of an international seminar*. Israel: Wingate Institute for Physical Education and Sport, 1975.

_____, & Day, J. Relationship between strength and work load in push-ups. *Res. Quart.*, 1967, *38*, 380-383.

_____, & Eichorn, D. H. Construct standards in skilled ation. *Child Develpm.*, 1974, *45*, 439-445.

_____, & _____. Developmental variability in reaction time. *Child Develpm.*, 1977, *48*, 452-458.

Edge, J. R.; Millard, F. J. C.; Reid, L.; Path, M. C.; & Simon, G. The radiographic appearances of the chest in persons of advanced age. *Brit. J. Radiol.*, 1964, *37* (442), 769-774.

Edgerton, V. R.; Smith, J. L.; & Simpson, D. R. Muscle fibre type populations of human leg muscles. *Histochemical J.*, 1975, *7*, 259-266.

Edington, D. D. & Edgerton, V. R. *The biology of physical activity*. Boston: Houghton Mifflin Co., 1976.

Eimas, P. D. Developmental aspects of speech perception. In R. Held; H. W. Leibowitz; and H. L. Teuber (Eds.), *Perception*. Berlin: Springer-Verlag, 1978.

Eisdorfer, C., & Wilkie, F. Auditory changes in the aged: A follow-up study *J. Amer. Geriatrics Soc.*, 1972, *20*, 377-382.

Ellis, J. D.; Carron, A. V.; & Bailey, D. A. Physical performance in boys from 10 through 16 years. *Hum. Biol.*, 1975, *47*, 263-281.

Ellis, R. W. B. Growth and health of Belgian children during and after the German occupation, 1940-1944. *Arch. Dis. Childh.*, 1945, *20*, 97-109.

_____. Age of puberty in the tropics. *Brit. Med. J.*, 1950, *1*, 85-89.

Engle, E. T.; Crafts, R. E.; & Zeithaml, C. E. First estrus in rats in relation to age, weight and length. *Proc. Soc. Exp. Biol.* (N.Y.), 1937, *37*, 427-432.

Engleman, D. M. Neutron-scattering studies of the ribosome. *Sci. Amer.*, 1976, *235* (4), 44-54.

Era, P., & Heikkinen, E. Postural sway during standing and unexpected disturbance of balance in random samples of men of different ages. *J. Geront.*, 1985, *40*, 287-295.

Erbaugh, S. J. The relationship of stability performance and the physical growth characteristics of pre-school children. *Res. Quart. for Exer. and Sport*, 1984, *55*, 8-16.

Ermini, M. Ageing changes in mammalian skeletal muscle: Biochemical studies. *Gerontology*, 1976, *22* (4), 301-316.

Epenschade, A. S. Motor performance in adolescence including the study of relationships with measures of physical growth and maturity. *Monogr. Soc. Res. Child Develpm.*, 1940, *5* (1), 1-126.

_____. Development of motor coordination in boys and girls. *Res. Quart.*, 1947, *18*, 30-43.

_____. Motor development. In W. R. Johnson (Ed.), *Science and medicine of exercise and sports*. New York: Harper & Row, Publishers, 1960.

_____. Restudy of relationships between physical performances of school children and age, height, and weight. *Res. Quart.*, 1963, *34* (2), 144-153.

_____; Dable, R. R.; & Schoendube, R. Dynamic balance in adolescent boys. *Res. Quart.*, 1953, *24*, 270-275.

_____, & Meleney, H. E. Motor performances of adolescent boys and girls of today in comparison with those of 24 years ago. *Res. Quart.*, 1961, *32*, 186-189.

Evans, H. J. Structure and organization of the human genome. In G. Obe (Ed.), *Mutations in Man*. Berlin: Springer-Verlag, 1984.

Eveleth, P. B., & Tanner, J. M. *Worldwide variation in human growth*. London: Cambridge University Press, 1976.

Farrar, R. P.; Martin, T. P.; & Ardies, C. M. The interaction of aging and endurance exercise upon the mitochondrial function of skeletal muscle. *J. Geront.*, 1981, *36*, 642-647.

Faucheux, B. A.; Baulon, A.; Poitrenaud, J.; Lille, F.; Moreaux, C.; Dupuis, C.; & Bourliere, F. Heart rate, urinary catecholamines and anxiety responses during mental stress in men in their fifties and seventies. *Age and Ageing*, 1983, *12*, 144-150.

Feldman, M. L., & Peters, A. Morphological changes in the aging brain. In G. J. Maletta (Ed.), *Survey* report on the aging nervous system (DHEW Publication No. (NIH) 74-296). Washington, D.C.: U.S. Government Printing Office (n.d.).

Feldman, W. M. *Principles of antenatal and postnatal child psychology, pure and applied.* New York: Longmans, Green & Co., 1920.

Fenn, W. O.; Brody, H.; & Petrilli, A. The tension developed by human muscles at different velocities of shortening. *Amer. J. Physiol.*, 1931, *97*, 1-14.

Fentress, J. C. The development of coordination. *J. Motor Behav.*, 1984, *16*, 99-134.

Fernie, G. R.; Gryfe, C. I.; Holliday, P. J.; & Llewellyn, A. The relationship of postural sway in standing to the incidence of falls in geriatric subjects. *Age and ageing*, 1982, *11*, 11-16.

Ferris, B. G., & Smith, C. W. Maximum breathing capacity and vital capacity in female children and adolescents. *Pediatrics*, 1953, *12*, 341-352.

_____; Whittenberger, J. L.; & Gallagher, J. R. Maximum breathing capacity and vital capacity of male children and adolescents. *Pediatrics*, 1952, *9*, 659-670.

Fiske, D. W., & Rice, L. Intra-individual response variability. *Psych. Bull.*, 1955, *52*, 217-250.

Fitzgerald, J. E., & Windle, W. F. Some observations on early human fetal movements. *J. Comp. Neurol.*, 1942, *76*, 159-167.

Flavell, J. H. *The developmental psychology of Jean Piaget.* Princeton, N.J.: D. Van Nostrand Co., Inc., 1963.

_____. Concept development. In P. Mussen (Ed.), *Carmichael's manual of child psychology,* New York: John Wiley & Sons, 1970.

Fleishman, A. E. *The structure and measurement of physical fitness.* Englewood Cliffs, N.J.: Prentice-Hall, Inc., 1964.

Fortney, V. L. The kinematics and kinetics of the running pattern of 2-, 4-, and 6-year-old children. *Res. Quart. for Exer. and Sport*, 1983, *54*, 126-135.

Frank, L. K. The cultural patterning of child development. In F. Falkner (Ed.), *Human development.* Philadelphia: W. B. Saunders Co., 1966.

Friedewald, W. T. Physical activity research and coronary heart disease. *Public Health Reports*, 1985, *100*, 115-117.

Frisch, R. E.; Gotz-Welbergen, A. V.; McArthur, J. W.; Albright, T.; Witschi, J.; Bullen, B.; Birnholz, J.; Reed, R. B.; & Hermann, H. Delayed menarche and amenorrhea of college athletes in relation to age of onset of training. *J. Amer. Med. Assoc.*, 1981, *246*, 1559-1563.

Frisch, R. E., & McArthur, J. W. Menstrual cycles: Fatness as a determinant of minimum weight for height necessary for their maintenance or onset. *Science*, 1974, *185*, 949-951.

Frisch, R. E.; Wyshak, G.; & Vincent, L. Delayed menarche and amenorrhea in ballet dancers. *New England J. Med.*, 1980, *303*, 17-19.

Froeschels, E., & Beebe, H. Testing the hearing of newborn infants. *Arch. Otolaryng.*, 1946, *44*, 710-714.

Frolkis, V. V.; Martynenko, O. A.; & Zamostyan, V. P. Aging of the neuromuscular apparatus. *Gerontology*, 1976, *22* (4), 224-279.

Fulop, T.; Worum, I.; Csongor, J.; Foris, G.; & Leovey, A. Body composition in elderly people. I. Determination of body composition by multiisotope method and the elimination kinetics of these isotopes in healthy elderly subjects. *Gerontology*, 1985, *31*, 6-14.

Gallagher, J. C.; Riggs, B. L.; Eisman, J.; Hamstra, A.; Arnaud, S. B.; & DeLuca, H. F. Intestinal calcium absorption and serum vitamin D metabolites in normal subjects and osteoporotic patients. Effect of age and dietary calcium. *J. Clinical Invest.*, 1979, *64*, 729-736.

Gallagher, J. D., & Thomas, J. R. Developmental effects of grouping and recoding on learning a movement series. *Res. Quart. for Exer. and Sport*, 1986, *57*, 117-127.

Gardener, E. B. The neuromuscular base of human movement: Feedback mechanism. *J. Health, Phys. Ed., and Rec.*, 1965, *36*, 61-62.

Garn, S. M. Fat accumulation and aging in males and females. In B. L. Strehler (Ed.), *The biology of aging.* Washington, D.C.: American Institute of Biological Sciences, 1960.

_____, & Clark, L. C. The sex difference in the basal metabolic rate. *Child Develpm.*, 1953, *24*, 215-224.

_____; _____; & Portray, R. Relationship between body composition and basal metabolic rate in children. *J. Appl. Physiol.*, 1953, *6*, 163-167.

Gates, A. I. The nature and educational significance of physical status and of mental, physiological, social and emotional maturity. *J. Educ. Psychol.*, 1924, *15*, 329-358.

Geschwind, N. Language and the brain. *Sci. Amer.* 1972, *226* (4), 76-83.

Gesell, A. *Infancy and human growth.* New York: Macmillan & Co., 1928.

_____. Maturation and the patterning of behavior. In C. Murchison, (Ed.), *A handbook of child psychology* (2nd ed)., Worcester: Clark University Press, 1933.

_____. The ontogenesis of infant behavior. In L. Carmichael, (Ed.), *Manual of child psychology* (2nd ed.), New York: John Wiley & Sons, Inc., 1954.

_____, & Ames, L. B. The ontogenetic organization of prone behavior in human infancy. *J. Genet. Psychol.*, 1940, *56*, 247-263.

_____, & _____. The development of handedness. *J. Genet. Psychol.*, 1947, *70*, 155-175.

_____, & Ilg, F. L. *The feeding behavior of infants: A pediatric approach to the mental hygiene of early life.* Philadelphia: J. B. Lippincott Co., 1937.

_____, & _____. *The child from five to ten.* New York: Harper & Row, Publishers, 1946.

_____, & Thompson, H. Learning and growth in identical infant twins: An experimental study of the method of co-twin control. *Genet. Psychol. Monogr.*, 1929, *6*, 1-124.

_____, & _____. *Infant behavior: Its genesis and growth.* New York: McGraw-Hill, 1934.

_____, & _____. *The psychology of early growth.* New York: Macmillan & Co., 1938.

Gibson, J. J. *The Senses Considered as Perceptual Systems.* Boston: Houghton Mifflin, 1966.

Gibson, J. J. *An Ecological Approach to Visual Perception.* Boston: Houghton Mifflin, 1979.

Gilliam, T. B.; Freedson, P. S.; Geenen, D. L.; & Shahraray, B. Physical activity patterns determined by heart rate monitoring in 6-7-year-old children. *Med. and Sci. in Sports and Exercise*, 1981, *13*, 65-67.

Glassow, R. B., & Kruse, P. Motor performance of girls age 6 to 14 years. *Res. Quart.*, 1960, *31* (3), 426-433.

Godin, G., & Shepard, R. J. Psychosocial factors influencing intentions to exercise of young students from grades 7 to 9. *Res. Quart. for Exer. and Sport*, 1986, *57*, 41-52.

Goetzinger, C. P. A reevaluation of the Health railwalking test. *J. Educ. Res.* 1961, *54*, 187-191.

Gogel, W. C. The adjacency principle in visual perception. *Sci. Amer.*, 1978, *238* (5), 126-139.

Golding, L. A. The effects of physical training upon total serum cholesterol levels. *Res. Quart.*, 1961, *32* (4), 499-506.

Gollnick, P. D.; Armstrong, R. B.; Saubert, C. W.; Piehl, K.; & Saltin, B. Enzyme activity and fiber composition in skeletal muscle of untrained and trained men. *J. Applied Physiol.*, 1972, *33*, 312-319.

Goodenough, F. L. *Developmental psychology: An introduction to the study of human behavior.* New York: Appleton-Century, 1945.

Goodwin, R. S., & Michel, G. F. Head orientation position during birth and in infant neonatal period, and hand preference at nineteen weeks. *Child Develpm.*, 1981, *52*, 819-826.

Goss, C. M. First contractions of the heart without cytological differentiation. *Anat. Rec.*, 1940, *76*, 19-27.

Gottfried, A. W.; Rose, S. A.; & Bridger, W. H. Cross-modal transfer in human infants. *Child Develpm.*, 1977, *48*, 305-312.

Granrud, C. E.; Yonas, A.; Smith, I. M.; Arterberry, M. E.; Glicksman, M. L.; & Sorknes, A. C. Infants' sensitivity to accretion and deletion of texture as information for depth at an edge. *Child Develpm.*, 1984, *55*, 1630-1636.

Graux, P.; Guazzi, G. C.; & Gesquiere, C. Spinal cord of the aged. *Rev. Neurol.*, 1962, *107* (4), 337-352.

Greulich, W. W., & Turner, M. L. The physical growth and development of children who survived the atomic bombing of Hiroshima and Nagasaki. *J. Pediat.*, 1953, *43*, 121-145.

Grimby, G.; Danneskiold-Samsoe, B.; Hvid, K.; & Saltin, B. Morphology and enzymatic capacity in arm and leg muscles in 78-81 year old men and women. *Acta Physiologica Scandinavica*, 1982, *115*, 125-134.

Gruber, J. J. Physical activity and self-esteem development in children: A meta-analysis. In G. A. Stull & H. M. Eckert (Eds.), *Effects of physical activity on children. The Academy Papers.* Champaign, IL: Human Kinetics, 1986.

Guedry, F. E., Jr. Age as a variable in post rotational phenomena. Project No. NM-001-063.01.19, Report No. 19. Pensacola, Florida: U.S. Naval School of Aviation Medicine, 1950.

Gutmann, E., & Hanzlikova, V. Fast and slow motor units in ageing. *Gerontology*, 1976, *22* (4), 280-300.

Guttridge, M. V. A study of motor achievements of young children. *Arch. Psych.*, 1939, *244*, 1-178.

Guyton, A. C. *Physiology of the human body* (5th ed.). Philadelphia: W. B. Saunders Co., 1979.

Haggmark, T.; Jansson, E.; & Svane, B. Cross-sectional area of the thigh muscle in man measured by computed tomography. *Scandinavian J. Clinical and Lab. Invest.* 1978, *38*, 355-360.

Haith, M. M. Visual competence in early infancy. In R. Held; H. W. Leibowitz; & H. L. Teuber (Eds.), *Perception.* Berlin: Springer-Verlag, 1978.

Hale, Creighton J. Physiological maturity of Little League Baseball players. *Res. Quart.*, 1956, *27*, 276-284.

Halverson, H. M. An experimental study of prehension in infants by means of systematic cinema records. *Gent. Psychol. Monogr.*, 1931, *10*, 107-286.

_____. Studies of the gasping responses of early infancy: I, II, III. *J. Genet. Psychol.*, 1939, *51*, 371-449.

_____. Genital and sphincter behavior of the male infant. *J. Genet. Psychol.*, 1940, *56*, 95-136.

_____. Variations in pulse and respiration during different phases of infant behavior. *J. Genet. Psychol.*, 1941, *59*, 259-330.

_____. Mechanisms of early infant feeding. *J. Genet. Psychol.*, 1944, *64*, 185-223.

Halverson, L. E., & Roberton, M. A. A study of motor pattern development in young children. Report at National Convention, American Association for Health, Physical Education and Recreation, 1966.

Halverson, L. E.; Roberton, M. A.; & Langendorfer, S. Development of the overarm throw: Movement and ball velocity changes by seventh grade. *Res. Quart. for Exer. and Sport*, 1982, *53*, 198-205.

Halverson, L., & Williams, K. Developmental sequences for hopping over distance: A prelongitudinal screening. *Res. Quart. for Exer. and Sport*, 1985, *56*, 37-44.

Hamill, P. V. V.; Johnston, F. E.; & Lemeshow, S. E. *Body weight, stature, and sitting height: White and Negro youths 12-17 years.* National Health Survey, Series 11, No. 126. Washington, D.C.: U.S. Government Printing Office, 1973.

Hammer, M., & Turkewitz, G. Relationship between effective intensity of auditory stimulation and directional eye turns in the human newborn. *Animal Behavior*, 1975, *23*, 287-290.

Harrison, R. G. The reaction of embryonic cells to solid surfaces. *J. Exp. Zool.*, 1914, *17*, 521-544.

Harrison, Virginia F. Review of the neuromuscular bases for motor learning. *Res. Quart.*, 1962, *33*, 59-69.

Hartman, C. G. *Time of ovulation in women.* Baltimore: Williams and Wilkins, 1936.

Hartman, D. M. The hurdle jump as a measure of the motor proficiency of young children. *Child Develpm.*, 1943, *14*, 201-211.

Harting, G. H.; Moore, C. E.; Mitchell, R.; & Kappus, C. Relationship of menopausal status and exercise level to HDL cholesterol in women. *Exper. Aging Res.*, 1984, *10*, 13-18.

Hartley, A. A., & Hartley, J. T. Performance changes in champion swimmers aged 30 to 84 years. *Exper. Aging Res.*, 1984, *10*, 141-147.

Haskell, W. L., & Fox, S. M. Physical activity in the prevention and therapy of cardiovascular disease. In W. R. Johnson & E. R. Buskirk (Eds.), *Science and medicine of exercise and sport.* New York: Harper & Row, 1974.

Haskell, W. L.; Montoye, H. J.; & Orenstein, D. Physical activity and exercise to achieve health-related physical fitness components. *Public Health Reports*, 1985, *100*, 202-212.

Hasselkus, B. R., & Shambes, G. M. Aging and postural sway in women. *J. Geront.*, 1975, *30*, 661-667.

Hatwell, Y. Form perception and related issues in blind humans. In R. Held; H. W. Leibowitz; and H. L. Teuber (Eds.), *Perception.* Berlin: Springer-Verlag, 1978.

Havighurst, R. J. *Developmental tasks and education.* New York: Longmans, Greens, 1950.

Hazen, N. L. Spatial exploration and spatial knowledge: Individual and developmental differences in very young children. *Child Develpm.*, 1982, *53*, 826-833.

Hazzard, W. R. Biological basis of the sex differential in longevity. *J. Amer. Geriat. Society*, 1986, *34*, 455-471.

Heath, B. H., & Carter, J. E. L. A modified somatotype method. *Amer. J. Phys. Anthrop.*, 1967, *27*, 57-74.

Heath, G. W.; Hagberg, J. M.; Ehsani, A. A.; & Holloszy, J. O. A physiological comparison of young and old endurance athletes. *J. Applied Physiol.: Respir., Environ. and Exer. Physiol.*, 1981, *51*, 634-640.

Heath, S. R. The rail walking test: Preliminary maturational norms for boys and girls. *Motor Skills Res. Exchg.*, 1949, *1*, 34-36.

Hebbelinck, M.; Duquet, W.; & Ross, W. A practical outline for the Heath-Carter Somatotyping Method applied to children. In O. Bar-Ord (Ed.), *Pediatric work physiology.* Israel: Wingate Institute, 1972.

Heikkinen, E. Health and socio-economic factors related to physical activity among the aged. In U. Simri (Ed.), *Physical exercise and activity for the aging: Proceedings of an international seminar.* Israel: Wingate Institute for Physical Education and Sport, 1975.

Hejinian, L., & Hatt, E. The stem-length: Recumbent-length as an index of body type in young children. *Amer. J. Phys. Anthrop.*, 1929, *13*, 287-307.

Held, R. Plasticity of sensory-motor systems. *Sci. Amer.*, 1965, *213* (5), 84-94.

Hellebrandt, F. A. & Braun, G. L. The influence of sex and age on the postural sway of man. *Amer. J. Physical Anthropology*, 1939, Series 1, *24*, 347-360.

_____; Rarick, G. L.; Glassow, R.; & Carns, M. L. Physiological analysis of basic motor skills. I. Growth and development of jumping. *Amer. J. Phys. Med.*, 1961, *40*, 14-25.

Hennessy, M. J.; Dixon, S. D.; & Simon, S. R. The development of gait: A study in African children ages one to five. *Child Develpm.*, 1984, *55*, 844-853.

Hensley, L. D.; East, W. B.; & Stillwell, J. L. Body fatness and motor performance during preadolescence. *Res. Quart. for Exer. and Sport*, 1982, *53*, 133-140.

Hess, J. H. *Premature and congenitally diseased infants.* Philadelphia: Lea and Febiger, 1922.

Herman, J. F.; Kolker, R. G.; & Shaw, M. L. Effects of motor activity on children's intentional and incidental memory in spatial locations. *Child Develpm.,* 1982, *53,* 239-244.

Herman, J. F.; Shiraki, J. H.; & Miller, B. S. Young children's ability to infer spatial relationships: Evidence from a large, familiar environment. *Child Develpm.,* 1985, *56,* 1195-1203.

Hershenson, M. Visual discrimination in the human newborn. *J. Compar. and Physiol. Psychol.,* 1964, *67,* 326-336.

Heyman, D. K., & Jeffers, F. C. Study of the relative influence of race and socio-economic status upon the activities and attitudes of a southern aged population. *J. Geront.,* 1964, *19* (2), 225-229.

Heyward, V. H.; Johannes-Ellis, S. M.; & Romer, J. F. Gender differences in strength. *Res. Quart. for Exer. and Sport,* 1986, *57,* 154-159.

Hicks, C. B. Why are twins so special? *Today's Health,* December 1963, pp. 18-21; 72-76.

Hildreth, G. Manual dominance in nursery school children. *J. Genet. Psychol.,* 1948, *73,* 29-45.

_____. The development and training of hand dominance: I. Characteristics of handedness; II. Developmental tendencies in handedness; III. Origin of handedness and lateral dominance. *J. Genet. Psychol.,* 1949, *75,* 197-275.

_____. The development and training of hand dominance; IV. Developmental problems associated with handedness; V. Training of handedness. *J. Genet. Psychol.,* 1950, *76,* 39-144.

Hilgard, J. R. Learning and maturation in preschool children. *J. Genet. Psychol.,* 1932, *41,* 36-56.

Hinchcliffe, R. Aging and sensory thresholds. *J. Geront.,* 1962, *17* (1), 45-50.

Hinton, G. Parallel computations for controlling an arm. *J. Motor Behav.,* 1984, *16,* 171-194.

Hoffman, S. J.; Imwold, C. H.; & Koller, J. A. Accuracy and prediction in throwing: A taxonomic analysis of children's performance. *Res. Quart. for Exer. and Sport,* 1983, *54,* 33-40.

Hogan, P. I., & Santomier, J. P. Effect of mastering swim skills on older adults' self-efficacy. *Res. Quart. for Exer. and Sport,* 1984, *55,* 294-296.

Hogberg, P. How do stride length and stride frequency influence the energy-output during running? *Arbeitsphysiologie,* 1952, *14,* 437-441.

Hogg, I. D. Sensory nerves and associated structures in the skin of human fetuses of 8 to 14 weeks of menstrual age correlated with functional capability. *J. Comp. Neurol.,* 1941, *75,* 371-410.

Hooker, D. Fetal behavior. *Res. Publ. Ass. Nerv. Ment. Dis.,* 1939, *19,* 237-243.

_____. The origin of overt behavior. Ann Arbor: University of Michigan Press, 1944.

Horrocks, J. E. The adolescent. In L. Carmichael (Ed.), *Manual of child psychology.* New York: John Wiley & Sons, Inc., 1954.

Hoshizaki, T. B., & Massey, B. H. Relationships of muscular endurance among specific muscle groups for continuous and intermittent static contractions. *Res. Quart. for Exer. and Sport,* 1986, *57,* 229-235.

Howe, P. E., & Schiller, M. Growth responses of the school child to changes in diet and environmental factors. *J. Appl. Physiol.,* 1952, *5,* 51-61.

Huggett, A. S. G. Foetal respiratory reflexes. *J. Physiol.,* 1930, *69,* 144-152.

Hughes, J. G.; Ehemann B.; & Brown, W.A. Electroencephalography of the newborn. III. Brain potentials of babies born of mothers given seconal sodium. *Amer. J. Dis. Child.,* 1948, *76,* 626-633.

Humphrey, T. Some correlations between the appearance of human fetal reflexes and the development of the nervous system. In D.P. Purpura and J. P. Schade (Eds.), *Growth and the maturation of the brain.* New York: Elsevier Publishing Co., 1964.

Hunsicker, P. A., & Reiff, G. G. A survey and comparison of youth fitness 1958-1965. *J. Health P.E. Rec.,* 1966, *37,* 23-25.

_____, & _____. Youth fitness report: 1958-1965-1975. *JOPER,* 1977, *48* (1), 31-32.

Hupprich, F. L., & Sigerseth, P. O. The specificity of flexibility in girls. *Res. Quart.,* 1950, *21,* 25-33.

Hurdle, A. D. F., & Rosin, A. J. Red cell volume and red cell survival in normal aged people. *J. Clin. Pathol.,* 1962, *15* (4), 343-345.

Hurlock, Elizabeth B. *Developmental physchology.* New York: McGraw-Hill Book Co., Inc., 1953.

Hurme, V. O. Ranges of normalcy in the eruption of the permanent teeth. *J. Dent. Child.,* 1949, *16,* 11-15.

Iliff, A., & Lee, V. A. Pulse rate, respiratory rate, and body temperature of children between two months and eighteen years of age. *Child Develpm.,* 1952, *23,* 237-245.

Imamura, K.; Ashida, H.; Ishikawa, T.; & Fujii, M. Human major psoas muscle and sacrospinalis muscle in relation to age: A study by computed tomography. *J. Geron.,* 1983, *38,* 678-681.

Irwin, O. C. The distribution of the amount of motility of young infants between two nursing periods. *J. Comp. Psychol.,* 1932, *14,* 429-445.

_____. Qualitative changes in a vertebral reaction pattern during infancy: A motion picture study. *Univ. Iowa Stud. Child Welfare*, 1936, *12*, 201-207.

_____. Effect of strong light on the body activity of newborns. *J. Comp. Psychol.*, 1941, *32*, 233-236.

_____. Can infants have IQ's? *Psychol. Rev.*, 1942, *49*, 68-79.

_____, & Weiss, A. P. A note on mass activity in newborn infants. *J. Genet. Psychol.*, 1930, *38*, 20-30.

_____, & Weiss, L. A. The effect of clothing on the general and vocal activity of the newborn infant. *Univ. Iowa Stud. Child Welfare*, 1934, *9*, 149-162.

Ito, P. K. Comparative biometrical study of physique of Japanese women born and reared under different environments. *Hum. Biol.*, 1942, *14*, 279-351.

Ives, W. Preschool children's ability to coordinate spatial perspectives through language and pictures. *Child Develpm.*, 1980, *51*, 1303-1306.

Jackson, A. S., & Frankiewicz, R. J. Factorial expressions of muscular strength. *Res. Quart.*, 1975, *46*, 206-217.

Jackson, C. M. Some aspects of form and growth. In W. J. Robbins; S. Brody; A. G. Hogan; C. M. Jackson; and C. W. Green, *Growth*. New Haven: Yale University Press, 1928.

Jenkins, L. M. *A comparative study of motor achievements of children five, six and seven years of age.* New York: Teachers College, Columbia University, 1930.

Jensen, K. Differential reactions to taste and temperature stimuli in newborn infants. *Genet. Psychol. Monogr.*, 1932, *12*, 263-479.

Jersild, A. T., & Tasch, R. *Children's interests and what they suggest for education.* New York: Bureau of Publications, Teachers College, Columbia University, 1949.

Johnell, O., & Sernbo, I. Health and social status in patients with hip fractures and controls. *Age and Ageing*, 1986, *15*, 285-291.

Johnson, B. *Mental growth of children in relation to the rate of growth in bodily development: A report of the bureau of educational experiments.* New York: Dutton, 1925.

Johnson, M. W. The effect on behavior of variation in the amount of play equipment. *Child Develpm.*, 1935, *6*, 56-68.

Jokl, E. *Alter und Leistung.* Berlin: Springer-Verlag, 1954.

Jones, H. E. *Motor performance and growth.* Berkeley: University of California Press, 1949.

_____, & Jones, M. C. *Adolescence.* Berkeley: University Extension, University of California, 1957.

Jones, T. D. The development of certain motor skills and play activities in young children. *Child Develpm. Monogr. Teachers College, Columbia University*, 1939, No. 26, 1-180.

Kagan, J. Do infants think? *Sci. Amer.*, 1972, *226* (3), 74-82.

Kane, R. J., & Meredith, H. V. Ability in the standing broad jump of school children 7, 9 and 11 years of age. *Res. Quart.*, 1952, *23*, 198-208.

Kannel, W. B. Habitual level of physical activity and risk of coronary heart disease: The Framingham study. *Canadian Med. Assoc. J.*, 1967, *96*, 811-812.

Kawin, E. *The wise choice of toys.* Chicago: The University of Chicago Press, 1934.

Kemsley, W. F. F. Changes in body weight from 1943 to 1950. *Ann. Eugen., Lond.*, 1953, *18*, 22-42.

Keogh, B. K. Pattern copying under three conditions of an expanded spatial field. *Developmental Psychol.*, 1971, *4*, 25-31.

Keogh, J. *Motor performance of elementary school children.* Los Angeles: Department of Physical Education, University of California, 1965.

Kiil, V. Stature and growth of Norwegian men during the past 200 years. *Skr. norske Vidensk Akad.*, 1939, No. 6.

Kirkendall, D. R. Effects of physical activity on intellectual development and academic performance. In G. A. Stull & H. M. Eckert (Eds.), *Effects of physical activity on children. The Academy Papers.* Champaign, IL: Human Kinetics, 1986.

Kirshenbaum, J. Assembly line for champions. *Sports Illus.*, 1976, *45* (2), 56-65.

Kleemeier, R. W. Behavior and the organization of the bodily and the external environment. In J. E. Birren (Ed.), *Handbook of aging and the individual.* Chicago: University of Chicago Press, 1959.

Kline, D. W.; Schieber, F.; Abusamra, L. C.; & Coyne, A. C. Age, the eye, and the visual channels: Contrast sensitivity and response speed. *J. Geron.*, 1983, *38*, 211-216.

Klissouras, V., Marisi, D. Q. Genetic basis of individual differences in physical performance, *McGill J. Education*, Olympic Edition, 1976, *11*(1), 15-28.

Kohn, R. R., & Rollerson, E. Age changes in swelling properties of human myocardium. *Proc. Soc. Exp. Biol., N.Y.*, 1959, *100*, 253-256.

Komi, P. V., & Karlsson, J. Physical performance, skeletal muscle enzyme activities, and fibre types in monozygous and dizygous twins of both sexes. *Acta Physiologica Scandinavica*, 1979, Suppl. *462*, 1.

Korcok, M. Add exercise to calcium in osteoporosis prevention. *J. Amer. Med. Assoc.*, 1982, *247*, 1106-1107.

Korner, A. F., & Grobstein, R. Visual alertness as related to soothing in neonates: Implications for maternal stimulation and early deprivation. In L. J. Stone; H. T. Smith; L. B. Murphy (Eds.), *The competent infant: Research and commentary.* New York: Basic Books, Inc., Publishers, 1973.

Kreutzfeldt, J.; Haim, M.; & Bach, E. Hip fracture among the elderly in a mixed urban and rural population. *Age and Ageing*, 1984, *13*, 111-119.

Kriska, A. M.; Bayles, C.; Cauley, J. A.; LaPorte, R. E.; Sandler, R. B.; & Pambianco, G. A randomized exercise trail in older women: Increased activity over two years and the factors associated with compliance. *Med. and Sci. in Sports and Exer.*, 1986, *18*, 557-562.

Krogman, W. M. A handbook of the measurement and interrelation of height and weight in the growing child. *Monogr. Soc. Res. Child Develpm.*, 1948, *13*(3).

_____. The concept of maturity from a morphological viewpoint. *Child Develpm.*, 1950, *21*, 25-32.

_____. The physical growth of children: An appraisal of studies 1950-1955. *Monogr. Soc. Res. Child Develpm.*, 1955, *20*(1), 1-91.

_____. Maturation age of 55 boys in the Little League World Series, 1957. *Res. Quart.*, 1959, *30*, 54-56.

Krolner, B., & Toft, B. Vertebral bone loss: An unheeded side effect of therapeutic bed rest. *Clinical Science*, 1983, *64*, 537-540.

Krolner, B.; Toft, B.; Nielson, S. P.; & Tondevold, E. Physical exercise as a prophylaxis against involutional vertebral bone loss: A controlled trial. *Clinical Science*, 1983, *64*, 541-546.

Lackner, J. R. Some mechanisms underlying sensory and postural stability in man. In R. Held; H. W. Leibowitz; and H. L. Teuber (Eds.), *Perception.* Berlin: Springer-Verlag, 1978.

Landis, C., & Hunt, W. A. *The startle pattern.* New York: Farrar and Rinehart, 1939.

Landiss, Carl W. Influences of physical education activities on motor ability and physical fitness of male freshmen. *Res. Quart.*, 1955, *26*(3), 295-307.

Landreth, C. *The psychology of early childhood.* New York: Alfred A. Knopf, 1958.

Langendorfer, S. A prelongitudinal test of motor stage theory. *Res. Quart. for Exer. and Sport*, 1987, *58*, 21-29.

Langley, J., & Anderson, H. The union of different kinds of nerve fibers. *J. Physiol.*, 1904, *31*, 365-391.

Langworthy, O. R. Development of behavior patterns and myelination of the nervous system in the human fetus and infant. *Contr. Embryol. Carn. Instn.*, 1933, *24*, 1-57.

Lansing, A. I. General biology of senescence. In J. E. Birren (Ed.), *Handbook of aging and the individual.* Chicago: The University of Chicago Press, 1959.

Larson, L. A. Some findings resulting from the Army Air Forces Physical Training Program. *Res. Quart.*, 1946, *17*, 144-164.

Larsson, L., & Karlsson, J. Isometric and dynamic endurance as a function of age and skeletal muscle characteristics. *Acta Physiologica Scandinavica*, 1978, *104*, 129-136.

Lasky, R. E., & Spiro, D. The processing of tachistoscopically presented visual stimuli by five-month-old infants. *Child Develpm.*, 1980, *51*, 1292-1294.

Lawson, K. R., & Turkewitz, G. Intersensory function in newborns: Effect of sound on visual preferences. *Child Develpm.*, 1980, *51*, 1295-1298.

Lawson, M. Champion cyclist is still an easy rider at age 72. *The Daily Californian.* University of California, Berkeley. October 24, 1977, p. 15.

Lee, W. A. Neuromotor synergies as a basis for coordinated intentional action. *J. Motor Behav.*, 1984, *16*, 135-170.

Leehey, S. C.; Moskowitz-Cook, A.; Brill, S.; & Held, R. Orientational anisotrophy in infant vision. *Science*, 1975, *190*, 900-902.

Lehman, Harvey C. *Age and achievement.* Published for the American Philosophical Society by Princeton University Press, Princeton, N.J., 1953.

Leon, A. S. Exercise and risk of coronary heart disease. In H. M. Eckert & H. J. Montoye (Eds.), *Exercise and health. The Academy Papers.* Champaign, IL: Human Kinetics, 1984.

Levin, I., & Gilat, I. A developmental analysis of early time concepts: The equivalence and additivity of the effect of interfering cues on duration comparisons of young children. *Child Develpm.*, 1983, *54*, 78-83.

Lewis, R. C.; Duval, A. M. & Iliff, A. Standards for the basal metabolism of children from 2 to 15 years of age, inclusive. *J. Pediat.*, 1943, *23*, 1-18.

Lewkowicz, D. J., & Turkewitz, G. Crossmodal equivalence in early infancy: Auditory-visual intensity matching. *Developmental Psychol.*, 1980, *16*, 597-607.

Ley, L. Über die Menarche der Frau und ihre Beziehungen zur Pigmentation: Unter uchungen am Schulkindern der Stadt Mainz. *Arch. Gynak.*, 1938, *165*, 489-503.

Liddell, E. G. T., & Sherrington, C. S. Recruitment and some other features of reflex inhibition. *Proc. Roy. Soc.; Series B. Biol. Sci.*, 1925, *97*, 488–518.

Liemohn, W. P. Strength and aging: An exploratory study. *Intl. J. Aging and Human Development*, 1975, *6*(4), 347-357.

Lindgren, G. Height, weight and menarche in Swedish urban school children in relation to socioeconomic and regional factors. *Annals of Hum. Biol.*, 1976, *3*, 510-528.

Ling, B. C. I. A genetic study of sustained visual fixation and associated behavior in the human infant from birth to six months. *J. Genet. Psychol.*, 1942, *61*, 227-277.

Linn, M. C., & Petersen, A. C. Emergence and characterization of sex differences in spatial ability: An meta-analysis. *Child Develpm.*, 1985, *56*, 1479-1498.

Lippman, H. S. Certain behavior responses in early infancy. *J. Genet. Psychol.*, 1927, *34*, 424-440.

Ljung, B.-O; Bergsten-Brucefors, A.; & Lindgren, G. The secular trend in physical growth in Sweden. *Annals of Hum. Biol.*, 1974, *1*(3), 245-256.

Lloyd, D. P. C. Principles of spinal reflex activity. In J. F. Fulton (Ed.), *Howell's textbook of physiology*. Philadelphia: W. B. Saunders, 1946.

Lloyd, T.; Triantafyllou, S. J.; Baker, E. R.; Houtz, P. S.; Whiteside, J. A.; Kalenak, A; & Stumpf, P. G. Women athletes with menstrual irregularity have increased musculoskeletal injuries. *Med. and Sci. in Sports and Exer.*, 1986, *18*, 374-379.

Lombard, O. M. Breadth of bone and muscle by age and sex in childhood. *Child Develpm.*, 1950, *21*, 229-239.

Long, D. M. Aging in the nervous system. *Neurosurgery*, 1985, *17*, 348-354.

Lorsbach, T. C., & Simpson, G. B. Age differences in the rate of processing in short-term memory. *J. Geron.*, 1984, *39*, 315-321.

Macht, M. L., & Buschke, H. Speed of recall in aging. *J. Geron.*, 1984, *39*, 439-443.

MacLennan, W. J.; Hall, M. R. P.; Timothy, J. I.; & Robinson, M. Is weakness in old age due to muscle wasting? *Age and Ageing*, 1980, *9*, 188-192.

Madison, L. S.; Madison, J. K.; & Adubato, S. A. Infant behavior and development in relation to fetal movement and habituation. *Child Develpm.*, 1986, *57*, 1475-1482.

Malina, R. M. Ethnic and cultural factors in the development of motor abilities and strength in American children. In G. L. Rarick (Ed.), *Physical activity: Human growth and development*. New York: Academic Press, 1973.

————; Hamill, P. V. V.; & Lemeshow, S. *Body dimensions and proportions: White and Negro children 6-11 years.* National Health Survey, Series 11, No. 143. Washington, D.C.: U.S. Government Printing Office, 1974.

————; Holman, J. D.; & Harper, A. B. Parent size and growth status of offspring. *Social Biology*, 1970, *17*, 120-123.

————; Johnston, F. E. Significance of age, sex, and maturity differences in upper arm composition. *Res. Quart.*, 1967, *38*, 219-230.

————; Mueller, W. H.; & Holman, J. D. Parent-child correlations and heritability of stature in Philadelphia black and white children 6 to 12 years of age. *Hum. Biol.*, 1976, *48*, 475-496.

————; & Rarick, G. L. Growth, physique, and motor performance. In G. L. Rarick (Ed.), *Physical activity: Human growth and development*. New York: Academic Press, 1973.

Mall, F. P. On the age of human embryos. *Amer. J. Anat.*, 1918, *23*, 397-422.

Mangarov, I. Physical development and capacity of Bulgarian students. *Bulletin d'information, Bulgarian Olympic Com.*, Year IX, 1964, No. 5.

Marcus, R.; Cann, C.; Madvig, P.; Minkoff, J.; Goddard, M.; Bayer, M.; Martin, M.; Gaudiani, L.; Haskell, W.; & Genant, H. Menstrual function and bone mass in elite women distance runners. *Annals of Intern. Med.*, 1985, *102*, 158-163.

Maresh, H. M. Growth of major long bones in healthy children. A preliminary report on successive roentgenograms of the extremities from early infancy to twelve years of age. *Amer. J. Dis. Child.*, 1943, *66*, 227-257.

Markus, E. J. Perceptual field dependence among aged persons. *Perceptual and Motor Skills*, 1971, *33*, 175-178.

Marloff, H. J. Werte des erythrocitären Systems bei 40 jungen Sporttreibenden Frauen. *Pflüg, Arch. ges. Physiol.*, 1949, *251*, 241-254.

Marshall, W. A. The relationship of variations in children's growth rates to seasonal climatic variations. *Annals of Hum. Biol.*, 1975, *2*, 243-250.

Martin, E. G. Muscular strength and muscular symmetry in human beings. *Amer. J. Physiol.*, 1918, *46*, 67-83.

Massaro, D. W. Preperceptual images, processing time, and perceptual units in auditory perception. *Psychol. Rev.*, 1972, *79*, 124-145.

Massaro, D. W. A comparison of forward versus backward recognition masking. *J. Exper. Psychol.*, 1973, *100*, 434-436.

Master, A. M. The two-step test of myocardial function. *Amer. Heart J.*, 1935, *10* (4), 495-510.

Mayer, R. F. Nerve conduction studies in man. *Neurology*, 1963, *13* (12), 1021-1030.

McCarthy, D. A. *The language development of the preschool child.* Minneapolis: University of Minnesota Press, 1930.

McCaskill, C. L., & Wellman, B. L. A study of common motor achievements at the preschool ages. *Child Develpm.*, 1938, *9*, 141-150.

McCloy, C. H. Appraising physical status: The selection of measurements. *Univ. Iowa Stud. Child Welfare*, 1936 *12*(2), 1-126.

_____. *Tests and measurements in health and physical education.* New York: Crofts, 1945.

McCormack, P. D. Coding of spatial information by young and elderly adults. *J. Geron.*, 1982, *37*, 80-86.

McDonagh, M. J. N.; White, M. J.; & Davies, C. T. M. Different effects of ageing on the mechanical properties of human arm and leg muscles. *Geron.*, 1984, *30*, 49-54.

McDonald, R.; Hegenauer, J.; & Saltman, P. Age-related differences in the bone mineralization pattern of rats following exercise. *J. Geron.*, 1986, *41*, 445-452.

McFarland, R. A.; Tune, G. S.; & Welford, A. T. On the driving of automobiles by older people. *J. Geron.*, 1964, *19*(2), 190-197.

McGinnis, J. M. Eye-movements and optic nystagmus in early infancy. *Genet. Psychol. Monogr.*, 1930, *8*, 321-430.

McGraw, M. B. *Growth: A study of Johnny and Jimmy.* New York: Appleton-Century, 1935.

_____. Behavior of the newborn infant and early neuromuscular development. *Res. Publ. Ass. Nerv. Ment. Dis.*, 1939a, *19*, 244-246.

_____. Later development of children specially trained during infancy. *Child Develpm.*, *10*, 1-19.

_____. Neuromuscular development of the human infant as exemplified in the achievement of erect locomotion. *J. Pediat.*, 1940a, *17*, 747-771.

_____. Neuromuscular mechanism of the infant. Development reflected by postural adjustments to an inverted position. *Amer. J. Dis. Child.*, 1940b, *60*, 1031-1042.

_____. Development of neuromuscular mechanisms as reflected in the crawling and creeping behavior of the human infant. *J. Genet. Psychol.*, 1941a, *58*, 83-111.

_____. Development of rotary-vestibular reactions of the human infant. *Child Develpm.*, 1941b, *12*, 17-19.

_____. *The neuromuscular maturation of the human infant* (reprinted). New York: Hafner Publishing Company, Inc., 1963.

_____. Maturation of behavior. In L. Carmichael (Ed.), *Manual of child psychology.* New York: John Wiley & Sons, Inc., 1954.

McKusick, V. A. The royal hemophelia. *Sci. Amer.*, 1965, *213*(2), 88-95.

McLaughlin, T. M.; Lardner, T. J.; & Dillman, C. J. Kinetics of the parallel squat. *Res. Quart.*, 1978, *49*, 175-189.

McMillen, M. M. Differential mortality by sex in fetal and neonatal deaths. *Science*, 1979, *204*, 89-91.

McWhirter, N. (Ed.). *Guinness book of world records.* New York: Sterling Publishing Co., 1978.

Mead, M. *Growing up in New Guinea.* New York: William Morrow & Co., 1930.

Mednick, B. R. Intellectual and behavioral functioning of ten- to twelve-year-old children who showed certain transient symptoms in the neonatal period. *Child Develpm.*, 1977, *48*, 844-853.

Mendelson, M. J., & Ferland, M. B. Auditory-visual transfer in four-month-old infants. *Child Develpm.*, 1982, *53*, 1022-1027.

Meredith, H. V. The rhythm of physical growth: A study of 18 anthropometric measures on Iowa City males ranging in age between birth and 18 years. *Univ. Iowa Stud. Child Welfare*, 1935, *11* (3).

_____. Order and age of eruption for the deciduous dentition. *J. Dent. Res.*, 1946, *25*, 43-66.

_____, & Boynton, B. The transverse growth of the extremities: An analysis of girth measurements for arm, forearm, thigh and leg taken on Iowa City white children. *Hum. Biol.*, 1937, *9*, 366-403.

Messier, S. P.; Franke, W. D.; & Rejeski, W. J. Effects of altered stride lengths on ratings of perceived exertion during running. *Res. Quart. for Exer. and Sport*, 1986, *57*, 273-279.

Metheny, E. Breathing capacity and grip strength of preschool children. *Univ. Iowa Stud. Child Welfare.*, 1941a, *18* (2), 1-207.

_____. The present status of strength testing for children of elementary school and preschool age. *Res. Quart.*, 1941b, 12, 115-130.

Metropolitan Life Insurance Co. Socioeconomic mortality differentials by leading cause of death. *Statistical Bulletin*, January 1977, *58*, 5-8.

Metropolitan Life Insurance Co. Trends in average weights and heights among insured men and women. *Statistical Bulletin*, October 1977, *58*, 2-6.

Meyer, M. H. A longitudinal study of certain motor activities of elementary school children. Unpublished study, University of Wisconsin, Madison, 1951.

Michael, E. D., & Gallon, A. Periodic changes in the circulation during athletic training as reflected by a step test. *Res. Quart.*, 1959, *30* (3), 303-311.

Michelson, N. Studies in physical development of Negroes. IV. Onset of puberty. *Amer. J. Phys. Anthrop.*, 1944, *2*, 151-166.

Miles, W. R. Simultaneous right- and left-hand grip. Vol. 3. In R. W. Gerard (Ed.), *Methods in medical research.* Chicago: Year Book Publishers, 1950.

Miles, W. R. Changes in motor ability during the life span. In R. G. Kuhlen & G. G. Thompson (Eds.), *Psychological studies of human development.* New York: Appleton-Century-Crofts, 1952. Meredith Publishing Co., 1963.

Milligan, W. L.; Powell, D. A.; Harley, C.; & Furchtgott, E. Physical health correlates of attitudes toward aging in the elderly. *Exper. Aging Res.*, 1985, *11*, 75-80.

Mills, C. A. Temperature dominance over human life. *Science*, 1949, *110*, 267-271.

_____. Temperature influence over human growth and development. *Hum. Biol.*, 1950, *22*, 71-74.

Milne, J. S., & Maule, M. M. A longitudinal study of handgrip and dementia in older people. *Age and Ageing*, 1984, *13*, 42-48.

Minkowski, M. Ueber Bewegungen und Reflexe des menschlichen Foetus während der ersten Hälfte seiner Entwicklung. *Schweiz. Arch. Neurol. Phychiat.*, 1921, *8*, 148-151.

_____. Ueber frühzeitige Bewegungen. Reflexe und muskuläre Reaktionen beim menschlichen Fötus und ihre Beziehungen zum fötalen Nerven- und Muskelsystem. *Schweiz. Med. Wschr.*, 1922, *52*, 721-724.

_____. Zum gengenwartigen Stand der Lehre von den Reflexen in entwicklungsgeschichtlicher und der anatomischphysiologischer Beziehung. *Schweiz. Arch. Neurol. Psychiat.*, 1924, *15*, 239-259.

_____. Sur les modalités et la localisation du réflexe plantaire au cours de son évolution du foetus à l'adulte. *C. R. Congr. Medecins. Alienistes et Neurologistes de France, Geneva*, 1926, *30*, 301-308.

_____. Neurobiologische Studien am munschenlichen Foetus. *Handb. Biol. ArbMeth.*, 1928, *5B*, 511-618.

Minot, C. S. *Human embryology.* New York: William Wood, 1892.

Miyashita, M., & Kanehisa, H. Dynamic peak torque related to age, sex, and performance. *Res. Quart.*, 1979, *50*, 249-255.

Molfese, D. L.; Freeman, R. B.; & Palermo, D. S. The ontogeny of brain lateralization for speech and nonspeech stimuli. *Brain and Language*, 1975, *2*, 356-368.

Monahan, T. Should women go easy on exercise? *The Physician and Sportsmed.*, 1986, *14*, 188-197.

Monckeberg, F. The effect of malnutrition on physical growth and brain development. In J. W. Prescott; M. S. Read; and D. B. Coursin (Eds.), *Brain function and malnutrition.* New York: John Wiley & Sons, 1975.

Montgomery, D. L. Physical activity as preventive medicine. *McGill J. Education*, Olympic Edition, 1976, *11*(1), 83-90.

Montoye, H. J. Exercise and osteoporosis. In H. M. Eckert & H. J. Montoye (Eds.), *Health and exercise. The Academy Papers.* Champaign, IL: Human Kinetics, 1984.

Montoye, H. J. Muscular strength in man: Has it changed in the last century. *Res. Quart. for Exer. and Sport*, 1985, *Centennial Issue*, 21-24.

Montoye, Henry J.; Van Huss, W. D.; Olson, H. W.; Pierson, W. R.; & Hudec, A. J. *The longevity and morbidity of college athletes.* Phi Epsilon Kappa Fraternity, 1957.

_____; Block, W.; Keller, J. B.; & Willis, P. W. III. Fitness, fatness, and serum cholesterol: An epidemiological study of an entire community. *Res. Quart.*, 1976, *47*, 400-408.

_____, & Lamphiear, D. E. Grip and arm strength in males and females, age 10 to 69. *Res. Quart.*, 1977, *48*, 109-120.

_____; Metzner, H. L.; & Keller, J. B. Familial aggregation of strength and heart rate response to exercise. *Hum. Biol.*, 1975, *47*, 17–36.

Montoye, H. J.; Smith, E. L.; Fardon, F. D.; & Howley, E. T. Bone mineral in senior tennis players. *Scandinavian J. Sports Sci.*, 1980, *2*, 26–32.

Montpetit, R. R.; Montoye, H. J.; & Leading, L. Grip strength of school children, Saginaw, Michigan: 1899 and 1964. *Res. Quart.*, 1967, *38*, 231–240.

Moore, T. E.; Richards, B.; & Hood, J. Aging and coding of spatial information. *J. Geron.*, 1984, *39*, 210–212.

Morgan, W. P. Selected psychological factors limiting performance: A mental health model. In D. H. Clarke & H. M. Eckert (Eds.), *Limits of human performance. The Academy Papers*, Champaign, IL: Human Kinetics, 1985.

Morris, A. M.; Atwater, A. E., Williams, J. M.; & Wilmore, J. H. *Preliminary report on the motor performance test battery for preschool children.* Paper presented at Western Society for Physical Education of College Women Conference, November 1978.

Morris, A. M.; Williams, J. M.; Atwater, A. E.; & Wilmore, J. H. Age and sex differences in motor performance of 3 through 6 year old children. *Res. Quart. for Exer. and Sport*, 1982, *53*, 214–221.

Morris, C. B. The measurement of the strength of muscle relative to the cross-section. *Res. Quart.*, 1948, *19*, 295–303.

Morris, J. N.; Heady, J. A.; Raffle, P. A. B.; Roberts, C. G.; & Parks, J. W.; Coronary heart disease and physical activity of work. *Lancet*, 1953, *265*, 1053–1057.

Morse, M.; Schultz, F. W.; & Cassels, D. E. The lung volume and its subdivisions in boys 10–17 year of age. *J. Clin. Invest.*, 1952, *31*, 380–391.

Mugrage, E. R., & Andresen, M. I. Values for red blood cells of average infants and children. *Amer. J. Dis. Child.*, 1936, *51*, 775–791.

_____, & _____. Red blood cell values in adolescence. *Amer. J. Dis. Child.*, 1938, *56*, 997–1003.

Mulligan, H. A. Inside E. Germany's sports factories. *S. F. Examiner & Chronicle*, September 12, 1976, Section C: 4–5.

Murakami, U. The effect of organic mercury on intrauterine life. In M. A. Klingberg; A. Abramovici; and J. Chemke (Eds.), *Drugs and fetal development.* New York: Plenum Press, 1972.

Murray, M. P.; Duthie, E. H.; Gambert, S. R.; Sepic, S. B.; & Mollinger, L. A. Age-related differences in knee muscle strength in normal women. *J. Geron.*, 1985, *40*, 275–280.

Mussen, P. Developmental psychology. In P. Mussen & M. R. Rosenzweig (Eds.), *Psychology.* Lexington, Mass.: D. C. Health, 1977.

Naeye, R. L.; Burt, L. S.; Wright, D. L.; Blanc, W. A.; & Tatter, D. Neonatal mortality, the male disadvantage. *Pediatrics*, 1971, *48*(6), 902–906.

_____; Diener, M. M.; Dellinger, W. S.; & Blanc, W. A. Urban poverty: Effects on prenatal nutrition. *Science*, 1969, *166* (3908), 1026.

Nagle, F. J., & Bassett, D. H. Metabolic requirements of distance running. In D. H. Clarke & H. M. Eckert (Eds.), *Limits of human performance. The Academy Papers.* Champaign, IL: Human Kinetics, 1985.

Nassau, E. Die Kitzelreaktion beim Säugling. *Jb.Kinderheilk.*, 1938, *151*, 46–49.

National Enquirer. Amazing Mom tells what it's like taking care of 6 babies, April 21, 1974.

National Foundation/March of Dimes. *Birth defects, tragedy and hope*, 1977.

National Foundation/March of Dimes. (Pamphlet) With best wishes for a happy birthday from the National Foundation.

Needham, J. *Chemical embryology.* Cambridge: University Press, 1931.

Neilson, N. P., & Cozens, F. W. *Achievement scales in physical education activities.* Sacramento State Dept. of Education, 1934.

Nelson, C. A., & Salapatek, P. Electrophysiological correlates of infant recognition memory. *Child Develpm.*, 1986, *57*, 1483–1497.

Nelson, J. K.; Thomas, J. R.; Nelson, K. R.; Abraham, P. C. Gender differences in children's throwing performance: Biology and environment. *Res. Quart. for Exer. and Sport*, 1986, *57*, 280–287.

Nelson, M. M.; Asling, C. W.; & Evans, H. M. Production of multiple congenital abnormalities in young by pteroyglutamic acid deficiency during gestation. *J. Nutrition*, 1952, *48*, 61–80.

Nelson, R. C., & Fahrney, R. A. Relationship between strength and speed of elbow flexion. *Res. Quart.*, 1965, *36*, 455–463.

Nevers, J. E. The effects of physiological age on motor achievement. *Res. Quart.*, 1948, *19*, 103–110.

Newbery, H. Studies in fetal behavior. IV. The measurement of three types of fetal activity. *J. Comp. Psychol.*, 1941, *32*, 521–530.

Nicolson, A. B., & Hanley, C. Indices of physiological maturity: Derivation and inter-relationships. *Child Develpm.*, 1953, *24*, 3–38.

Nordgren, R. A.; Hirsch, G. P.; Menzies, R. A.; Hendley, D. D.; Kutsky, R.; Strehler, B. L. Evidence of long-lived components in developing mouse tissues labeled with leucine. *Exp. Gerontology*, 1969, *4*, 7–16.

Norman, J. R.; Schweppe, I. H.; Salazar, E.; & Knowles, J. H. Lung changes and aging: A review of a report of changes in 43 Spanish-American War Veterans. *J. Amer. Geriat. Soc.*, 1964, *12*(1), 38–49.

Norris, A. H., & Shock, N. W. Exercise in the adult years—with special reference to the advanced years. In W. R. Johnson (Ed.), *Science and medicine of exercise and sports.* New York: Harper & Row, 1960.

————; ————; & Yiengst, M. J. Age changes in heart rate and blood pressure responses to tilting and standardized exercise. *Circulation*, 1953, *8*, 521–526.

Norris, A. H., & Shock, N. W. Exercise in the adult years. In W. R. Johnson & E. R. Buskirk (Eds.), *Science and medicine of exercise and sport.* New York: Harper & Row, 1974.

Norton, W. T. Recent developments in the investigation of purified myelin. In R. Paoletti, and A. N. Davison (Eds.), *Chemistry and brain development.* New York: Plenum Press, 1971.

Norval, M. A. Relationship of weight and length of infants at birth to the age at which they begin to walk alone. *J. Pediat.*, 1947, *30*, 676–678.

Nylin, G. The physiology of the circulation during puberty. *Acta. Med. Scand.*, 1935, *69* (Suppl.).

Oakland Tribune. Septuplets born to mother, 24. October 3, 1966, p. 10.

Olmsted, J. M. D. The nerve as a formative influence in the development of taste-buds. *J. Comp. Neurol.*, 1931, *31*, 465–468.

Orma, E. J., & Koshenoja, M. Postural dizziness in the aged. *Geriatrics*, 1957, *12*, 49–50.

Oscai, L. B. Recent progress in understanding obesity. In H. M. Eckert & H. J. Montoye (Eds.), *Exercise and health. The Academy Papers.* Champaign, IL: Human Kinetics, 1984.

Ostrow, A. C., & Dzewaltowski, D. A. Older adults' perceptions of physical activity participation based on age-role and sex-role appropriateness. *Res. Quart. for Exer. and Sport*, 1986, *57*, 167–169.

Paffenbarger, R. S.; Hyde, P. H.; Wing, A. L.; & Hsieh, C. Physical activity, all-cause mortality, and longevity of college alumni. *New England J. Med.*, 1986, *314*, 605–613.

Palmer, C. E. Seasonal variations of average growth in weight of elementary school children. *Pbl. Hlth. Rep., Wash.*, 1933, *18*, 211–233.

Palti, H., & Adler, B. Anthropometric measurements of the newborn, sex differences, and correlations between measurements. *Hum. Biol.*, 1975, *47*, 523–530.

Panek, P. E. Age differences in field-dependence/independence. *Exper. Aging Res.*, 1985, *11*, 97–99.

Parizkova, J. Body composition and exercise during growth and development. In G. L. Rarick (Ed.), *Physical activity: Human growth and development.* New York: Academic Press, 1973.

Park, D. C.; Puglisi, J. T.; & Sovacool, M. Memory for pictures, words, and spatial location in older adults: Evidence for pictorial superiority. *J. Geron.*, 1983, *38*, 582–588.

Parmelee, A. H., & Sigman, M. D. Perinatal brain development and behavior. In M. M. Haith & J. J. Campos (Eds.), *Infancy and developmental psychobiology.* Volume II of P. H. Mussen (Ed.), *Handbook of child psychology.* New York: John Wiley & Sons, 1983.

Parnell, R. W. *Behavior and physique. An introduction to practical and applied somatometry.* London: Arnold, 1958.

Pate, R. R.; Barnes, C.; & Miller, W. A physiological comparison of performance-matched female and male distance runners. *Res. Quart. for Exer. and Sport*, 1985, *56*, 245–250.

Pearson, K. The control of walking. *Sci. Amer.*, 1976, *235*(6), 72–86.

Peiper, A. Ueber die Helligkeits und Farbenempfindungen der Fruhgeburten. *Arch Kinderheilk.*, 1926, *80*, 1–20.

————. Die Fuhrung des Saugzentrums durch das Schluckzentrum. *Pflüg. Arch. Ges. Physiol.*, 1939, *242*, 751–755.

————. Die Schnappatmung in Filmausschnitten. *Kinderarztliche Praxis*, 1951, *19*, 272–279.

Perlmutter, M.; Metzger, R.; Nezworski, T.; & Miller, K. Spatial and temporal memory in 20 and 60 year olds. *J. Geron.*, 1981, *36*, 59–65.

Phelps, M. E., & Mazziotta, J. C. Positron emission tomography: Human brain function and biochemistry. *Science*, 1985, *228*, 799–809.

Phillips, S.; King, S.; & DuBois, L. Spontaneous activities of female versus male newborns. *Child Develpm.*, 1978, *49*, 590–597.

Piaget, Jean. *Plays, dreams and imitation in childhood.* New York: W. W. Norton & Co., Inc., 1962.

Piaget, J. *The child's conception of time.* London: Routledge & Kegan Paul, 1969.

Piatt, J. Nerve-muscle specificity in Amblystoma, studied by means of heterotopic cord grafts. *J. Exp. Zool.*, 1940, *85*, 211–237.

———. Transplantation of aneurogenic forelimbs in Amblystoma punctatum. *J. Exp. Zool.*, 1942, *91*, 79–101.

Pierson, I. M., & Montoye, H. J. Movement time, reaction time, and age. *J. Gerontol.*, 1958, *13*, 418–421.

Pigott, R. E., & Shapiro, D. C. Motor schema: The structure of the variability session. *Res. Quart. for Exer. and Sport*, 1984, *55*, 41–55.

Pikler, E. Some contributions to the study of gross motor development in children. *J. Genet. Psychol.*, 1968, *113*, 27–39.

Plagenhoef, S. The joint force and moment analysis of all body segments when performing a non-symmetrical, three-dimensional motion. *Medicine and Sport*, 1973, *8* (Biomechanics III); 165–171.

Poe, A. (1976) Description of the movement characteristics of two-year-old children performing the jump and reach. *Res. Quart.*, 1976, *47*, 260–268.

Pollock, M. L.; Dimmick, J.; Miller, H. S.; Kendrick, A.; & Linnerud, A. C. Effects of mode of training on cardiovascular function and body composition of adult men. *Med. and Sci. in Sports*, 1975, *7*, 139–145.

Pollock, S. Manganese-deficient diet linked to osteoporosis. *UC Clip Sheet*, 1987, *62*(14), February 3.

Porcari, J.; McCarron, R.; Kline, G.; Freedson, P. S.; Ward, A.; Ross, A. R.; & Rippe, J. M. Is fast walking an adequate aerobic stimulus for 30 to 69-year-old men and women? *The Physician and Sportsmed.*, 1987, *15*, 119–129.

Pratt, K. C. Note on the relation of temperature and humidity on the activity of young infants. *J. Genet. Psychol.*, 1930, *38*, 480–484.

———. The neonate. In L. Carmichael (Ed.), *Manual of child psychology* (2nd ed.). New York: John Wiley & Sons, 1954.

———; Nelson, A. K.; & Sun, K. H. The behavior of the newborn infant. *Ohio State Univ. Stud. Contr. Psychol.*, No. 10, 1930.

Prechtl, H. F. R. The behavioral states of the newborn infant (a review). *Brain Res.*, 1974, *76*, 185–212.

Pressey, S. L., & Kuhlen, R. G. *Psychological development through the life span.* New York: Harper & Row, Publishers, 1957.

Pryor, H. B. Certain physical and physiological aspects of adolescent development in girls. *J. Pediat.*, 1936, *8*, 52–62.

———, & Stolz, H. R. Determining appropriate weight for body build. *J. Pediat.*, 1933, *3*, 608–622.

Puhl, J.; Case, S.; Fleck, S.; & Van Handel, P. Physical and physiological characteristics of elite volleyball players. *Res. Quart. for Exer. and Sport*, 1982, *53*, 257–262.

Ramsay, D. S., & Weber, S. L. Infants' hand preference in a task involving complementary roles for the two hands. *Child Develpm.*, 1986, *57*, 300–307.

Ramsey, G. V. Sexual growth of Negro and White boys. *Hum. Biol.*, 1950, *22*; 146–149.

Rarick, G. L. *Motor development during infancy and childhood.* Mimeographed monograph. Madison, Wis.: University of Wisconsin, 1954.

Rarick, G. L., & Dobbins, D. A. Basic components in the motor performance of children six to nine years of age. *Med. and Sci. in Sports*, 1975, *7*, 105–110.

———, & McKee, R. A study of twenty third grade children exhibiting extreme levels of achievements on tests of motor proficiency. *Res. Quart.*, 1949, *20*, 142–150.

———, & Oyster, N. Physical maturity, muscular strength, and motor performance of young school-age boys. *Res. Quart.*, 1964, *35*, 523–531.

———, & Thompson, J. A. Reontgenographic measurements of leg muscle size and ankle extensor strength of seven-year-old children. *Res. Quart.*, 1956, *27*, 321–322.

Read, M. S. Behavioral correlates of malnutrition. In M. A. B. Brazier (Ed.), *Growth and brain development.* New York: Raven Press, 1975.

Reilly, F. J. *New rational athletics for boys and girls.* Boston: Heath, 1917.

Reynolds, E. L. Degree of kinship and pattern of ossification. *Amer. J. Phys. Anthrop.*, 1943, *1*, 405–416.

———. Differential tissue growth in the leg during childhood. *Child Develpm.*, 1944, *15*, 181–205.

———. The bony pelvic girdle in early infancy. *Amer. J. Phys. Anthrop.*, 1945, *3*, 321–354.

———. The bony pelvis in prepuberal childhood. *Amer. J. Phys. Anthrop.*, 1947, *5*, 165–200.

———, & Schoen, G. Growth patterns of identical triplets from eight through eighteen years. *Child Develpm.*, 1947, *18*, 130–151.

———, & Sontag, L. W. Seasonal variations in weight, height and appearance of ossification centers. *J. Pediat.*, 1944, *24*, 524–535.

_____, & Wines, J. V. Individual differences in physical changes associated with adolescence in girls. *Amer. J. Dis. Child.*, 1948, *75*, 329–350.

_____, & _____. Physical changes associated with adolescence in boys. *Amer. J. Dis. Child.*, 1951, *82*, 529–547.

Rich, A., & Kim, S. H. The three-dimensional structure of transfer RNA. *Sci. Amer.*, 1978, *238* (1), 52–62.

Richards, T. W., & Irwin, O. C. Plantar responses of infants and young children: An examination of the literature and reports of new experiments. *Univ. Iowa Stud. Child Welfare*, 1934, No. 11.

_____; Newbery, H.; & Fallgatter, R. Studies in fetal behavior. II. Activity of the human fetus *in utero* and its relation to other prenatal conditions, particularly the mother's basal metabolic rate. *Child Develpm.*, 1938, *9*, 69–78.

Richey, H. G. The blood pressure in boys and girls before and after puberty. Its relation to growth and to maturity. *Amer. J. Dis. Child.*, 1931, *42*, 1281–1330.

_____. Relation of accelerated, normal and retarded puberty to the height and weight of school children. *Monog. Soc. Res. Child Develpm.*, 1937, *2*(1), 1–67.

Richter, C. P. The grasp reflex of the newborn infant. *Amer. J. Dis. Child.*, 1934, *48*, 327–332.

Rikli, R., & Busch, S. Motor performance of women as a function of age and physical activity level. *J. Geron.*, 1986, *41*, 645–649.

Roberton, M. A. Stability of stage categorizations across trails: Implications for the 'stage theory.' *J. Human Movement Studies.* 1977, *3*(1), 49–59.

_____. Stages in motor development. In M. V. Ridenour (Ed.), *Motor development: Issues and application.* Princeton, N.J.: Princeton Book Company, 1978.

Robertson, S. S. Intrinsic temporal patterning in the spontaneous movement of awake neonates. *Child Develpm.*, 1982, *53*, 1016–1021.

Robinow, M.; Richards, T. W.; & Anderson, M. The eruption of deciduous teeth. *Growth*, 1942, *6*, 127–133.

Robinson, H. P. Sonar measurement of fetal crown-rump length as means of assessing maturity in first trimester of pregnancy. *British Med. J.*, 1973, *4*, 28–31.

Robinson, S. Experimental studies of physical fitness in relation to age. *Arb. Physiol.*, 1938, *10*, 251–323.

Rochelle, R. H. Blood plasma cholesterol changes during a physical training program. *Res. Quart.*, 1961, *32*(4), 538–550.

Romanes, G. J. The prenatal medullation of the sheep's nervous system. *J. Anat. Lond.*, 1947, *81*, 64–81.

Rosensweig, M. R.; Bennett, E. L.; & Diamond, M. C. Brain changes in response to experience. *Sci. American*, 1972, *226*, 22–29.

Ruff, H. A. The development of perception and recognition of objects. *Child Develpm.*, 1980, *51*, 981–992.

Ruja, H. Relation between neonate crying and length of labor. *J. Genet. Psychol.*, 1948, *73*, 53–55.

Rundgren, A.; Eklund, S.; & Jonson, R. Bone mineral content in 70- and 75-year-old men and women: An analysis of some anthropometric background factors. *Age and Ageing*, 1984, *13*, 6–13.

Rydzynski, Z. Clinical observations on late effects of early malnutrition. In R. Paoletti & A. N. Davison (Eds.), *Chemistry and brain development.* New York: Plenum Press, 1971.

Sager, R. Genes outside the chromosomes. *Sci. Amer.*, 1965, *212*(1), 71–79.

Saunders, J. W. The proximo-distal sequence of origin of wing parts and the role of the ectoderm. *Anat. Rec.*, 1947, *99*, 11.

Schaie, K. W.; Baltes, P.; & Strother, C. R. A study of auditory sensitivity in advanced age. *J. Gerontol.*, 1964, *19*(4), 453–457.

Schaub, M. C. The aging of collagen in the heart muscle. *Gerontologia*, 1964/5, *10*(1), 38–41.

Scheinfeld, Amram. *You and heredity.* New York: Frederick A. Stokes Co., 1939.

Schmidt, L. Der "erste" Atemzug. *Mschr. Kinderheilk.*, 1950, *98*, 213–217.

Schmidt, R. A. A schema theory of discrete motor skill learning. *Psychol. Rev.*, 1975, *82*, 225–260.

Scott, K. E., & Usher, R. Epiphyseal development in fetal malnutrition syndrome. *New England J. Med.*, 1964, *270*, 822–824.

Scott, R. B.; Cardozo, W. W.; Smith, A. DeG.; & DeLilly, M. R. Growth and development of Negro infants: III. Growth during the first year of life as observed in private pediatric practice. *J. Pediat.*, 1950, *37*, 885–893.

Seashore, H. G. The development of a beam walking test and its use in measuring development of balance in children. *Res. Quart.*, 1947, *18*, 246–259.

Seils, L. G. The relationship between measures of physical growth and gross motor performance of primary-grade school children. *Res. Quart.*, 1951, *22*, 244–260.

Severson, J. A. Neurotransmitter receptors and aging. *J. Amer. Geriat. Society*, 1984, *31*, 24–27.

Sexton, M., & Hebel, J. R. A clinical trial of change in maternal smoking and its effect on birth weight. *J. Amer. Med. Assoc.*, 1984, *251*, 911–915.

Shapiro, S.; Weinblatt, E.; Frank, C. W.; & Sager, R. V. Incidence of coronary heart disease in a population insured for medical care (HIP). *Amer. J. Public Health and the Nation's Health*, 1969, *59*(6), Suppl. to June, 1.

Sheldon, J. H. Medical-social aspects of the aging process. In M. Derber (Ed.), *The aged and society*. Champaign, Ill.: Industrial Relations Research Association, 1950.

_____. The effect of age on the control of sway. *Gerontol. Clin. (Basel)*, 1963, *5*(3), 129–138.

Sheldon, W. H.; Stevens, S. S.; & Tucker, W. B. *The varieties of human physique*. New York: Harper & Row, Publishers, 1940.

Shelton, M. D.; Parsons, O. A.; & Leber, W. R. Verbal and visuospatial performance and aging: A neuro-psychological approach. *J. Geron.*, 1982, *37*, 336–341.

Shepard, G. M. Microcircuits in the nervous system. *Sci. Amer.*, 1978, *238*(2), 92–103.

Shepard, S. B., & Martz, L. (Eds.). The graying of America. *Newsweek*, February 28, 1977, pp. 50–65.

Sherman, E. D., & Robillard, E. Sensitivity to pain in relationship to age. *J. Amer. Geriat. Soc.*, 1964, *12*(11), 1037–1044.

Sherman, M., & Sherman, I. C. Sensorimotor responses in infants. *J. Comp. Psychol.*, 1925, *5*, 53–68.

_____; _____; & Flory, C. D. Infant behavior. *Comp. Psychol. Monogr.*, 1936, *12*(4).

Shirkey, H. C. Human experiences related to adverse drug reactions to the fetus or neonate from some maternally administered drugs. In M. S. Klingberg; A. Abramovici; and J. Chemke (Eds.), *Drugs and fetal development*. New York: Plenum Press, 1972.

Shirley, M. M. *The first two years: A study of twenty-five babies. Vol. I. Postural and locomotor development*. Minneapolis: University of Minnesota Press, 1931.

_____. *The first two years: A study of twenty-five babies. Vol. II. Intellectual development*. Minneapolis: University of Minnesota Press, 1933.

Shock, N. W. Age changes and sex differences in alveolar CO_2 tension. *Amer. J. Physiol.*, 1941, *133*, 610–616.

_____. Basal blood pressure and pulse rate in adolescents. *Amer. J. Dis. Child.*, 1944, *68*, 16–22.

_____. Physiological responses of adolescents to exercise. *Texas Rep. Biol. Med.*, 1946, *4*, 368–386.

_____ (Ed.). *Problems of aging*. New York: Josiah Macy, Jr., Foundation, 1952.

_____ (Ed.). *Aging . . . some social and biological aspects*. American Assoc. for the Advancement of Science, Washington, D.C., 1960.

_____. The physiology of aging. *Sci. Amer.*, 1962, *206*(1), 100–110.

_____, & Soley, M. H. Average values for basal respiratory functions in adolescents and adults. *J. Nutr.*, 1939, *18*, 143–153.

Shuttleworth, F. K. The physical and mental growth of girls and boys age six to nineteen in relation to age at maximum growth. *Monogr. Soc. Res. Child Develpm.*, 1939, *4*(3), 1–291.

_____. The adolescent period: a graphic atlas. *Monogr. Soc. Res. Child Develpm.*, 1949, *14*, Serial No. 49, No. 1.

Siegel, J. S., & Hoover, S. L. *International Trends and Perspectives: Aging*. International Research Document No. 12, U.S. Department of Commerce, Bureau of the Census, 1984.

Simmons, K. The Brush Foundation study of child growth and development. II. Physical growth and development. *Mongr. Soc. Res. Child Develpm.*, 1944, *9*(1), 1–87.

_____, & Todd, T. W. Growth of well children: Analysis of stature and weight, 3 months to 13 years. *Growth*, 1938, *2*, 93–143.

Simonson, E. Changes in physical fitness and cardiovascular functions with age. *Geriatrics*, 1957, *12*, 28–39.

_____; Kearns, W. M.; & Enzer, N. Effect of oral administration of methyltestosterone on fatigue in eunuchoids and castrates. *Endocrinology*, 1941, *28*, 506–512.

Simowitz, C. Two old guys who jog. *California Living Magazine, San Francisco Sunday Examiner & Chronicle*, March 13, 1977, pp. 16–19.

Sinclair, C. B. *Movement and movement patterns of early childhood*. Richmond, Virginia: State Department of Education, 1971.

Sinclair, H. Sensorimotor action patterns as a condition for the acquisition of syntax. In R. Huxley & E. Ingram (Eds.), *Language acquisition: Models and methods*. New York: Academic Press, 1971.

Sinning, W. E. Body composition and athletic performance. In D. H. Clarke & H. M. Eckert (Eds.), *Limits of human performance. The Academy Papers*. Champaign, IL: Human Kinetics, 1985.

Sjöstrand, T. Volume and distribution of blood and their significance in regulating the circulation. *Physiol. Rev.*, 1953, *33*, 202–228.

Skinner, J. S., & Morgan, D. W. Aspects of anaerobic performance. In D. H. Clarke & H. M. Eckert (Eds.), *Limits of human performance. The Academy Papers.* Champaign, IL: Human Kinetics, 1985.

Slaughter, M. H.; Lohman, T. G.; & Misner, J. E. Relationship of somatotype and body composition to physical performance in 7- to 12-year-old boys. *Res. Quart.*, 1977, *48*, 159–168.

Slava, S.; Laurie, D. R.; & Corbin, C. B. Long-term effects of a conceptual physical education program. *Res. Quart. for Exer. and Sport*, 1984, *55*, 161–168.

Sloan, A. W. Physical fitness of college students in South Africa, United States of America and England. *Res. Quart.*, 1963, *34*(2), 244–248.

Smith, D. L.; Akhtar, A. J.; & Garraway, W. M. Proprioception and spatial neglect after stroke. *Age and Ageing*, 1983, *12*, 63–69.

Smith, E. L., Jr. Bone, changes with age and physical activity. Unpublished Ph.D. thesis. University of Wisconsin, Madison, 1971.

Smith, E. L.; Reddan, W.; & Smith, P. E. Physical activity and calcium modalities for bone mineral increase in aged women. *Med. and Sci. in Sports and Exer.*, 1981, *13*, 60–64.

Sonies, B. C.; Baum, B. J.; & Shawker, T. H. Tongue motion in elderly adults: Initial in situ observations. *J. Geron.*, 1984, *39*, 279–283.

Sontag, L. W., & Wallace, R. F. Changes in the rate of the human fetal heart in response to vibratory stimuli. *Amer. J. Dis. Child.*, 1936, *51*, 583–589.

Sophian, C., & Huber, A. Early developments in children's causal judgments. *Child Develpm.*, 1984, *55*, 512–526.

Southard, D. Interlimb movement control and coordination in children. In J. E. Clark & J. H. Humphrey (Eds.), *Motor development. Current selected research.* Princeton, NJ: Princeton Book, 1985.

Spalding, D. A. Instinct; with original observations on young animals. *Macmillan's Mag.*, 1873, *27*, 282–293.

_____. Instinct and acquisition. *Nature*, 1875, *12*, 507–508.

Speidel, C. C. Prolonged histories of vagus nerve regeneration patterns, sterile distal stumps and sheath cell outgrowths. *Anat. Rec.*, 1946, *94*, 55.

_____. Correlated studies of sense organs and nerves of the lateral-line in living frog tadpoles. II. The trophic influence of specific nerve supply as revealed by prolonged observations of denervated and reinnervated organs. *Amer. J. Anat.*, 1948, *82*, 277–320.

Spelt, D. K. The conditioning of the human fetus *in utero. J. Exp. Psychol.*, 1948, *38*, 338–346.

Sperry, R. W. Reestablishment of visuomotor coordinations by optic nerve regeneration, *Anat. Rec.*, 1942, *84*, 470.

_____. Visuomotor coordination in the newt (*Triturus viridescens*) after regeneration of the optic nerve. *J. Comp. Neurol.*, 1943, *79*, 33–55.

_____. Optic nerve regeneration with return of vision in anurans. *J. Neurophysiol.*, 1944, *7*, 57–69.

_____. Mechanisms of neural maturation. In S. S. Stevens (Ed.), *Handbook of experimental psychology.* New York: John Wiley & Sons, Inc., 1951.

Sperry, R. W. The growth of nerve circuits. *Sci. Amer.*, 1959, *201* (5), 68–75.

Spiegelman, M. Factors in human mortality. In B. L. Strehler (Ed.), *The biology of aging.* Washington, D.C.: American Institute of Biological Sciences, 1960.

Spirduso, W. W. Reaction and movement time as a function of age and physical activity level. *J. Geront.*, 1975, *30*, 435–440.

Spirduso, W. W. Exercise as a factor in aging motor behavior plasticity. In H. M. Eckert & H. J. Montoye (Eds.), *Exercise and health. The Academy Papers.* Champaign, IL: Human Kinetics, 1984.

Spirduso, W. W. Age as a limiting factor in human neuromuscular performance. In D. H. Clarke & H. M. Eckert (Eds.), *Limits of human performance. The Academy Papers.* Champaign, IL: Human Kinetics, 1985.

Staehelin, L. A., & Hull, B. E. Junctions between living cells. *Sci. Amer.*, 1978, *238*(5), 140–152.

Stein, G. S.; Stein, J. S.; & Kleinsmith, L. J. Chromosomal proteins and gene regulation. *Sci. Amer.*, 1975, *232* (2), 47–49, 57.

Stein, S.; Linn, M. W.; Slater, E.; & Stein, E. M. Future concerns and recent life events of elderly community residents. *J. American Geriat. Society*, 1984, *32*, 431–434.

Sternberg, R. J. Human intelligence: The model is the message. *Science*, 1985, *230*, 1111–1118.

Stillman, R. J.; Lohman, T. G.; Slaughter, M. H.; & Massey, B. H. Physical activity and bone mineral content in women aged 30 to 85 years. *Med. and Sci. in Sports and Exer.*, 1986, *18*, 576–580.

Stirnimann, F. Versuche über die Reaktionen Neugeborener auf Wärme-und Kältereize. Z. Kinderpsychiat., 1939, 5, 143–150.

_____. Ueber das Farbempfinden Neugeborener. Ann. Paediat., 1944, 163, 1–25.

Stolz, H. R., & Stolz, L. M. Somatic development of adolescent boys. A study of the growth of boys during the second decade of life. New York: Macmillan, 1951.

Strandell, T. Heart rate and work load at minimal working intensity in old men. Acta Med. Scand., 1964, 176(3); 301–318.

Streeter, G. L. Weight, sitting height, head size, foot length, and menstrual age of the human embryo. Contr. Embryol., Carnegie Inst. Wash., 1920, 11(55), 143–170.

Strehler, Bernard L. (Ed.). The biology of aging. Washington, D.C., American Institute of Biological Sciences, 1960.

Strong, E. K. Changes of interest with age. Stanford, Calif.: Stanford University Press, 1931.

Stubbs, E. M. The effect of the factors of duration, intensity, and pitch of sound stimuli on the responses of newborn infants. Univ. Iowa Stud. Child Welfare, 1934, 9(4), 75–135.

_____, & Irwin, O. C. Laterality of limb movements of four newborn infants. Child Develpm., 1933, 4, 358-359.

Sullivan, F. J.; Bender, A. D.; & Horvath, S. M. The aging cell. J. Amer. Geriat. Soc., 1963, 11(10), 923–932.

Susanne, C. Genetic and environmental influence on morphological characteristics. Annals of Hum. Biol., 1975, 2, 279–288.

Takeda, S., & Matsuzawa, T. Brain atrophy during aging: A quantitative study using computed tomography. J. Amer. Geriat. Society, 1984, 32, 520–524.

Talmage, R. V.; Stinnett, S. S.; Landwehr, J. T.; Vincent, L. M.; & McCartney, W. H. Age-related loss of bone mineral density in non-athletic and athletic women. Bone and Mineral, 1986, 1, 115–125.

Tanner, J. M. The relationships between the frequency of the heart, oral temperature and rectal temperature in man at rest. J. Physiol., 1951, 115, 391–409.

_____. Growth at adolescence. Oxford: Blackwell Scientific Publications, 1955.

_____. Trend towards earlier menarche in London, Oslo, Copenhagen, the Netherlands and Hungary. Nature, 1973, 243, 95–96.

_____. Foetus into man. Cambridge, Mass.: Harvard University Press, 1978.

_____, & Taylor, G. R. Growth. New York: Time Inc., 1965.

Taylor, D. J.; Crowe, M.; Bore, P. J.; Arnold, D. L.; & Radda, G. K. Examination of the energetics of aging skeletal muscle using nuclear magnetic resonance. Geron., 1984, 30, 2–7.

Taylor, R. Hunger in the infant. Amer. J. Dis. Child., 1917, 14, 233–257.

Teeple, J., & Massey, B. Force-time parameters and physical growth of boys ages 6 to 12 years. Res. Quart., 1976, 47, 464–471.

Terman, L. M., & Merrill, M. A. Measuring intelligence. New York: Houghton Mifflin & Co., 1937.

Teuber, H. L. The brain and human behavior. In R. Held; H. W. Leibowitz; & H. L. Teuber (Eds.), Perception. Berlin: Springer-Verlag, 1978.

Thelen, E. Learning to walk is still an "old" problem: A reply to Zelazo (1983). J. Motor Behav., 1983, 15, 139–161.

Thelen, E. Treadmill-elicited stepping in seven-month-old infants. Child Develpm., 1986, 57, 1498–1506.

This World. Healthy sextuplets are born. San Francisco: Chronicle Publishing Co. September 25, 1977a.

This World. San Francisco: Chronicle Publishing Co. April 17; October 16, 1977b.

This World. Test-tube baby is called a 'threat.' San Francisco: Chronicle Publishing Co. August 6, 1978a, p. 20.

This World. Alarming genetic data. San Francisco: Chronicle Publishing Co. August 27, 1978b, p. 26.

This World. San Francisco: Chronicle Publishing Co. August 6, 1978c, pg. 25.

This World. San Francisco: Chronicle Publishing Co. March 26, 1978d.

Thomas, B. Early toy preferences of four-year-old readers and nonreaders. Child Develpm., 1984, 55, 424-430.

Thompson, J. S.; Wekstein, D. R.; Rhoades, J. L.; Kirkpatrick, C.; Brown, S. A.; Roszman, T.; Straus, R.; & Tietz, N. The immune status of healthy centenarians. J. Amer. Geriat. Society, 1984, 30, 274–281.

Thompson, H. Physical growth. In L. Carmichael (Ed.), Manual of child psychology. New York: John Wiley & Sons, Inc. 1954.

Thorland, W. G.; Johnson, G. O.; Cisar, C. J.; Housh, T. J.; & Tharp, G. D. Strength and anaerobic responses of elite young female sprint and distance runners. Med. and Sci. in Sports and Exer., 1987, 19, 56–61.

Timiras, P. S.; Vernadakis, A.; & Sherwood, N. M. Development and plasticity of the nervous system. In N. S. Assali (Ed.), *Biology of gestation*. New York: Academic Press, 1968.

Tinetti, M. E. Performance-oriented assessment of mobility problems in elderly patients. *J. Amer. Geriat. Society*, 1986, *34*, 119–126.

Tisserand-Perrier, M. Etude comparative de certains processus de croissance chez les jumeaux. *J. Genet. Hum.*, 1953, *2*, 87–102.

Tollefsbol, T. O., & Cohen, H. J. Role of protein molecular and metabolic aberrations in aging, in the physiological decline of the aged, and in age-associated diseases. *J. Amer. Geriat. Society*, 1986, *34*, 282–294.

Tomasello, M., & Farrar, M. J. Joint attention and early language. *Child Develpm.*, 1986, *57*, 1454–1463.

Tomikawa, S. A., & Dodd, D. H. Early word meanings: Perceptually or functionally based? *Child Develpm.*, 1980, *51*, 1103–1109.

Ulrich, B. D. Perceptions of physical competence, motor competence, and participation in organized sport: Their interrelationships in young children. *Res. Quart. for Exer. and Sport*, 1987, *58*, 57–67.

Ulrich, B. D., & Ulrich, D. A. The role of balancing ability in performance of fundamental skills in 3-, 4-, and 5-year-old children. In J. E. Clark & J. H. Humphrey (Eds.), *Motor development. Current selected research*. Princeton, NJ: Princeton Book, 1985.

Ungerer, J. A., & Sigman, M. The relation of play and sensorimotor behavior to language in the second year. *Child Develpm.*, 1984, *55*, 1448–1455.

University Bulletin. Study of newborn babies' eyes, 1964, *12* (25), 151–152.

University Bulletin. Many newborns need special hospital care, 1972a, *21*(11), 59.

University Bulletin. UC medical schools saving newborns from often-fatal respiratory distress, 1972b, *21*(6), 31–32.

Updegraff, R. Preferential handedness in young children. *J. Exp. Educ.*, 1932, *1*, 134–139.

Upton, S. J.; Hagan, R. D.; Rosentsweig, J.; & Gettman, L. R. Comparison of the physiological profiles of middle-aged women distance runners and sedentary women. *Res. Quart. for Exer. and Sport*, 1983, *54*, 83–87.

U.S. Bureau of the Census. *Statistical abstract of the United States: 1977* (98th ed.). Washington, D.C., 1977.

U.S. Bureau of the Census. *Statistical abstract of the United States: 1978* (99th Ed.). Washington, D.C., 1978.

Vaccaro, P.; Ostrove, S. M.; Vandervelden, L.; Goldfarb, A. H.; Clarke, D. H.; & Dummer, G. M. Body composition and physiological responses of masters female swimmers 20 to 70 years of age. *Res. Quart. for Exer. and Sport*, 1984, *55*, 278–284.

Valentine, W. L., & Wagner, I. Relative arm motility in the newborn infant. *Ohio State Univ. Stud.*, 1934, *12*, 53–68.

Van Alstyne, D. *Play behavior and choice of play materials of preschool children*. Chicago: The University of Chicago Press, 1932.

Vasta, R.; Regan, K. G.; & Kerley, J. Sex differences in pattern copying: Spatial cues or motor skills? *Child Develpm.*, 1980, *51*, 932–934.

Verhaegen, P., & Ntumba, A. Note on the frequency of left-handedness in African children. *J. Educ. Psychol.*, 1964, *55*, 89–90.

Verzár, F. The aging of collagen. *Sci. Amer.*, 1963, *208*(4), 104–114.

Victors, E. E. A cinematographical analysis of catching behavior of a selected group of seven and nine year old boys. *Dissert. Abstracts*, 1961, *22*, 1903–1904.

Vincent, M. F. Motor performance of girls from 12–18 years of age. *Res. Quart.*, 1968, *39*, 1094–1100.

Visser, H. Gait and balance in senile dementia of Alzheimer's type. *Age and Ageing*, 1983, *12*, 296–301.

von Mering, O., & Weniger, F. L. Social-cultural background of the aging individual. In J. E. Birren (Ed.), *Handbook of aging and the individual*. Chicago: The University of Chicago Press, 1959.

von Muralt, A. Influence of early protein-calorie malnutrition on the intellectual development: The point of view of a physiologist. In M. A. B. Brazier (Ed.), *Growth and brain development*. New York: Raven Press, 1975.

Waddington, C. H. *New patterns in genetics and development*. New York: Columbia University Press, 1962.

Wallon, H.; Evart-Chmielniski, E.; & Sauterey, R. Equilibre statique, équilibre en mouvement: double latéralisation. *Enfance*, 1958, *11*, 1–29.

Warren, M. P.; Brooks-Gunn, J.; Hamilton, L. H.; Warren, L. F.; & Hamilton, W. G. Scoliosis and fractures in young ballet dancers. *New England J. Med.*, 1986, *314*, 1348–1353.

Watson, J. B. *Psychology from the standpoint of a behaviorist*. Philadelphia: Lippincott, and Co., 1919.

Wayner, M. J., & Emmers, R. Spinal synaptic delay in young and aged rats. *Am. J. Physiol.*, 1958, *194*, 403–405.

Webb, W. B., & Agnew, H. W. Sleep deprivation, age, and exhaustion time in the rat. *Science*, 1962, *136* (3522), 1122.

Weiss, A. D. Sensory functions. In J. E. Birren (Ed.), *Handbook of aging and the individual*. Chicago: The University of Chicago Press, 1959.

Weiss, L. A. Differential variations in the amount of activity of newborn infants under continuous light and sound stimulation. *Univ. Iowa Stud. Child Welfare*, 1934, *9*, 1–74.

Weiss, P. A. Selectivity controlling the central-peripheral relations in the nervous system. *Biol. Rev.*, 1936, *11*, 494–531.

———. Further experimental investigations on the phenomenon of homologous response in transplanted amphibian limbs. I. Functional observations. *J. Comp. Neurol.*, 1937a, *66*, 181–209.

———. Further experimental investigations on the phenomenon of homologous response in transplanted amphibian limbs. II. Nerve regeneration and the innervation of transplanted limbs. *J. Comp. Neurol.*, 1937b, *66*, 481–535.

———. Further experimental investigations on the phenomenon of homologous response in transplanted amphibian limbs. III. Homologous response in the absence of sensory innervation. *J. Comp. Neurol.*, 1937c, *66*, 537–548.

———. Nerve patterns: The mechanics of nerve growth. *Third Growth Symposium*, 1941a, *5*, 163–203.

———. Self-differentiation of the basic patterns of coordination. *Comp. Psychol. Monogr.*, 1941b, *17*, 1–96.

———, & Edds, M. Sensory-motor nerve crosses in the rat. *J. Neurophysiol.*, 1945, *8*, 173–194.

Welford, A. T. Psychomotor performance. In J. E. Birren (Ed.), *Handbook of aging and the individual*. Chicago: The University of Chicago Press, 1959.

Wellman, B. L. Motor achievements of preschool children. *Child. Educ.*, 1937, *13*, 311–316.

Wells, C. L. The limits of female performance. In D. H. Clarke & H. M. Eckert (Eds.), *Limits of human performance. The Academy Papers*. Champaign, IL: Human Kinetics, 1985.

West, R. L., & Cohen, S. L. The systematic use of semantic and acoustic processing in younger and older adults. *Exper. Aging Res.*, 1985, *11*, 81–86.

Wetzel, N. C. Physical fitness in terms of physique, development and basal metabolism. *J. Amer. Med. Assoc.*, 1941, *116*, 1187–1195.

———. Assessing the physical condition of children: I. Case demonstration of failing growth and the determination of "par" by the grid method. II. Simple malnutrition: A problem of failing growth and development. III. The components of physical status and physical progress and their evaluation. *J. Pediat.*, 1943, *22*, 82–110, 208–225, 329–361.

Whitbourne, S. K. *The Aging Body. Physiological Changes and Psychological Consequences*. New York: Springer-Verlag, 1985.

Whitley, J. D., & Smith, L. E. Velocity curves and static strength-action in relation to the mass moved by the arm. *Res. Quart.*, 1963, *34*, 379–395.

Whittle, H. D. Effects of elementary school physical education upon aspects of physical, motor, and personality development. *Res. Quart.*, 1961, *32*, 249–260.

Wickstrom, R. *Fundamental movement patterns*. Philadelphia: Lea & Febiger, 1970.

Wild, Monica R. The behavior pattern of throwing and some observations concerning its course of development in children. *Res. Quart.*, 1938, *9*(3), 20–24.

Willerman, L., & Plomin, R. Activity level in children and their parents. *Child Develpm.*, 1973, *44*(4), 854–858.

Williams, J. W. *Obstetrics*. New York: Appleton-Century-Crofts, 1931.

Williams, M. H. Weight control through exercise and diet for children and young athletes. In G. A. Stull & H. M. Eckert (Eds.), *Effects of physical activity on children. The Academy Papers*. Champaign, IL: Human Kinetics, 1986.

Willmott, M. The effect of vinyl floor surface and carpeted floor surface upon walking in elderly hospital in-patients. *Age and Ageing*, 1986, *15*, 119–120.

Wilmore, J. H. Alterations in strength, body composition and anthropometric measurements consequent to a 10-week weight training program. *Med. and Sci. in Sports*, 1974, *6*, 133–138.

Wilmore, J. H. Appetite and body composition consequent to physical activity. *Res. Quart. for Exer. and Sport*, 1983, *54*, 415–425.

Wilson, D. C., & Sutherland, I. Further observations on the age of the menarche. *Brit. Med. J.*, 1950, *2*, 862–866.

_____, & _____. The age of menarche in the tropics. *Brit. Med. J.*, 1953, *2*, 607–608.

Wilson, M. U. Biological changes in American women in the last fifty years. *Res. Quart.*, 1957, *28*(4), 413–421.

Wilson, V. J. Inhibition in the central nervous system. *Sci. Amer.*, 1966, *214*(5), 102–110.

Winchester, A. M. *Heredity: An introduction to genetics.* New York: Barnes & Noble, Inc., 1961.

_____. *Human genetics* (3rd ed.). Columbus, Ohio: Charles E. Merrill, 1979.

Windle, W. F. Physiology and anatomy of the respiratory system in the fetus and newborn infant. *J. Pediat.*, 1941, *19*, 437–444.

_____, & Fitzgerald, J. E. Development of the spinal reflex mechanism in human embryos. *J. Comp. Neurol.*, 1937, *67*, 493–509.

Winick, M. Cellular growth of the human placenta. III. Intrauterine growth failure. *J. Pediat.*, 1967, *71*, 390–395.

_____. Cellular growth in intra-uterine malnutrition. *Pediat. Clin. N. Amer.*, 1970, *17*, 69–78.

Witelson, S. F. Sex and the single hemisphere: Specialization of the right hemisphere for spatial processing. *Science*, 1976, *193*, 425–427.

_____. Developmental dyslexia: Two right hemispheres and none left. *Science*, 1977, *195*, 309–311.

Witelson, S. F. The brain connection: The corpus callosum is larger in left-handers. *Science*, 1985, *229*, 665–668.

Winter, D. A. Biomechanical motor patterns in normal walking. *J. Motor Behav.*, 1983, *15*, 302–330.

Woodward, D. O., & Woodward, V. W. *Concepts of molecular genetics.* New York: McGraw-Hill, 1977.

Woolf, Charles M. Paternal age effect for cleft lip and palate. *Amer. Jour. Human Genet.*, 1963, *15*(4), 389–393.

Worden, P. E., & Meggison, D. L. Aging and the category-recall relationship. *J. Geron.*, 1984, *39*, 322–324.

Working Group. Relation of nutrition to fetal growth and development. In Committee on Maternal Nutrition, National Research Council, *Maternal nutrition and the course of pregnancy.* Washington, D.C.: National Academy of Sciences, 1970.

Woyciechowski, B. Ruchy zarodka ludzkiego 42 mm. *Polsk. Gazeta Lekarska*, 1928, *7*, 409–411.

Wright, I. S., & Blass, J. P. Longevity and aging research: An analysis of reality. *J. Amer. Geriat. Society*, 1984, *32*, 91.

Wyrick, W. Biophysical perspectives. In E. W. Gerber; J. Felshin; P. Berlin; & W. Wyrick, *The American woman in sport.* Reading, Mass.: Addison-Wesley Publishing Co., 1974.

Yarmolenko, A. The motor sphere of school age children. *J. Genet. Psychol.*, 1933, *42*, 298–318.

Yerkes, R. M., & Bloomfield, D. Do kittens instinctively kill mice? *Psychol. Bull.*, 1910, *7*, 253–263.

Yonas, A.; Pettersen, L.; & Granrud, C. E. Infants' sensitivity to familiar size as information for distance. *Child Develpm.*, 1982, *53*, 1285–1290.

Young, A.; Stokes, M.; & Crowe, M. The relationship between quadriceps size and strength in elderly women. *Clinical Science*, 1982, *63*, 35P–36P.

Younger, L. A comparison of reaction and movement times of women athletes and non-athletes. *Res. Quart.*, 1959, *30* (3), 349–355.

Zacharias, L.; Wurtman, R. J.; & Schatzoff, M. Sexual maturation in contemporary American girls. *Amer. J. Obstet. Gynec.*, 1970, *108*(5), 833–846.

Zelazo, P. R. The development of walking: New findings and old assumptions. *J. Motor Behav.*, 1983, *15*, 99–137.

Zimmerman, Helen M. Characteristic likenesses and differences between skilled and non-skilled performance of standing broad jump. *Res. Quart.*, 1956, *27*, 352–362.

Index

AAHPER Youth Fitness Test, 318-321, 344-345
Acoustopalpebral reflex, 82
Aging: exercise and, 352-353, 355-357, 360-361, 371, 373-376, 383, 386-387, 392, 395-398, 403, 415-416, 417-428; cardiorespiratory changes and, 380-381, 383, 418-422; elimination and, 383; immune systems and, 427; metabolic changes in, 377-378, 387-388; molecular changes in, 376-377; muscle changes in, 388-393; neurological changes in, 377, 409-417; strength and, 384-393; work rates and, 379-381
Ahlfeld breathing movements, 58, 63
Alameda County, CA study, 353-354
Alcohol, 353; during pregnancy, 31
Alleles, 4
Amaurotic family idiocy, 11
Ambidexterity, 124
Amenorrhea, 287; training and, 358-359; weight and, 357, 362
Amniocentesis, 12
Andorgen, 251, 304, 310, 331, 378, 388
Androgeny: classifications of, 330; ratings of, 329-331
Anorexia, 359
Apgar evaluation, 92
Apposition, 393
Arm pull torque, 256
Arm strength, 249
Arthritis, 422-423
Asphixia, fetal, 92
Aspirin: during pregnancy, 30-31
Atherosclerosis, 356
Athletes, 374; aging, 344; body size differences in, 335-337; longevity and, 375-376; training of, 342-343
Auditory evoked responses (AER), 163, 164
Autism, 163
Autonomic systems, 74-76
Axillary hair growth, 283
Babinski reflex, 65, 77
Babkin reflex, 77
Balance: adolescence, 315-317; aging and, 402, 421-422; early childhood, 220-222, 227-228; floor surfaces and, 409; later childhood, 264-267, 268-269; sensory inputs for, 405-406
Ball bouncing, 214-216, 227, 311
Ball catching. See Catching
Ball throwing. See Throwing
Ballet dancing, 357-358
Basal metabolic rate, 304-305
Bayley Scales of Infant Development, 59
Benson, Jaqueline, 23
Binocular vision, 81, 142
Birth defects, 24, 29-30, 31, 33-35, 36
Birth experience, 71-74
Birth weight, 28, 36
Blastocyst, 20-21
Blindness, 24, 30, 85-86, 88
Blood pressure, 356

Body build, 242-248, 296, 361; height, 243; motor performance and, 340-342; weight, 243
Body composition: aging and, 378-379; physical performance and, 336-337, 356-357, 358; sex differences in, 332-333. See also, Weight
Body proportions, 293-297
Body size: historical trends, 337-340; in adulthood, 334-337
Body strength, 261
Body temperature, 298
Bone mineral content: aging and, 378, 397-402, 422, 429; amenorrhea and, 359, 362; exercise and, 360; in marathon runners, 336; spinal, 358. See also, Osteoporosis
Brace test, 269-270, 316, 319
Brachyphalangy, 6, 11-12
Brain, 161; development, 21; left hemisphere, 161-164; processing of motor information, 158; right hemisphere, 163-164
Brain atrophy index (BAI), 409-410
Brain damage: neonate, 93
Brazelton Neonatal Behavior Assessment Scale, 59, 93
Breast development, 279-281
Bruininks-Oseretsky Test of Motor Proficiency, 221
Calcium, 395-397
California Infant Scale of Motor Development, 226-227
Cardiovascular disease: age and, 353-355, 417; exercise and, 355-356, 360, 362, 371-376, 417-418; socioeconomic levels and, 354-355
Cataracts, 29
Catching, 211-214, 227-228, 269
Cell division, 4-6, 39
Center of gravity, 157
Center of movement, 156-159
Cerebral palsy, 24
Chapman, Marion, 23
Chemie Club, 247-248
Chubbiness, 243
Cleft lip and palate, 33
Climatic effects on growth. See Seasonal effects
Climbing, 192-195, 198
Club foot, 33, 36
Collagen, 381, 388
Color blindness, 12-13
Comaneci, Nadia, 247, 342
Commissural neurons, 42
Congenital deformities, 30
Continuous Positive Airway Pressure, 24
Coordination, 267-271, 315-317
Creeping, 128
Cretinism, 34
Crossing over of genes, 4-6
Cultural influences, 99, 125-126, 273, 324
Cutaneous sensitivity, 84-86
Deafness, 29, 30
Dean, Penny, 340
Death rates, 368-369, 373, 418
Defecation, 76
Delano, Ed, 421